Current Practices in Ophthalmology

Series Editor
Parul Ichhpujani, Department of Ophthalmology
Government Medical College and Hospital
Chandigarh, India

This series of highly organized and uniform handbooks aims to cover the latest clinically relevant developments in ophthalmology. In the wake of rapidly evolving innovations in the field of basic research, pharmacology, surgical techniques and imaging devices for the management of ophthalmic disorders, it is extremely important to invest in books that help you stay updated. These handbooks are designed to bridge the gap between journals and standard texts providing reviews on advances that are now part of mainstream clinical practice. Meant for residents, fellows-in-training, generalist ophthalmologists and specialists alike, each volume under this series covers current perspectives on relevant topics and meets the CME requirements as a go-to reference guide. Supervised and reviewed by a subject expert, chapters in each volume provide leading-edge information most relevant and useful for clinical ophthalmologists. This series is also useful for residents and fellows training in various subspecialties of ophthalmology, who can read these books while at work or during emergency duties. Additionally, these handbooks can aid in preparing for clinical case discussions at various forums and examinations.

Aparna Ramasubramanian
Editor

Pediatric Ophthalmology

Springer

Editor
Aparna Ramasubramanian
Phoenix Children's Hospital
Phoenix, AZ, USA

ISSN 2523-3807 ISSN 2523-3815 (electronic)
Current Practices in Ophthalmology
ISBN 978-981-19-4962-3 ISBN 978-981-19-4963-0 (eBook)
https://doi.org/10.1007/978-981-19-4963-0

This Springer imprint is published by the registered company Springer Nature Singapore Pte Ltd.
The registered company address is: 152 Beach Road, #21-01/04 Gateway East, Singapore 189721, Singapore

Preface

The specialty of pediatric ophthalmology has seen a paradigm shift in the last decade with the advent of multiple subspecialities which has improved the patient outcome and have improved the family's experience. The World Health Organization (WHO), Geneva, Switzerland, with the International Agency for the Prevention of Blindness (IAPB), launched the VISION 2020: The Right to Sight initiative in 1999. One of their focuses was on childhood blindness. This brought much needed attention to pediatric eye conditions—their early detection and management. Also, the profile of ocular conditions has changed in the modern world. It is estimated that 32% of the world's population is myopic currently and that has been projected to increase to 60% by 2050. This requires a better understanding of pediatric eye conditions and early intervention measures. The advent of newer technologies including vision screeners, widefield fundus imaging, and optical coherence tomography have advanced the screening and early detection of diseases. A major stride has also been made in the field of genetic disorders with genomic testing and gene therapies.

We have ventured to capture this advancement in the field of pediatric ophthalmology in this book. We hope that it would give an oversight on the current management of pediatric eye conditions and open up more avenues for collaboration and development.

Phoenix, AZ   Aparna Ramasubramanian

Contents

About the Author

Aparna Ramasubramanian is an ocular oncologist and pediatric ophthalmologist and is the Director of the retinoblastoma program at Phoenix Children's Hospital. After her ophthalmology residency at Indiana University, she did an ocular oncology fellowship at Wills Eye Institute, Philadelphia, and a pediatric ophthalmology fellowship at Boston Children's Hospital. She is the author of the leading textbook *Retinoblastoma* and is the program developer for the "Cure Retinoblastoma" campaign by the Children's Eye Foundation. She received the American Academy of Ophthalmology Achievement Award in 2018 and treats both adults and kids with eye cancer.

Epidemiology and Pathogenesis of Myopia

1

Swapnil Thakur, Rohit Dhakal, Satish K. Gupta, and Pavan K. Verkicharla

1.1 Trends in Myopia Epidemics

1.1.1 Global

Myopia has currently become a global epidemic issue, affecting nearly 34% (2.6 billion) of the total world's population as of the year 2020 [1]. It has been predicted that half of the world's population (nearly five billion) will become myopic by the year 2050. With regards to the regional differences, the estimated prevalence of myopia is reported to be lowest in East Africa with a prevalence rate of 8.4% in 2020, which is predicted to rise to 22.7% by 2050. In contrast, myopia prevalence in the developed countries of the Asia-Pacific regions, East Asia, and South-East Asia is estimated to be 53.4%, 51.6%, and 46.1% in the year 2020, and will rise to 66.4%, 65.3%, and 62.0%, respectively, by the year 2050.

1.1.2 East Asia

East Asian countries such as Singapore, China, Korea, and Taiwan have witnessed a steep rise in the prevalence of myopia in the last few decades. The prevalence of myopia was as high as 96.5% among 19-year-old teenagers in Korea [2], 79.3%

S. Thakur · R. Dhakal · S. K. Gupta · P. K. Verkicharla (✉)
Myopia Research Lab & Infor Myopia Centre, Brien Holden Institute of Optometry and Vision Sciences, Prof. Brien Holden Eye Research Centre, L V Prasad Eye Institute, Hyderabad, India
e-mail: swapnil.thakur@lvpei.org; rohitdhakal@lvpei.org; satish.gupta@lvpei.org; pavanverkicharla@lvpei.org

A. Ramasubramanian (ed.), *Pediatric Ophthalmology*, Current Practices in Ophthalmology, https://doi.org/10.1007/978-981-19-4963-0_1

among 17–19 years young adults in Singapore [3], and 86.1% among 18–24 years young military conscripts in Taiwan [4]. The prevalence has increased by fivefold in 7-year old (5.37–25.41%), and two to threefold in 12- (30.66–76.67%) and 15-year-old (44.3–92.9%) children from 1983 to 2016 in Taiwan [5]. In China, myopia prevalence among young adults aged 18.46 ± 0.69 years has increased from 79.54% to 87.7% in the urban regions over a period of 15 years (between 2001 and 2015) [6], and in university students aged 20.20 ± 2.80 years, it has escalated to 95% [7]. It has been predicted that nearly 84% of children between 3 and 19 years old will become myopic by the year 2050 in China [8].

1.1.3 South Asia

The South Asian region has observed relatively lower myopia prevalence in school-aged children below 20 years compared to the East Asian region in the last decade, ranging from as low as 2% in Nepal [9], 4.8% in Sri Lanka [10], 6.6% in Bhutan [11], 5.8% in Bangladesh [12], 12.7% in Pakistan [13], and as high as 35.5% in India [14]. A meta-analysis reporting the pooled prevalence of myopia in the last four decades in India revealed an increment of two-fold, from 6.6% between 1980 and 2008 to 14.2% between 2009 and 2019 in children aged 11–15 years [15]. According to a recent study from North India, 21.1% of schoolchildren aged 5–15 years had myopia [16]. If the current incidence rate of myopia continues, the prevalence in such urban regions is estimated to rise to 32% in 2030, 40% in 2040, and 48.14% in 2050 [17].

1.1.4 Middle East, Europe, Africa, and America

Although the epidemic of myopia is high in East Asian countries, other parts of the world also testify to the growing prevalence of myopia. In an age group below 21 years, the myopia prevalence ranged from 3.4 to 7% in Africa [18, 19], 6.5–9% in the Middle East [20, 21], 1.4–14.7% in South America [22–25], 14.8–17.3% in Australia [26], 29% in Canada [27], and 2.4–42.7% in Europe [28–30]. In the United States, the myopic population aged 25–54 years almost doubled (25.0 vs. 41.6%) in a period of three decades between 1971 and 72 to 1999 and 2004 [31]. Fig. 1.1 depicts the trend of increasing myopia prevalence at different time points in different countries.

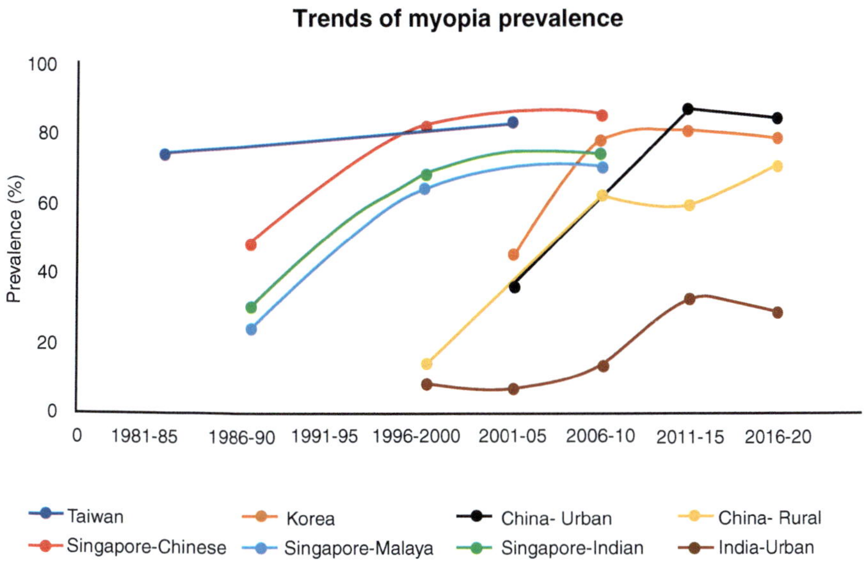

Fig. 1.1 Trends of myopia prevalence within different time points between 1981 and 2020 in different countries

1.2 High Myopia

1.2.1 Definition

High myopia is defined based on the magnitude of myopic refractive error. The World Health Organization (WHO) has indicated a threshold of ≤−5.00 D to define high myopia based on the diagnostic approach, as the predicted uncorrected distance visual acuity due to −5.00 D myopia would approximately equate to <20/400 which is considered as a threshold for blindness. However, to maintain consistency, the International Myopia Institute has proposed ≤−6.00 D as a threshold to define high myopia, considering most of the epidemiological and intervention studies applied this threshold [32].

1.2.2 Influence of Age and Urbanization

The prevalence of high myopia is reported to be higher in adults than in children, in urban regions than in rural regions. A study conducted in China in 2009, which included 5083 university students, showed 23% of students aged 24 ± 2.5 years had high myopia (≤−6.00 D) compared to 18.12% in students aged 18.8 ± 0.8 years [7]. Likewise, another study has found high myopia in 1.39% in 12-year-old, 4.37% in

15-year-old, and 24.16% in 18-year-old Taiwanese children [5]. The epidemiological studies reported high myopia of 0.3% in children aged 3–10 years [33] and 19.3% of young teenagers aged 18 years [6] in urban regions compared to 0.1% in 3–6 years [34] and 8.6% in 6–18 years old young children in rural regions [35].

1.2.3 Current and Predicted Trends of High Myopia

Bullimore and Brennan reported that each diopter increase in myopia increases the likelihood of developing myopic maculopathy by 40%, irrespective of the degree of myopic refractive error [36]. This indicates the alarming condition that can arise due to high myopia. Globally, 5.2% of the total world's population is predicted to have high myopia in 2020, and these estimates are likely to rise to nearly 9.8% (938 million people) by the year 2050 [1].

The temporal prevalence of high and very high myopia (defined as SER ≤ -10.00 D) among adults aged 18.5 ± 0.7 years showed an increment of greater than twofold (7.9% from 16.6%) and greater than 11-fold (0.92% from 0.08%) respectively, over a period of 15 years (2001–2015) in China [6]. A similar trend was reported from Taiwan, where the high myopia prevalence rate increased from 1.39% to 4.26% in 12-year-old children, 4.37–15.36% in 15-year-old children, and 16.87–24.16% in 18-year-old children within a period of three decades [5]. In the Korean population aged 18–35 years, there was a minimal increase in high myopia prevalence (from 11.3% in 2009 to 12.9% in 2013) over a period of 5 years [37]. In the US, the prevalence of high myopia (≤ -8.00 D) increased eightfold in a period of three decades, from 0.2% to 1.6%, between 1971 and 1972 to 1999 and 2004 [31].

1.3 Pathological Myopia

1.3.1 Definition

Pathological myopia is sometimes interchangeably used with high myopia; however, both of these terminologies have different meaning. High myopia is solely defined based on the degree of myopia (≤ -6.00 D) and is not necessarily associated with the presence of any pathological signs [32]. The International Myopia Institute has defined pathological myopia as "excessive axial elongation associated with myopia that leads to structural changes in the posterior segment of the eye (including posterior staphyloma, myopic maculopathy, and high myopia-associated optic neuropathy) and that can lead to loss of best-corrected visual acuity. The META-PM (Meta-analysis of Pathological Myopia) study has defined and classified pathological myopia based on the presence of signs associated with myopic maculopathy as (i) Category 0—no macular lesions, (ii) Category 1—tessellated fundus, (iii) Category 2—diffuse chorioretinal atrophy, (iv) Category 3—patchy chorioretinal atrophy, and (v) Category 4—macular atrophy [38]. The plus signs are lacquer cracks, myopic choroidal neovascularization, and Fuch's spot. Pathological myopia is defined if fundus photographs reveal any of these signs with and above category 2.

1.3.2 Current and Predicted Trends of Pathologic Myopia

The prevalence of pathological myopia ranges from 0.9 to 3.1% in China [39, 40], 1.2% in Australia [41], 1.7% in Japan, 3% in Taiwan [42], and 2.2% in India [43] (Fig. 1.2). Pathologic myopia lesions are reported to be equally prevalent in both low and high myopes (2.2% in low vs. 2.5% in high myopes); however, serious complications such as retinal detachment and posterior staphyloma were found to be higher in high myopes [44]. Among only high myopes, pathologic myopia lesions are found in 28.7%–72.7% of adults or older aged people >30 years in East Asian countries and Australia [39–41, 45, 46]. A systematic review and meta-analysis that included four population-based and three clinic/school-based studies reported the pooled prevalence of myopic macular degeneration (MMD) to be 0.4% in rural India, 0.5% in Beijing, 1.5% in Russia, and 5.2% in Singapore [47]. Another systematic review has indicated a nearly threefold increase in the pooled prevalence of MMD (1.3–3.5%) from 1993–2006 to 2007–2017 [48].

Vision impairment or blindness due to sight-threatening complications of pathologic myopia is known to affect one in one thousand to one in one hundred individuals of different ethnicities [49]. Although there is no direct evidence predicting the future epidemic of pathological myopia, given that 10% of myopes globally will be high myopic by the year 2050 [1] and the manifestation of pathologic lesions even in low grades of myopia, the epidemic of myopia associated with sight-threatening complications might upsurge in the future.

1.3.3 Myopia Incidence and Progression

Myopia incidence and progression are found to be associated with ethnicity. Unlike myopia prevalence, the evidence on myopia incidence is scarce owing to the need for longitudinal studies. The incidence of myopia among 6-year-old

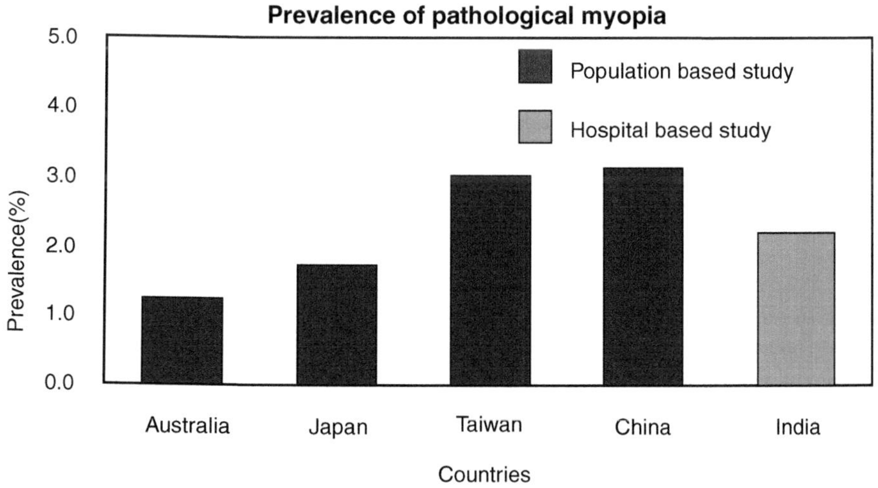

Fig. 1.2 Prevalence of pathological myopia in different countries

Chinese children was 39.5% over a period of 3 years [50]. In Singapore, the cumulative 3-year myopia incidence ranged from 32.4% to 47.7% in children aged 7–9 years [51]. The Northern Ireland Childhood Errors of Refraction (NICER) study conducted in the UK during 2012–2014 (baseline data from 2006–2008) reported an annual incidence rate of 2.2% in the younger cohort (6–7 years at baseline) and 0.7% in the older (12–13 years at baseline) cohort. Conversely, in the same age group of Australian children, an opposite trend was seen where only 1.3% of children aged 6–7 years and 2.9% of children aged 12–13 years developed myopia [52].

Annual incidence rates were higher in East-Asian ethnicity in both younger (6.6% in East Asians vs. 0.7% in European Caucasians) and older (3.2% vs. 1.2%, respectively) cohort of children than European Caucasians [52]. A significantly lower number of Indian and Malayan children (27.2%) developed myopia compared to Chinese children (49.5%) of a similar age group in Singapore, indicating higher incidence rates in individuals of Chinese ethnicity [51]. In the South Asian region, urban schoolchildren aged 5–15 years had an annual incidence rate of 3.4% [16].

With regards to myopia progression, the shift in myopic refractive error in Chinese children aged 6 years was reported to be −1.59 D over a period of 3 years, whereas the annual rate of progression ranged from −0.28 to −0.30 D among 6–13 years old school-aged children [53]. The amount of progression was higher in Australian children (baseline) that ranged from −0.31 to −0.41 D/year in children aged 6–13 years [54]. Compared to this, Irish children showed a lesser annual shift in myopia (ranging from −0.09 to −0.18 D/year) in the NICER study across the same age cohorts [55]. Mean annual change in myopic refractive error in North Indian urban children aged 5–15 years (who were already myopic at baseline) was reported to −0.27 ± 0.42 D/year [16]. Another retrospective study involving Indian children and young adults aged 1–30 years indicated an annual progression of −0.07 D to −0.51 D/year [56].

1.3.4 Emmetropisation and Refractive Development

Emmetropia refers to a refractive condition when the incident parallel rays of light from distant objects focus on the retina while accommodation is at rest. Emmetropisation is an active process where refractive components and the axial length of the eye (the linear distance from the anterior surface of the cornea to the retina along the visual axis) come into balance to achieve the emmetropic condition [57, 58]. Any disruption in this process or emmetropisation leads to the development of refractive errors [58].

Myopia can be broadly classified into two qualitative categories as either a) axial myopia—refractive state that can be attributed to excessive axial elongation or b) refractive myopia—refractive state that can be attributed to changes in the structure or location of the image forming structures, i.e., the cornea and/or lens [32]. Similar to the axial growth observed in a variety of animal experiments [59, 60], myopic eyes in children [25, 61], young adults [62], and the elderly [63, 64] were reported to have a deeper vitreous chamber depth, indicating that axial myopia is primarily due to elongation of the vitreous chamber, with nominal changes in corneal curvature and crystalline lens power [65].

1.4 Ocular Expansion Models

Ocular stretching causes structural changes in the myopic eye, notably in the posterior region of the eye (vitreous chamber depth, retina, choroid, and sclera). The ocular stretching is observed not just along the visual axis but in a variety of ways (Fig. 1.3), such as (a) "Global expansion" where ocular expansion occurs in all directions from the limbus towards the posterior pole [66], (b) "Equatorial expansion" where ocular stretching occurs parallel to the optic axis and is limited to the equatorial region of the eye [67], (c) "Posterior pole expansion" where ocular elongation is limited to the posterior pole typically owing to increased tension at the level of zonules and ciliary body [68], (d) "Axial expansion" or the hybrid model of elongation where the globe expands along both posterior pole and equatorial directions [69], and (e) "Asymmetrical expansion" where the eyeball could follow the global expansion model, but undergo unequal/uneven stretching from anterior to posterior pole [70].

1.4.1 Role of the Retina in Regulating the Ocular Growth

The retina is the light-sensitive layer located as the innermost layer of the posterior coat [71, 72]. The fovea (central region of the retina) is a depression in the inner retinal surface about 1.5 mm wide, whereas the rest is referred to as the peripheral retina (approximately about 21 mm from the fovea to ora-serrata) [73].

Humans [74–78] and various animal species such as chicks [59, 79–85], monkeys [86–91], tree shrews [92, 93], mice [94, 95], guinea pigs [96], marmosets [60], kittens [97, 98], and squids [99] are capable of detecting the retinal image defocus and accordingly regulating ocular growth [58, 100]. This retinal image defocus detection system appears to operate independently and locally within the eye. Despite an absence of input from the accommodative system (induced via cycloplegia, ciliary nerve section, or damage to the Edinger-Westphal nucleus) [82, 101] or higher visual centers (induced

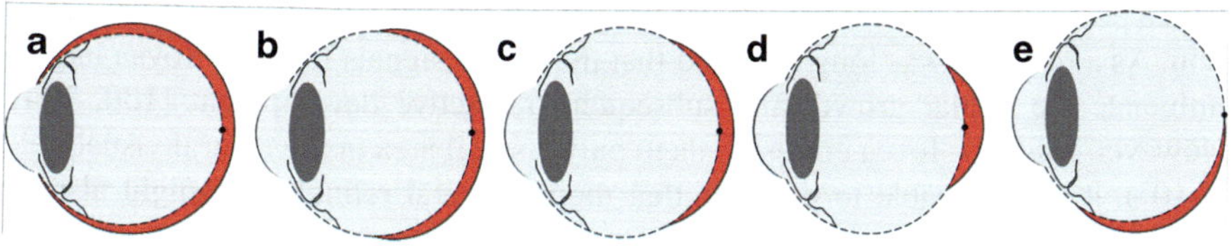

Fig. 1.3 The figure above shows various globe expansion models for myopic eyes. Global expansion (**a**), equatorial expansion (**b**), axial expansion (**c**), posterior pole expansion (**d**), and asymmetrical expansion (**e**)

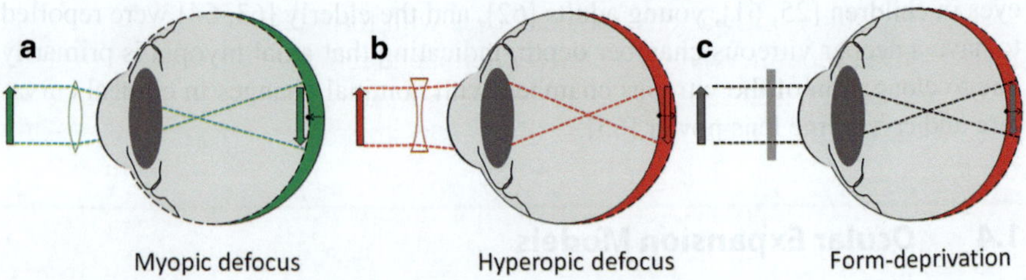

Fig. 1.4 The figure above shows the directional change in axial length in response to myopic defocus (**a**), hyperopic defocus (**b**), and form-deprivation (**c**). The green and red color indicates decrease and increase in axial length, respectively

via optic nerve section) [102], the eye still responds to the imposed form-deprivation (retinal image quality degradation) [81, 102], and detects the sign of optical defocus (Fig. 1.4) [82, 85, 101–103]. This suggets that the blur signal at the retinal level may initiate complex signaling cascades responsible for cellular and biochemical changes in retinal structures for refractive development [71, 100, 104, 105].

Morphologically, the thickness profile of the ganglion cell-inner plexiform layer and retinal nerve fiber layer (RNFL) in children with myopic refractive error is reported to be thinner compared to that of non-myopes [106, 107]. The total thickness of the peripheral retina was found to be thinner in high myopic eyes compared to emmetropes, attributable to a thinner inner nuclear layer, combined Henle fiber layer, outer nuclear layer, and outer segment of the photoceptor layer [108]. High myopic eyes were shown to have thinner RNFL and Ganglion cell complex (GCC) thickness compared to low and moderate myopia [109].

Overall, axial growth is associated with retinal thinning, mainly in the equatorial and pre-equatorial regions, with no changes in foveal retina thickness [110]. It is noteworthy that the changes in macular retinal thickness in mild to moderate myopia are relatively small (6 microns) and unlikely to be of clinical significance [111]. More importantly, the proportion of the decline in sub-foveal choroidal thickness is higher than the retinal thickness, indicating that changes in choroid thickness occur earlier and more rapidly during myopia development or progression [111–113].

1.4.2 Central vs. Peripheral Retina

Fovea possesses high-contrast visual acuity, cone-receptor density, and high resolution. As a result, it was long assumed that the visual signals from the fovea largely influence the ocular growth and subsequent refractive development [100, 104]. However, since the fovea corresponds to only a small area in the central visual field (≈10°), it is reasonable to presume that the peripheral retinal area might also be important in driving the refractive status.

In animal studies, it was observed that eyes with form-deprivation (induced via diffusers/Bangerter filters) imposed on the peripheral retina and having unrestricted clear central vision led to an increase in axial length and resulted in form-deprivation myopia (FDM) [87, 114]. Furthermore, ablating the central 10° diameter of the retina around the fovea while leaving the periphery intact resulted in an emmetropic refractive state [91] and also compensated for form-deprivation (FDM), optically induced hyperopic [115], and myopic defocus [89]. These studies indicated that the visual signals from the retinal periphery are also indeed critical for visually guided eye growth and that refractive development is susceptible to local and regionally selective mechanisms in the peripheral retina [90].

1.4.3 Theories Related to Peripheral Optics and Retinal Shape in Myopia

Various animal and human studies have reported that myopes exhibit relative peripheral hyperopia (the peripheral retinal image is focused behind relative to the central focus), and emmetropes and hyperopes exhibit relative peripheral myopia (the peripheral retinal image is focused in front relative to the central focus) [69, 100, 104, 116, 117]. The optically induced peripheral hyperopic and myopic defocus, respectively, accelerated and decelerated the eye growth, indicating the role of that relative peripheral hyperopic defocus in the development of myopia (myopiagenesis) and myopia progression [100, 118–124]. When the form-deprivation [125–128] or optically induced peripheral hyperopic defocus is imposed to a specific retinal region of chick and guinea pig eyes, only the region imposed by the hyperopic defocus exhibited maximum elongation of axial length [125, 127, 128], and resulted in alteration of posterior eye shape, indicating a local regulation of ocular growth [69, 117, 126].

Considering that the refractive state of the eye is always based on the presence of the focal plane in relation to the retinal plane, several studies have attempted to anticipate the peripheral retinal shape variations based on the type and magnitude of refractive error in the periphery of the eye. As shown in Fig. 1.5, myopic eyes with relative peripheral hyperopia are known to exhibit a steeper or prolate retinal shape, whereas hyperopic or emmetropic eyes with relative peripheral myopia exhibit a flatter or oblate retinal shape [69, 118, 129–132]. Retinal shapes have been shown to differ depending on factors such as ethnicity and primary refractive meridians [117, 133], with the East Asian myopes exhibiting steeper (prolate) retinal shape and greater relative peripheral hyperopia than Caucasians, along horizontal than in vertical meridian.

In high myopic eyes, the baseline shape of the posterior pole had a substantial impact on the speed with which the posterior pole shape changed. Eyes having a flatter shape at baseline tended to change shape more slowly, whereas an eye with restrained shape deformation tended to change shape rapidly [134].

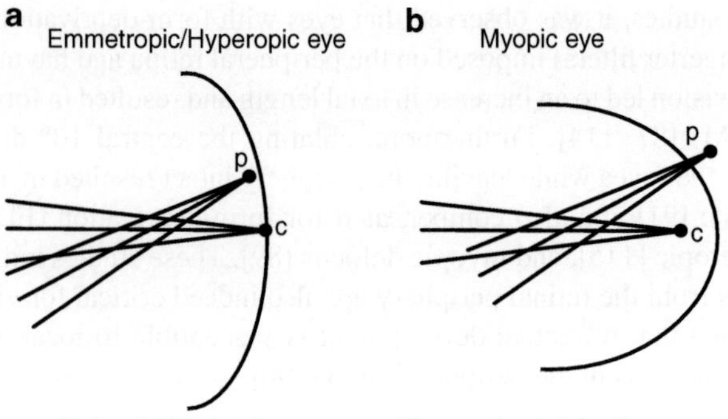

Fig. 1.5 The figure above shows the comparison of central and peripheral optics in the emmetropic eye (**a**) and myopic eye (**b**). Note that the peripheral rays may not always be hyperopic as shown in panel **b**

1.4.4 Changes in the Choroid

The choroid, a highly vascular tissue that lies between the retina and sclera, is the primary source of oxygen and nutrients to the outer retina and is considered to play a major role in the regulation of ocular temperature, intraocular pressure, modulation of vascularization, and growth of the sclera [135]. Experiments in a wide range of animal species [136–139] and humans [74, 77, 140–142] investigating the effect of retinal defocus on choroidal response indicated that the choroid plays a critical role in the regulation of ocular growth and refractive development. Overall, thickening of the choroid has been observed in response to myopic defocus, whereas thinning has been observed in response to hyperopic defocus. Studies have also demonstrated that thinning of the choroid is a structural hallmark feature of human myopia [143], with a negative correlation between choroidal thickness and axial length, suggesting that the change in choroidal thickness may be a predictive biomarker for long-term changes in ocular elongation. Choroidal thickness has been shown to decrease approximately by 26 microns with each additional millimeter increase in axial length [144]. Since the choroid is primarily a vascular structure capable of rapidly changing blood flow, variations of choroidal thickness are considered to be associated with changes in choroidal vascularity [145].

However, the underlying mechanism of how the choroid plays a role in ocular growth and refractive development is still unknown. It has been suggested that since the choroid lies between the retina and sclera, it acts as a channel to transfer the retinal signalling molecules or growth factors from the retina to the choroid. Apart from the effect of defocus, several other factors like muscarinic antagonists such as homatropine and atropine [146, 147], dopamine agonists such as apomorphine and quinpirole [148], accommodation [149, 150], and increased light exposure [151, 152] have resulted in changes to the choroidal thickness.

1.4.5 Changes in the Sclera

The sclera is considered as the skeleton of the eye, which forms the outer coat of the eyeball. It comprises the fibrous shell of collagen and fibroblasts, which helps in the production and maintenance of extracellular matrix (ECM) [153], serves as an attachment for the extraocular muscles, allows passage for the optic nerve, channels for arterial blood supply, venous drainage, nerves for interocular structures, and drainage of aqueous humour [153]. It is also known to neutralize the short-term fluctuation in intraocular pressure and act as a mechanical barrier [153]. The disturbance in the structure and function of the sclera can lead to an alteration in refractive development. Ocular enlargement in myopic eyes is shown to be associated with progressive thinning of the sclera [70, 154]. Overall thinning of the sclera is associated with thinning of the collagen fiber bundles along with the reduction in the glycosaminoglycan and collagen contents and the size of the individual collagen fibrils particularly the small diameter fibrils, rendering the sclera biochemically weaker in myopic eyes [155, 156]. Given that longitudinal fibers of the ciliary body run adjacent and parallel to the sclera with tendons connecting equatorial sclera and choroid extending anteriorly to the sclera spur [157], sustained accommodation during close distance near work is shown to result in thinning of the anterior sclera, mainly 3 mm posterior to the scleral spur [158]. Furthermore, high myopes are shown to exhibit a greater sagittal height of the anterior sclera in the nasal region than emmetropes, indicating high myopes have a different anterior eye shape [159]. Adding to the evidence, inferior anterior scleral thickness was found to decrease with an increasing degree of myopia [70].

1.4.6 Optical, Biomechanical, and Neural Mechanisms in Myopiageneis

Accommodation is the fundamental part of any near work activity, which is defined as "the ability of the eye to change its optical power to focus on objects at different distances." The structural changes that occur during accommodation include the shape of the crystalline lens (principally the anterior surface), where the anterior surface becomes more curved with little changes in the posterior surface, the central thickness of the crystalline lens increases, the equatorial diameter decreases, and lens volume remains constant with the decrease in surface area [160, 161]. Accommodative response reflects the change in the dioptric power of the crystalline lens in response to a stimulus (accommodative demand). If the accommodative response is lower than the accommodative demand during near-viewing conditions, this results in an error known as the lag of accommodation. And if the accommodative response is higher than the accommodative demand, this results in an error known as the lead of accommodation.

Given that near work plays a major role in myopiagenesis, accommodation during near work has been considered to be the potential cause for ocular growth. Moreover, several other non-accommodative mechanisms explain the role of near work and myopia. All proposed theories related to near work and myopia are discussed below (Fig. 1.6).

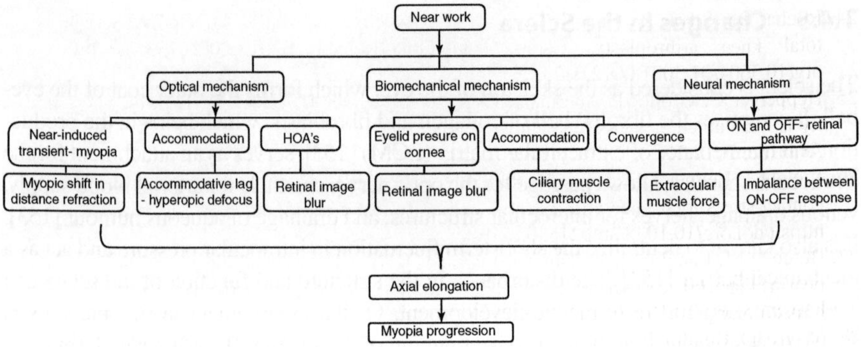

Fig. 1.6 The flowchart above shows the various theories proposed related to near work and myopia

1.4.6.1 Accommodative Lag Theory

Myopia has been linked to central hyperopic retinal defocus associated with the lag of accommodation during near-work activities, and the lag theory indicates *that* such a hyperopic defocus could trigger ocular growth (Fig. 1.7). This is based on the findings from studies in a wide range of animal species, including guinea pigs [162], chicks [81], and monkeys [86] that chronic hyperopic retinal blur triggered axial elongation to compensate for the blur stimulus. The fact that myopic eyes have a higher lag of accommodation (i.e., reduced accommodative response to blur) compared to non-myopic eyes [163, 164], supports the theory that myopic eyes experience a greater amount of hyperopic blur during near work, which might lead to excessive axial growth. Evidence suggests that children who use bifocals [165, 166] and progressive addition lens (PALs) [167, 168] showed less myopia progression compared to children wearing single vision spectacle lenses. However, the consensus regarding the association between the lag of accommodation and the progression of myopia has so far been conflicting. Few studies have shown that lag of accommodation is associated with progression of myopia [169, 170], few suggest that greater myopia progression in adults is associated with a low lag of accommodation [171], and others found no significant association between lag of accommodation and myopia [172, 173]. It is indicated that lag of accommodation can be the consequence rather than a cause of myopia, since lag of accommodation was not significantly different before the onset or during the onset of myopia between children who became myopic and emmetropic children [174].

While it has been considered that stimuli presented to the foveal area can elicit an accommodative response, there is also evidence suggesting that stimuli presented at the peripheral retina can also produce accommodative responses (in the absence of a central stimulus), termed as peripheral accommodation [175–177]. It is shown that the accommodative response to the target decreased with the increase in the eccentricity (5°, 10°, and 15°) of the target [177]. Furthermore, It has been speculated that although the image is well focused on the retina accompanied with image-focused in front of the perifoveal retina, the eye will relax to bring the image closer to the retina, which in turn, causes lag of accommodation and may trigger myopia [176].

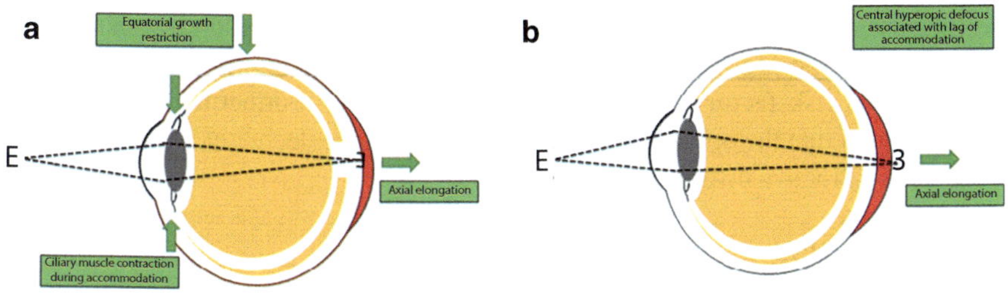

Fig. 1.7 Illustration of mechanical tension theory (**a**) and accommodative lag theory (**b**)

1.4.6.2 Mechanical Tension Theory

This theory explains the role of "mechanical stress" or "force" created by the ciliary body or the crystalline lens at the anterior part of the globe during accommodation in accelerating axial ocular growth by restricting the equatorial ocular growth to a point where proportional globe expansion is no longer possible (Fig. 1.7) [178, 179]. Accommodation can promote ocular growth by choroidal or scleral action, or with a combination of both. Because the fibers of the ciliary body extend posteriorly till the choroid, contraction of the ciliary body during accommodation (ciliary-choroidal tension) causes forward pulling of the choroid with a reduction in the circumference of the sclera and results in axial elongation [180]. Several human studies have found a significant transient increase in axial length and thinning of the choroid associated with short-term near work, supporting the mechanical tension theory [150, 181, 182]. Sustained accommodation has been found to induce a hyperopic shift in relative peripheral refraction, implying that the ciliary muscle's mechanical influence on the choroid can result in a more prolate ocular shape during accommodation [183]. Adding further evidence, accommodation was found to cause significant thinning of the anterior sclera, particularly 3 mm posterior to the scleral spur [158]. These changes were found to be more prominent in myopes compared to emmetropes.

1.4.6.3 Higher-Order Aberrations

Accommodative response and higher-order aberrations have been demonstrated to be influenced by downward gaze during near work [184–186]. A shift in corneal optics during near work has been postulated as a possible connection between near work and myopia development [187–189]. Changes in corneal astigmatism and higher-order aberrations have been found to occur after a near task in the downward gaze, which significantly affects retinal image quality. These changes are likely to be caused by the eyelid pressure on the corneal surface.

The magnitude and sign of HOA, particularly negative spherical aberration, are thought to provide a directional cue to the retina, leading to compensatory eye growth to improve image quality. Positive spherical aberration, on the other hand, has been considered to be protective against myopia progression due to its action in reducing the hyperopic defocus associated with the lag of accommodation during near work, and improve the retinal image quality. In a study of Chinese schoolchildren, higher-order aberrations were reported to be significantly higher in children with faster myopia progression (≥0.50 D/year) compared to children with a slower rate of myopia progression (<0.50 D/year), suggesting that higher-order aberrations could be the risk factor for myopia progression [190]. Furthermore, it has been demonstrated that the optical quality of the retinal image decreases with an increase in myopic refractive error [191].

1.4.6.4 Near-Induced Transient Myopia (NITM)

It is defined as a myopic shift in distance refraction (far-point) immediately after a period of extended or sustained near work [192–195]. It has been suggested that NITM acts as a myopic blur for distance vision immediately after a sustained period of near work and delayed decay to the baseline, which could lead to permanent myopia. Myopes show a greater level of myopic shift compared to emmetropes. Late-onset myopes have a longer NITM decay time to reach their baseline level than early-onset myopes following a shorter period of near work [196]. Progressive myopes tend to have a greater level of NITM than stable myopes and emmetropes [196, 197]. The manifestation of NITM was found to be associated with the sympathetic pathway of the autonomic nervous system. The autonomic nervous system has two pathways: (a) the parasympathetic pathway which innervates the synaptic muscarinic receptors (M3) in the iris sphincter and ciliary body and results in contraction of the ciliary body, (b) the sympathetic pathway which has alpha 1 and alpha 2 receptors resulting in pupillary mydriasis, and b1 and b2 receptors resulting in inhibition of accommodation. The present hypotheses indicate that NITM could be either due to a deficit in sympathetic input (resulting in delayed decay to the baseline), or it could be a deficit in both parasympathetic and sympathetic pathways, given that they function in a complementary manner [198].

1.4.6.5 Role of Convergence and Extraocular Muscles

This theory suggests that stress generated by extraocular muscles during near work could potentially cause an increase in axial length. Mechanical pressure from the rectus and oblique muscles during convergence has been proposed as a possible cause for ocular growth [199]. Given, the scleral stiffness at the posterior pole is only 62% of that of the anterior pole [200], the oblique muscles might exert enough localized tension on the posterior sclera to elicit axial elongation due to their attachment site at the posterior part of the globe (in proximity to the optic nerve). It has also been hypothesized that the extraocular muscle's mechanical stress at the equator is than the ciliary muscle contraction during accommodation [199]. The axial length of the eye was shown to increase in inferonasal gaze, and this change was greater in myopic than emmetropic participants [201]. During downward gaze, the axial length increased for eye movement without head movement compared with primary gaze, suggesting that changes in axial length in downgaze are due to the influence of the extraocular muscles, particularly oblique muscles [201]. Recently, it has been found that the medial rectus was significantly thinner in myopic eyes compared to emmetropes, and the sustained stress during binocular viewing conditions could affect the anterior scleral shape [202] which could in turn lead to asymmetrical growth of the eye associated with myopia development or progression.

1.4.6.6 Role of ON-OFF Pathway

Retinal ganglion cells have circular fields which are organized into ON-center/OFF-surround and OFF-center/ON-surround pattern. The properties of ON-center cells show that when a small annulus of light falls at the center of the cell, it leads to the depolarization of the cell membrane resulting in activation of the cells, whereas hyperpolarization (i.e., inhibition of the cell) occurs when light is presented on the surrounding field of the cell, sparing the center. Conversely, the OFF-center cells depolarize by the light stimulus in the surrounding field of the cell (i.e., offset of stimulus in the center). Experiments in chickens and mice with deficient ON- or OFF-pathway signalling suggest that ON-pathway activity represents an inhibitory signal for eye growth, while the OFF-pathway may be stimulatory [203, 204]. Based on this information, recent studies in humans have reported that reading black text on a white background overstimulated the OFF-pathway, resulting in significant thinning of the choroid, whereas reading white text on a black background overstimulated the ON-pathway, resulting in significant thickening of the choroid [205].

1.4.7 Role of Genetics and Other Factors in the Refractive Development

The risk factors responsible for the development and progression of myopic refractive error can be broadly categorized into genetic and environmental factors [206]. There is a strong line of evidence indicating the role of hereditary etiology in myopia development [207]. It has been suggested that the heritability of myopia could be between 60% and 80% [207]. MYP1—a myopia-related gene locus, was one of the first recognized gene loci to be associated with high myopia [208]. To date, 200 gene loci have been identified related to myopic refractive error [207]. Parental history of myopia has been considered to be a risk factor for myopia development and faster progression in myopic children [209, 210]. The risk of developing myopia was reported to be two to threefold higher in children with two myopic parents compared to 1.5 times higher in children with one myopic parent, and lowes with no myopic parents [211]. Children with two myopic parents have been shown to have rapid myopia progression with single vision spectacles and atropine treatment, and children having one myopic parent progress less than the former but faster than the children with no myopic parents [209, 212].

Despite several indications of a relationship between genetics and myopia, the rapid rise in the prevalence of myopia over the last several decades cannot be just attributed to genetic influence, especially when such a dramatic rise in the prevalence is observed in a specific population or specific region. Apart from nearwork [213–215], several other factors such as closer reading distance (less than 30 cm) and longer periods of continuous near work (more than 30–45 min) [214, 216], posture and gaze angle during reading [217–220], time spent in outdoor activities [221–223], education level [224–227], intelligence [228–231], location (rural vs. urban) [232], digital screen time [233–235], level of physical activity [236], socio-economic status [237], body stature [238], and low birth weight [239] have been identified to be associated with the development and/or progression of myopia.

Key Points

1. Prevalence, incidence, and progression of myopia vary with region and ethnicity.
2. The retina is capable of detecting the retinal image defocus and regulate ocular growth independently and locally within the eye via a series of complex cellular and biochemical mechanisms.
3. The visual signals from the retinal periphery are indeed critical for visually guided eye growth and corresponding refractive development.
4. The shape of the retina and the type and magnitude of peripheral retinal defocus may have a potential role in myopia development and progression.
5. Optical, biomechanical, and neural mechanisms are known to play role in myopiageneis.
6. The ocular growth is not just observed along the visual axis, but the expansion of eye can happen following any of the proposed models.

References

1. Holden BA, Fricke TR, Wilson DA, et al. Global prevalence of myopia and high myopia and temporal trends from 2000 through 2050. Ophthalmology. 2016;123:1036–42.
2. Jung S-K, Lee JH, Kakizaki H, Jee D. Prevalence of myopia and its association with body stature and educational level in 19-year-old male conscripts in Seoul, South Korea. Invest Ophthalmol Vis Sci. 2012;53:5579–83.
3. Wu H-M, Seet B, Yap EP-H, et al. Does education explain ethnic differences in myopia prevalence? A population-based study of young adult males in Singapore. Optom Vis Sci. 2001;78:234–9.
4. Lee Y-Y, Lo C-T, Sheu S-J, Lin JL. What factors are associated with myopia in young adults? A survey study in Taiwan Military Conscripts. Invest Ophthalmol Vis Sci. 2013;54:1026–33.
5. Tsai T-H, Liu Y-L, Ma IH, et al. Evolution of the prevalence of Myopia among Taiwanese schoolchildren: a review of survey data from 1983 through 2017. Ophthalmology. 2021;128:290–301.
6. Chen M, Wu A, Zhang L, et al. The increasing prevalence of myopia and high myopia among high school students in Fenghua city, eastern China: a 15-year population-based survey. BMC Ophthalmol. 2018;18:159.
7. Sun J, Zhou J, Zhao P, et al. High prevalence of myopia and high myopia in 5060 Chinese University Students in Shanghai. Invest Ophthalmol Vis Sci. 2012;53:7504–9.
8. Dong L, Kang YK, Li Y, Wei WB, Jonas JB. Prevalence and time trends of myopia in children and adolescents in China: a systemic review and meta-analysis. Retina. 2020;40:399–411.
9. Pant SR, Awasthi S, Bhatta RC, Poudel M, Shrestha MK. Refractive error among public and private school children in Dhangadhi city of far West Nepal. J Ophthalmol Res. 2021;4:174–82.
10. Wimalasundera S. Astigmatism among other refractive errors in children of Southern Sri Lanka. Global J Med Res. 2015;15(1-F)
11. Sharma IP, Lepcha NT, Lhamo T, et al. Visual impairment and refractive error in school children in Bhutan: the findings from the Bhutan School Sight Survey (BSSS 2019). PLoS One. 2020;15:e0239117.
12. Kader MA, Tarafder S, Anwar AA, et al. Study of refractive errors on school going children in North West Zone of Bangladesh. TAJ J Teachers Assoc. 2016;29:1–6.

13. Latif MZ, Khan MA, Afzal S, Gillani SA, Chouhadry MA. Prevalence of refractive errors; an evidence from the public high schools of Lahore, Pakistan. J Pak Med Assoc. 2019;69:464–7.
14. Sankaridurg P, Philip K, Konda N, et al. Prevalence of refractive errors in urban schoolchildren in India: The Hyderabad Eye Study. Invest Ophthalmol Vis Sci. 2015;56:2936.
15. Agarwal D, Saxena R. Prevalence of myopia in Indian school children: Meta-analysis of last four decades. PLoS One. 2020;15:e0240750.
16. Saxena R, Vashist P, Tandon R, et al. Incidence and progression of myopia and associated factors in urban school children in Delhi: The North India Myopia Study (NIM Study). PLoS One. 2017;12:e0189774.
17. Priscilla JJ, Verkicharla PK. Time trends on the prevalence of myopia in India - a prediction model for 2050. Ophthalmic Physiol Opt. 2021;41:466–74.
18. Kumah BD, Ebri A, Abdul-Kabir M, et al. Refractive error and visual impairment in private school children in Ghana. Optom Vis Sci. 2013;90:1456–61.
19. Wajuihian SO, Hansraj R. Refractive error in a sample of black high school children in South Africa. Optom Vis Sci. 2017;94:1145–52.
20. Aldebasi YH. Prevalence of correctable visual impairment in primary school children in Qassim Province, Saudi Arabia. J Optom. 2014;7:168–76.
21. Al Wadaani FA, Amin TT, Ali A, Khan AR. Prevalence and pattern of refractive errors among primary school children in Al Hassa, Saudi Arabia. Global J Health Sci. 2013;5:125.
22. Galvis V, Tello A, Otero J, et al. Prevalence of refractive errors in Colombia: MIOPUR study. Br J Ophthalmol. 2018;102:1320–3.
23. Galvis V, Tello A, Otero J, et al. Refractive errors in children and adolescents in Bucaramanga (Colombia). Arq Bras Oftalmol. 2017;80:359–63.
24. Carter MJ, Lansingh VC, Schacht G, et al. Visual acuity and refraction by age for children of three different ethnic groups in Paraguay. Arq Bras Oftalmol. 2013;76:94–7.
25. Lira RPC, Arieta CEL, Passos THM, et al. Distribution of ocular component measures and refraction in Brazilian school children. Ophthalmic Epidemiol. 2017;24:29–35.
26. French AN, Morgan IG, Mitchell P, Rose KA. Risk factors for incident myopia in Australian schoolchildren: the Sydney adolescent vascular and eye study. Ophthalmology. 2013;120:2100–8.
27. Yang M, Luensmann D, Fonn D, et al. Myopia prevalence in Canadian school children: a pilot study. Eye. 2018;32:1042–7.
28. Tideman JWL, Polling JR, Hofman A, et al. Environmental factors explain socioeconomic prevalence differences in myopia in 6-year-old children. Br J Ophthalmol. 2018;102:243–7.
29. Matamoros E, Ingrand P, Pelen F, et al. Prevalence of myopia in France: a cross-sectional analysis. Medicine. 2015;94
30. McCullough SJ, O'Donoghue L, Saunders KJ. Six year refractive change among white children and young adults: evidence for significant increase in myopia among white UK Children. PLoS One. 2016;11:e0146332.
31. Vitale S, Sperduto RD, Ferris FL III. Increased prevalence of myopia in the United States between 1971-1972 and 1999-2004. Arch Ophthalmol. 2009;127:1632–9.
32. Flitcroft DI, He M, Jonas JB, et al. IMI–Defining and classifying myopia: a proposed set of standards for clinical and epidemiologic studies. Invest Ophthalmol Vis Sci. 2019;60:M20–30.
33. Ma Y, Qu X, Zhu X, et al. Age-specific prevalence of visual impairment and refractive error in children aged 3–10 years in Shanghai, China. Invest Ophthalmol Vis Sci. 2016;57:6188–96.
34. Lan W, Zhao F, Lin L, et al. Refractive errors in 3–6 year-old Chinese children: a very low prevalence of myopia? PLoS One. 2013;8:e78003.
35. Guo Y, Duan JL, Liu LJ, et al. High myopia in greater Beijing school children in 2016. 2017, 12:e0187396.
36. Bullimore MA, Brennan NA. Myopia control: why each diopter matters. Optom Vis Sci. 2019;96:463–5.
37. Lee DC, Lee SY, Kim YC. An epidemiological study of the risk factors associated with myopia in young adult men in Korea. Sci Rep. 2018;8:1–7.

38. Ohno-Matsui K, Kawasaki R, Jonas JB, et al. International photographic classification and grading system for myopic maculopathy. Am J Ophthalmol. 2015;159(877–883):e877.
39. Liu HH, Xu L, Wang YX, et al. Prevalence and progression of myopic retinopathy in Chinese adults: the Beijing Eye Study. Ophthalmology. 2010;117:1763–8.
40. Gao LQ, Liu W, Liang YB, et al. Prevalence and characteristics of myopic retinopathy in a rural Chinese adult population: the Handan Eye Study. Arch Ophthalmol. 2011;129:1199–204.
41. Vongphanit J, Mitchell P, Wang JJ. Prevalence and progression of myopic retinopathy in an older population. Ophthalmology. 2002;109:704–11.
42. Chen SJ, Cheng CY, Li AF, et al. Prevalence and associated risk factors of myopic maculopathy in elderly Chinese: the Shihpai eye study. Invest Ophthalmol Vis Sci. 2012;53:4868–73.
43. Dhakal R, Goud A, Narayanan R, Verkicharla PK. Patterns of posterior ocular complications in myopic eyes of Indian population. Sci Rep. 2018;8:13700.
44. Ohno-Matsui K, Wu PC, Yamashiro K, et al. IMI pathologic myopia. Invest Ophthalmol Vis Sci. 2021;62:5.
45. Asakuma T, Yasuda M, Ninomiya T, et al. Prevalence and risk factors for myopic retinopathy in a Japanese population: the Hisayama Study. Ophthalmology. 2012;119:1760–5.
46. Wong Y-L, Sabanayagam C, Ding Y, et al. Prevalence, risk factors, and impact of myopic macular degeneration on visual impairment and functioning among adults in Singapore. Invest Ophthalmol Vis Sci. 2018;59:4603–13.
47. Wong YL, Zhu X, Tham YC. Prevalence and predictors of myopic macular degeneration among Asian adults: pooled analysis from the Asian Eye Epidemiology Consortium. Br J Ophthalmol. 2021;105:1140–8.
48. Zou M, Wang S, Chen A, et al. Prevalence of myopic macular degeneration worldwide: a systematic review and meta-analysis. Br J Ophthalmol. 2020;104:1748–54.
49. Wong TY, Ferreira A, Hughes R, Carter G, Mitchell P. Epidemiology and disease burden of pathologic myopia and myopic choroidal neovascularization: an evidence-based systematic review. Am J Ophthalmol. 2014;157(9–25):e12.
50. Choi HK, Lin W, Loon SC, et al. Facial scanning with a digital camera: a novel way of screening for primary angle closure. J Glaucoma. 2015;24:522–6.
51. Saw S-M, Tong L, Chua W-H, et al. Incidence and progression of myopia in singaporean school children. Invest Ophthalmol Vis Sci. 2005;46:51–7.
52. Rose KA, French A, Morgan IG, Mitchell P. Incidence of myopia in Australian adolescents: the Sydney Childhood Eye Study (SCES). Invest Ophthalmol Vis Sci. 2012;53:2307.
53. Wang J, Li Y, Musch DC, et al. Progression of myopia in school-aged children after COVID-19 home confinement. JAMA Ophthalmol. 2021;139:293–300.
54. Rose KA, French A, Morgan IG, Mitchell PJIO, Science V. Incidence of myopia in Australian adolescents: the Sydney Childhood Eye Study (SCES). Investig Ophthalmol Vis Sci. 2012;53:–2307.
55. Breslin KM, O'Donoghue L, Saunders KJ. A prospective study of spherical refractive error and ocular components among Northern Irish schoolchildren (the NICER study). Invest Ophthalmol Vis Sci. 2013;54:4843–50.
56. Verkicharla PK, Kammari P, Das AV. Myopia progression varies with age and severity of myopia. PLoS One. 2020;15:e0241759.
57. Smith EL 3rd. Spectacle lenses and emmetropization: the role of optical defocus in regulating ocular development. Optom Vis Sci. 1998;75:388–98.
58. Wallman J, Winawer J. Homeostasis of eye growth and the question of myopia. Neuron. 2004;43:447–68.
59. Irving EL, Sivak JG, Callender MG. Refractive plasticity of the developing chick eye. Ophthalmic Physiol Opt. 1992;12:448–56.
60. Graham B, Judge SJ. The effects of spectacle wear in infancy on eye growth and refractive error in the marmoset (Callithrix jacchus). Vis Res. 1999;39:189–206.
61. Ramamurthy D, Lin Chua SY, Saw SM. A review of environmental risk factors for myopia during early life, childhood and adolescence. Clin Exp Optom. 2015;98:497–506.

62. McBrien NA, Millodot M. A biometric investigation of late onset myopic eyes. Acta Ophthalmol. 1987;65:461–8.
63. Xie R, Zhou XT, Lu F, et al. Correlation between myopia and major biometric parameters of the eye: a retrospective clinical study. Optom Vis Sci. 2009;86:E503–8.
64. Wong TY, Foster PJ, Ng TP, et al. Variations in ocular biometry in an adult Chinese population in Singapore: the Tanjong Pagar Survey. Invest Ophthalmol Vis Sci. 2001;42:73–80.
65. Jiang BC, Woessner WM. Vitreous chamber elongation is responsible for myopia development in a young adult. Optom Vis Sci. 1996;73:231–4.
66. van Alphen GW. Choroidal stress and emmetropization. Vis Res. 1986;26:723–34.
67. Cheng HM, Singh OS, Kwong KK, et al. Shape of the myopic eye as seen with high-resolution magnetic resonance imaging. Optom Vis Sci. 1992;69:698–701.
68. Sorsby A, Benjamin B, Sheridan M, Stone J, Leary GA. Refraction and its components during the growth of the eye from the age of three. Memo Med Res Counc. 1961;301(Special):1–67.
69. Verkicharla PK, Mathur A, Mallen EA, Pope JM, Atchison DA. Eye shape and retinal shape, and their relation to peripheral refraction. Ophthalmic Physiol Opt. 2012;32:184–99.
70. Dhakal R, Vupparaboina KK, Verkicharla PK. Anterior sclera undergoes thinning with increasing degree of myopia. Invest Ophthalmol Vis Sci. 2020;61:6.
71. Chakraborty R, Pardue MT. Molecular and biochemical aspects of the retina on refraction. In: Hejtmancik JF, Nickerson JM, editors. Progress in molecular biology and translational science. Burlington: Academic Press; 2015. p. 249–67.
72. Masland RH. Neuronal diversity in the retina. Curr Opin Neurobiol. 2001;11:431–6.
73. Kolb H, Fernandez E, Webvision RN. The organization of the retina and visual system. Salt Lake City, UT: University of Utah Health Sciences Center; 2020.
74. Chakraborty R, Read SA, Collins MJ. Monocular myopic defocus and daily changes in axial length and choroidal thickness of human eyes. Exp Eye Res. 2012;103:47–54.
75. Chakraborty R, Read SA, Collins MJ. Hyperopic defocus and diurnal changes in human choroid and axial length. Optom Vis Sci. 2013;90:1187–98.
76. Moderiano D, Do M, Hobbs S, et al. Influence of the time of day on axial length and choroidal thickness changes to hyperopic and myopic defocus in human eyes. Exp Eye Res. 2019;182:125–36.
77. Wang D, Chun RK, Liu M, et al. Optical defocus rapidly changes choroidal thickness in schoolchildren. PLoS One. 2016;11:e0161535.
78. Phillips JR. Monovision slows juvenile myopia progression unilaterally. Br J Ophthalmol. 2005;89:1196–200.
79. Irving EL, Callender MG, Sivak JG. Inducing myopia, hyperopia, and astigmatism in chicks. Optom Vis Sci. 1991;68:364–8.
80. Nickla DL, Wildsoet C, Wallman J. Visual influences on diurnal rhythms in ocular length and choroidal thickness in chick eyes. Exp Eye Res. 1998;66:163–81.
81. Schaeffel F, Glasser A, Howland HC. Accommodation, refractive error and eye growth in chickens. Vis Res. 1988;28:639–57.
82. Schmid KL, Wildsoet CF. Effects on the compensatory responses to positive and negative lenses of intermittent lens wear and ciliary nerve section in chicks. Vis Res. 1996;36:1023–36.
83. Wallman J, Wildsoet C, Xu A, et al. Moving the retina: choroidal modulation of refractive state. Vis Res. 1995;35:37–50.
84. Wildsoet C, Wallman J. Choroidal and scleral mechanisms of compensation for spectacle lenses in chicks. Vis Res. 1995;35:1175–94.
85. Schaeffel F, Troilo D, Wallman J, Howland HC. Developing eyes that lack accommodation grow to compensate for imposed defocus. Vis Neurosci. 1990;4:177–83.
86. Hung L-F, Crawford MLJ, Smith EL. Spectacle lenses alter eye growth and the refractive status of young monkeys. Nat Med. 1995;1:761–5.
87. Smith EL, Huang J, Hung LF, et al. Hemiretinal form deprivation: evidence for local control of eye growth and refractive development in infant monkeys. Invest Ophthalmol Vis Sci. 2009;50:5057–69.

88. Smith EL, Hung L-F. The role of optical defocus in regulating refractive development in infant monkeys. Vis Res. 1999;39:1415–35.
89. Smith EL, Hung LF, Huang J, Arumugam B. Effects of local myopic defocus on refractive development in monkeys. Optom Vis Sci. 2013;90:1176–86.
90. Smith EL, Hung LF, Huang J, et al. Effects of optical defocus on refractive development in monkeys: evidence for local, regionally selective mechanisms. Invest Ophthalmol Vis Sci. 2010;51:3864–73.
91. Smith EL, Ramamirtham R, Qiao-Grider Y, et al. Effects of foveal ablation on emmetropization and form-deprivation myopia. Invest Ophthalmol Vis Sci. 2007;48:3914–22.
92. Norton TT, Essinger JA, McBrien NA. Lid-suture myopia in tree shrews with retinal ganglion cell blockade. Vis Neurosci. 1994;11:143–53.
93. Norton TT, Siegwart JT Jr, Amedo AO. Effectiveness of hyperopic defocus, minimal defocus, or myopic defocus in competition with a myopiagenic stimulus in tree shrew eyes. Invest Ophthalmol Vis Sci. 2006;47:4687–99.
94. Barathi VA, Boopathi VG, Yap EPH, Beuerman RW. Two models of experimental myopia in the mouse. Vis Res. 2008;48:904–16.
95. Tkatchenko TV, Shen Y, Tkatchenko AV. Mouse Experimental Myopia Has Features of Primate Myopia. Invest Ophthalmol Vis Sci. 2010;51:1297–303.
96. Howlett MHC, McFadden SA. Spectacle lens compensation in the pigmented guinea pig. Vis Res. 2009;49:219–27.
97. Nathan J, Crewther SG, Crewther DP, Kiely PM. Effects of retinal image degradation on ocular growth in cats. Invest Ophthalmol Vis Sci. 1984;25:1300–6.
98. Smith EL, Maguire GW, Watson JT. Axial lengths and refractive errors in kittens reared with an optically induced anisometropia. Invest Ophthalmol Vis Sci. 1980;19:1250–5.
99. Turnbull PRK, Backhouse S, Phillips JR. Visually guided eye growth in the squid. Curr Biol. 2015;25:R791–2.
100. Chakraborty R, Ostrin LA, Benavente-Perez A, Verkicharla PK. Optical mechanisms regulating emmetropisation and refractive errors: evidence from animal models. Clin Exp Optom. 2020;103:55–67.
101. Schwahn HN, Schaeffel F. Chick eyes under cycloplegia compensate for spectacle lenses despite six-hydroxy dopamine treatment. Invest Ophthalmol Vis Sci. 1994;35:3516–24.
102. Choh V, Lew MY, Nadel MW, Wildsoet CF. Effects of interchanging hyperopic defocus and form deprivation stimuli in normal and optic nerve-sectioned chicks. Vis Res. 2006;46:1070–9.
103. Chung KM. Critical review: effects of optical defocus on refractive development and ocular growth and relation to accommodation. Optom Vis Sci. 1993;70:228–33.
104. Chakraborty R, Read SA, Vincent SJ. Understanding myopia: pathogenesis and mechanisms. In: Ang M, Wong TY, editors. Updates on myopia: a clinical perspective. Singapore: Springer; 2020. p. 65–94.
105. Troilo D, Smith EL 3rd, Nickla DL, et al. IMI - report on experimental models of emmetropization and myopia. Invest Ophthalmol Vis Sci. 2019;60:M31–m88.
106. Lu B, Wang Y, Zhang P, et al. Evaluation of the association of macular ganglion cell-inner plexiform layer thickness and myopia in Chinese young adults. Eye (Lond). 2021;35:393–9.
107. Malakar M, Askari SN, Ashraf H, et al. Optical coherence tomography assisted retinal nerve fibre layer thickness profile in high myopia. J Clin Diagn Res. 2015;9:Nc01–3.
108. Liu X, Shen M, Yuan Y, et al. Macular thickness profiles of intraretinal layers in myopia evaluated by ultrahigh-resolution optical coherence tomography. Am J Ophthalmol. 2015;160:53–61.e52.
109. Sezgin Akcay BI, Gunay BO, Kardes E, Unlu C, Ergin A. Evaluation of the ganglion cell complex and retinal nerve fiber layer in low, moderate, and high myopia: a study by RTVue spectral domain optical coherence tomography. Semin Ophthalmol. 2017;32:682–8.
110. Jonas JB, Xu L, Wei WB, et al. Retinal thickness and axial length. Invest Ophthalmol Vis Sci. 2016;57:1791–7.
111. Read SA, Alonso-Caneiro D, Vincent SJ. Longitudinal changes in macular retinal layer thickness in pediatric populations: myopic vs non-myopic eyes. PLoS One. 2017;12:e0180462.

112. Read SA, Alonso-Caneiro D, Vincent SJ, Collins MJ. Longitudinal changes in choroidal thickness and eye growth in childhood. Invest Ophthalmol Vis Sci. 2015;56:3103–12.
113. Read SA, Collins MJ, Vincent SJ, Alonso-Caneiro D. Choroidal thickness in myopic and nonmyopic children assessed with enhanced depth imaging optical coherence tomography. Invest Ophthalmol Vis Sci. 2013;54:7578–86.
114. Smith EL, Kee CS, Ramamirtham R, Qiao-Grider Y, Hung LF. Peripheral vision can influence eye growth and refractive development in infant monkeys. Invest Ophthalmol Vis Sci. 2005;46:3965–72.
115. Smith EL, Hung LF, Huang J. Relative peripheral hyperopic defocus alters central refractive development in infant monkeys. Vis Res. 2009;49:2386–92.
116. Seidemann A, Schaeffel F, Guirao A, Lopez-Gil N, Artal P. Peripheral refractive errors in myopic, emmetropic, and hyperopic young subjects. J Opt Soc Am. 2002;19:2363–73.
117. Verkicharla PK, Suheimat M, Schmid KL, Atchison DA. Peripheral refraction, peripheral eye length, and retinal shape in myopia. Optom Vis Sci. 2016;93:1072–8.
118. Charman WN, Radhakrishnan H. Peripheral refraction and the development of refractive error: a review. Ophthalmic Physiol Opt. 2010;30:321–38.
119. Morgan IG. Brief periods of exposure to myopic defocus block the effects of prolonged periods of hyperopic defocus on axial elongation in the chick. Invest Ophthalmol Vis Sci. 2003;44:1988.
120. Morgan IG, Ambadeniya MP. Imposed Peripheral Myopic Defocus Can Prevent the Development of Lens–Induced Myopia. Invest Ophthalmol Vis Sci. 2006;47:–3328.
121. Schippert R, Schaeffel F. Peripheral defocus does not necessarily affect central refractive development. Vis Res. 2006;46:3935–40.
122. Benavente-Perez A, Nour A, Troilo D. Axial eye growth and refractive error development can be modified by exposing the peripheral retina to relative myopic or hyperopic defocus. Invest Ophthalmol Vis Sci. 2014;55:6765–73.
123. Liu Y, Wildsoet C. The effect of two-zone concentric bifocal spectacle lenses on refractive error development and eye growth in young chicks. Invest Ophthalmol Vis Sci. 2011;52:1078–86.
124. Bowrey H, Zeng G, Tse D, et al. The effect of spectacle lenses containing peripheral defocus on refractive error and horizontal eye shape in the guinea pig. Invest Ophthalmol Vis Sci. 2017;58:2705–14.
125. Gottlieb MD, Fugate-Wentzek LA, Wallman J. Different visual deprivations produce different ametropias and different eye shapes. Invest Ophthalmol Vis Sci. 1987;28:1225–35.
126. Stone RA, Pendrak K, Sugimoto R, et al. Local patterns of image degradation differentially affect refraction and eye shape in chick. Curr Eye Res. 2006;31:91–105.
127. Wallman J, Adams JI. Developmental aspects of experimental myopia in chicks: susceptibility, recovery and relation to emmetropization. Vis Res. 1987;27:1139–63.
128. Wallman J, Gottlieb MD, Rajaram V, Fugate-Wentzek LA. Local retinal regions control local eye growth and myopia. Science. 1987;237:73–7.
129. Atchison DA, Charman WN. Can partial coherence interferometry be used to determine retinal shape? Optom Vis Sci. 2011;88:E601–7.
130. Atchison DA, Pritchard N, Schmid KL, et al. Shape of the retinal surface in emmetropia and myopia. Invest Ophthalmol Vis Sci. 2005;46:2698–707.
131. Gilmartin B, Nagra M, Logan NS. Shape of the posterior vitreous chamber in human emmetropia and myopia. Invest Ophthalmol Vis Sci. 2013;54:7240–51.
132. Schmid GF. Association between retinal steepness and central myopic shift in children. Optom Vis Sci. 2011;88:684–90.
133. Verkicharla PK, Suheimat M, Schmid KL, Atchison DA. Differences in retinal shape between East Asian and Caucasian eyes. Ophthalmic Physiol Opt. 2017;37:275–83.
134. Wakazono T, Yamashiro K, Miyake M, et al. Time-course change in eye shape and development of staphyloma in highly myopic eyes. Invest Ophthalmol Vis Sci. 2018;59:5455–61.
135. Nickla DL, Wallman J. The multifunctional choroid. Prog Retin Eye Res. 2010;29:144–68.
136. Zhu X, Wallman J. Temporal properties of compensation for positive and negative spectacle lenses in chicks. Invest Ophthalmol Vis Sci. 2009;50:37–46.

137. Park TW, Winawer J, Wallman J. Further evidence that chick eyes use the sign of blur in spectacle lens compensation. Vis Res. 2003;43:1519–31.
138. Hung LF, Wallman J, Smith EL 3rd. Vision-dependent changes in the choroidal thickness of macaque monkeys. Invest Ophthalmol Vis Sci. 2000;41:1259–69.
139. Troilo D, Nickla DL, Wildsoet CF. Choroidal thickness changes during altered eye growth and refractive state in a primate. Invest Ophthalmol Vis Sci. 2000;41:1249–58.
140. Hoseini-Yazdi H, Vincent SJ, Read SA, Collins MJ. Astigmatic defocus leads to short-term changes in human choroidal thickness. Invest Ophthalmol Vis Sci. 2020;61:48.
141. Hoseini-Yazdi H, Vincent SJ, Collins MJ, Read SA. Regional alterations in human choroidal thickness in response to short-term monocular hemifield myopic defocus. Ophthalmic Physiol Opt. 2019;39:172–82.
142. Chiang ST, Phillips JR, Backhouse S. Effect of retinal image defocus on the thickness of the human choroid. Ophthalmic Physiol Opt. 2015;35:405–13.
143. Read SA, Fuss JA, Vincent SJ, Collins MJ, Alonso-Caneiro D. Choroidal changes in human myopia: insights from optical coherence tomography imaging. Clin Exp Optom. 2019;102:270–85.
144. Flores-Moreno I, Lugo F, Duker JS, Ruiz-Moreno JM. The relationship between axial length and choroidal thickness in eyes with high myopia. Am J Ophthalmol. 2013;155:314–319.e311.
145. Liu Y, Wang L, Xu Y, Pang Z, Mu G. The influence of the choroid on the onset and development of myopia: from perspectives of choroidal thickness and blood flow. Acta Ophthalmol. 2021;99:730–8.
146. Sander BP, Collins MJ, Read SA. The interaction between homatropine and optical blur on choroidal thickness. Ophthalmic Physiol Opt. 2018;38:257–65.
147. Zhang Z, Zhou Y, Xie Z, et al. The effect of topical atropine on the choroidal thickness of healthy children. Sci Rep. 2016;6:34936.
148. Nickla DL, Totonelly K, Dhillon B. Dopaminergic agonists that result in ocular growth inhibition also elicit transient increases in choroidal thickness in chicks. Exp Eye Res. 2010;91:715–20.
149. Woodman-Pieterse EC, Read SA, Collins MJ, Alonso-Caneiro D. Regional changes in choroidal thickness associated with accommodation. Invest Ophthalmol Vis Sci. 2015;56:6414–22.
150. Woodman EC, Read SA, Collins MJ. Axial length and choroidal thickness changes accompanying prolonged accommodation in myopes and emmetropes. Vis Res. 2012;72:34–41.
151. Lan W, Feldkaemper M, Schaeffel F. Bright light induces choroidal thickening in chickens. Optom Vis Sci. 2013;90:1199–206.
152. Ulaganathan S, Read SA, Collins MJ, Vincent SJ. Daily axial length and choroidal thickness variations in young adults: Associations with light exposure and longitudinal axial length and choroid changes. Exp Eye Res. 2019;189:107850.
153. Trier K. The sclera. J Adv Organ Biol. 2005;10:353–73.
154. Rada JA, Shelton S, Norton TT. The sclera and myopia. Exp Eye Res. 2006;82:185–200.
155. Markov PP, Eliasy A, Pijanka JK, et al. Bulk changes in posterior scleral collagen microstructure in human high myopia. Mol Vis. 2018;24:818–33.
156. Curtin BJ, Iwamoto T, Renaldo DP. Normal and staphylomatous sclera of high myopia. An electron microscopic study. Arch Ophthalmol. 1979;97:912–5.
157. Ishikawa T. Fine structure of the human ciliary muscle. Investig Ophthalmol. 1962;1:587–608.
158. Woodman-Pieterse EC, Read SA, Collins MJ, Alonso-Caneiro D. Anterior scleral thickness changes with accommodation in myopes and emmetropes. Exp Eye Res. 2018;177:96–103.
159. Niyazmand H, Read SA, Atchison DA, Collins MJ. Anterior eye shape in emmetropes, low to moderate myopes, and high myopes. Cont Lens Anterior Eye. 2021;44:101361.
160. Martinez-Enriquez E, Pérez-Merino P, Velasco-Ocana M, Marcos S. OCT-based full crystalline lens shape change during accommodation in vivo. Biomed Opt Express. 2017;8:918–33.
161. Brown N. The change in shape and internal form of the lens of the eye on accommodation. Exp Eye Res. 1973;15:441–59.
162. Lu F, Zhou X, Jiang L, et al. Axial myopia induced by hyperopic defocus in guinea pigs: A detailed assessment on susceptibility and recovery. Exp Eye Res. 2009;89:101–8.

163. McBrien NA, Millodot M. The effect of refractive error on the accommodative response gradient. Ophthalmic Physiol Opt. 1986;6:145–9.
164. Gwiazda J, Thorn F, Bauer J, Held R. Myopic children show insufficient accommodative response to blur. Invest Ophthalmol Vis Sci. 1993;34:690–4.
165. Fulk GW, Cyert LA. Can bifocals slow myopia progression? J Am Optom Assoc. 1996;67:749–54.
166. Fulk GW, Cyert LA, Parker DE. A randomized trial of the effect of single-vision vs. bifocal lenses on myopia progression in children with esophoria. Optom Vis Sci. 2000;77:395–401.
167. Berntsen DA, Sinnott LT, Mutti DO, Zadnik K. A randomized trial using progressive addition lenses to evaluate theories of myopia progression in children with a high lag of accommodation. Invest Ophthalmol Vis Sci. 2012;53:640–9.
168. Gwiazda JE, Hyman L, Norton TT, et al. Accommodation and related risk factors associated with myopia progression and their interaction with treatment in COMET children. Invest Ophthalmol Vis Sci. 2004;45:2143–51.
169. Price H, Allen PM, Radhakrishnan H, et al. The Cambridge anti-myopia study: variables associated with myopia progression. Optom Vis Sci. 2013;90:1274–83.
170. Allen PM, O'Leary DJ. Accommodation functions: co-dependency and relationship to refractive error. Vis Res. 2006;46:491–505.
171. Rosenfield M, Desai R, Portello JK. Do progressing myopes show reduced accommodative responses? Optom Vis Sci. 2002;79:268–73.
172. Weizhong L, Zhikuan Y, Wen L, Xiang C, Jian G. A longitudinal study on the relationship between myopia development and near accommodation lag in myopic children. Ophthalmic Physiol Opt. 2008;28:57–61.
173. Chen Y, Drobe B, Zhang C, et al. Accommodation is unrelated to myopia progression in Chinese myopic children. Sci Rep. 2020;10:12056.
174. Mutti DO, Mitchell GL, Hayes JR, et al. Accommodative lag before and after the onset of myopia. Invest Ophthalmol Vis Sci. 2006;47:837–46.
175. Gu Y, Legge GE. Accommodation to stimuli in peripheral vision. JOSA A. 1987;4:1681–7.
176. Labhishetty V, Cholewiak SA, Banks MS. Contributions of foveal and non-foveal retina to the human eye's focusing response. J Vis. 2019;19:18.
177. Hartwig A, Charman WN, Radhakrishnan H, Optics P. Accommodative response to peripheral stimuli in myopes and emmetropes. Ophthalmic Physiol Opt. 2011;31:91–9.
178. Mutti DO, Zadnik K, Fusaro RE, et al. Optical and structural development of the crystalline lens in childhood. Invest Ophthalmol Vis Sci. 1998;39:120–33.
179. Zadnik K, Mutti DO, Fusaro RE, Adams AJ. Longitudinal evidence of crystalline lens thinning in children. Invest Ophthalmol Vis Sci. 1995;36:1581–7.
180. Drexler W, Findl O, Schmetterer L, Hitzenberger CK, Fercher AF. Eye elongation during accommodation in humans: differences between emmetropes and myopes. Invest Ophthalmol Vis Sci. 1998;39:2140–7.
181. Read SA, Collins MJ, Woodman EC, Cheong SH. Axial length changes during accommodation in myopes and emmetropes. Optom Vis Sci. 2010;87:656–62.
182. Mallen EA, Kashyap P, Hampson KM. Transient axial length change during the accommodation response in young adults. Invest Ophthalmol Vis Sci. 2006;47:1251–4.
183. Walker TW, Mutti DO. The effect of accommodation on ocular shape. Optom Vis Sci. 2002;79:424–30.
184. Takeda T, Neveu C, Stark L. Accommodation on downward gaze. Optom Vis Sci. 1992;69:556–61.
185. Ghosh A, Collins MJ, Read SA, Davis BA, Iskander DR. The influence of downward gaze and accommodation on ocular aberrations over time. J Vis. 2011;11:17.
186. Ghosh A, Collins MJ, Read SA, Davis BA, Iskander DR. Measurement of ocular aberrations in downward gaze using a modified clinical aberrometer. Biomed Opt Express. 2011;2:452–63.

187. Collins MJ, Buehren T, Bece A, Voetz SC. Corneal optics after reading, microscopy and computer work. Acta Ophthalmol Scand. 2006;84:216–24.
188. Vincent SJ, Collins MJ, Read SA, Carney LG, Yap MK. Corneal changes following near work in myopic anisometropia. Ophthalmic Physiol Opt. 2013;33:15–25.
189. Buehren T, Collins MJ, Carney L. Corneal aberrations and reading. Optom Vis Sci. 2003;80:159–66.
190. Zhang N, Yang XB, Zhang WQ, et al. Relationship between higher-order aberrations and myopia progression in schoolchildren: a retrospective study. Int J Ophthalmol. 2013;6:295–9.
191. Paquin MP, Hamam H, Simonet P. Objective measurement of optical aberrations in myopic eyes. Optom Vis Sci. 2002;79:285–91.
192. Jaschinski-Kruza W. Transient myopia after visual work. Ergonomics. 1984;27:1181–9.
193. Ciuffreda KJ, Wallis DM. Myopes show increased susceptibility to nearwork aftereffects. Invest Ophthalmol Vis Sci. 1998;39:1797–803.
194. Ciuffreda KJ, Lee M. Differential refractive susceptibility to sustained nearwork. Ophthalmic Physiol Opt. 2002;22:372–9.
195. Ong E, Ciuffreda KJ. Nearwork-induced transient myopia: a critical review. Doc Ophthalmol. 1995;91:57–85.
196. Ciuffreda KJ, Vasudevan B. Nearwork-induced transient myopia (NITM) and permanent myopia—is there a link? Ophthalmic Physiol Opt. 2008;28:103–14.
197. Vera-Díaz FA, Strang NC, Winn B. Nearwork induced transient myopia during myopia progression. Curr Eye Res. 2002;24:289–95.
198. Mallen EA, Gilmartin B, Wolffsohn JS. Sympathetic innervation of ciliary muscle and oculomotor function in emmetropic and myopic young adults. Vis Res. 2005;45:1641–51.
199. Bayramlar H, Cekiç O, Hepşen IF. Does convergence, not accommodation, cause axial-length elongation at near? A biometric study in teens. Ophthalmic Res. 1999;31:304–8.
200. Friberg TR, Lace JW. A comparison of the elastic properties of human choroid and sclera. Exp Eye Res. 1988;47:429–36.
201. Ghosh A, Collins MJ, Read SA, Davis BA. Axial length changes with shifts of gaze direction in myopes and emmetropes. Invest Ophthalmol Vis Sci. 2012;53:6465–71.
202. Niyazmand H, Read SA, Atchison DA, Collins MJ. Effects of accommodation and simulated convergence on anterior scleral shape. Ophthalmic Physiol Opt. 2020;40:482–90.
203. Crewther DP, Crewther SG, Xie RZ. Changes in eye growth produced by drugs which affect retinal ON or OFF responses to light. J Ocul Pharmacol Ther. 1996;12:193–208.
204. Chakraborty R, Park HN, Hanif AM, et al. ON pathway mutations increase susceptibility to form-deprivation myopia. Exp Eye Res. 2015;137:79–83.
205. Aleman AC, Wang M, Schaeffel F. Reading and myopia: contrast polarity matters. Sci Rep. 2018;8:10840.
206. Morgan IG, Wu PC, Ostrin LA, et al. IMI risk factors for myopia. Invest Ophthalmol Vis Sci. 2021;62:3.
207. Tedja MS, Haarman AEG, Meester-Smoor MA, et al. IMI - myopia genetics report. Invest Ophthalmol Vis Sci. 2019;60:M89–m105.
208. Zhang Q, Guo X, Xiao X, et al. Novel locus for X linked recessive high myopia maps to Xq23-q25 but outside MYP1. J Med Genet. 2006;43:e20.
209. Kurtz D, Hyman L, Gwiazda JE, et al. Role of parental myopia in the progression of myopia and its interaction with treatment in COMET children. Invest Ophthalmol Vis Sci. 2007;48:562–70.
210. Jiang X, Tarczy-Hornoch K, Cotter SA, et al. Association of parental myopia with higher risk of myopia among multiethnic children before school age. JAMA Ophthalmol. 2020;138:501–9.
211. Zhang X, Qu X, Zhou X. Association between parental myopia and the risk of myopia in a child. Exp Ther Med. 2015;9:2420–8.

212. Loh KL, Lu Q, Tan D, Chia A. Risk factors for progressive myopia in the atropine therapy for myopia study. Am J Ophthalmol. 2015;159:945–9.
213. Huang HM, Chang DS, Wu PC. The association between near work activities and myopia in children-a systematic review and meta-analysis. PLoS One. 2015;10:e0140419.
214. Ip JM, Saw SM, Rose KA, et al. Role of near work in myopia: findings in a sample of Australian school children. Invest Ophthalmol Vis Sci. 2008;49:2903–10.
215. Saw SM, Chua WH, Hong CY, et al. Nearwork in early-onset myopia. Invest Ophthalmol Vis Sci. 2002;43:332–9.
216. Li SM, Li SY, Kang MT, et al. Near work related parameters and myopia in Chinese children: the anyang childhood eye study. PLoS One. 2015;10:e0134514.
217. Pärssinen O, Kauppinen M. Associations of reading posture, gaze angle and reading distance with myopia and myopic progression. Acta Ophthalmol. 2016;94:775–9.
218. Charman WN. Aniso-accommodation as a possible factor in myopia development. Ophthalmic Physiol Opt. 2004;24:471–9.
219. Bez D, Megreli J, Bez M, et al. Association between type of educational system and prevalence and severity of myopia among male adolescents in Israel. JAMA Ophthalmol. 2019;137:887–93.
220. Bao J, Drobe B, Wang Y, et al. Influence of near tasks on posture in myopic Chinese Schoolchildren. Optom Vis Sci. 2015;92:908–15.
221. Sherwin JC, Reacher MH, Keogh RH, et al. The association between time spent outdoors and myopia in children and adolescents: a systematic review and meta-analysis. Ophthalmology. 2012;119:2141–51.
222. Xiong S, Sankaridurg P, Naduvilath T, et al. Time spent in outdoor activities in relation to myopia prevention and control: a meta-analysis and systematic review. Acta Ophthalmol. 2017;95:551–66.
223. French AN, Ashby RS, Morgan IG, Rose KA. Time outdoors and the prevention of myopia. Exp Eye Res. 2013;114:58–68.
224. Nickels S, Hopf S, Pfeiffer N, Schuster AK. Myopia is associated with education: results from NHANES 1999-2008. PLoS One. 2019;14:e0211196.
225. Mirshahi A, Ponto KA, Hoehn R, et al. Myopia and level of education: results from the Gutenberg Health Study. Ophthalmology. 2014;121:2047–52.
226. Tay MT, Au Eong KG, Ng CY, Lim MK. Myopia and educational attainment in 421,116 young Singaporean males. Ann Acad Med Singap. 1992;21:785–91.
227. Au Eong KG, Tay TH, Lim MK. Education and myopia in 110,236 young Singaporean males. Singap Med J. 1993;34:489–92.
228. Verma A, Verma A. A novel review of the evidence linking myopia and high intelligence. J Ophthalmol. 2015;2015:271746.
229. Saw SM, Tan SB, Fung D, et al. IQ and the association with myopia in children. Invest Ophthalmol Vis Sci. 2004;45:2943–8.
230. Saw SM, Cheng A, Fong A, et al. School grades and myopia. Ophthalmic Physiol Opt. 2007;27:126–9.
231. Mirshahi A, Ponto KA, Laubert-Reh D, et al. Myopia and cognitive performance: results from the gutenberg health study. Invest Ophthalmol Vis Sci. 2016;57:5230–6.
232. He M, Zheng Y, Xiang F. Prevalence of myopia in urban and rural children in mainland China. Optom Vis Sci. 2009;86:40–4.
233. McCrann S, Loughman J, Butler JS, Paudel N, Flitcroft DI. Smartphone use as a possible risk factor for myopia. Clin Exp Optom. 2021;104:35–41.
234. Yang GY, Huang LH, Schmid KL, et al. Associations between screen exposure in early life and myopia amongst Chinese preschoolers. Int J Environ Res Public Health. 2020;17:1056.
235. Liu S, Ye S, Xi W, Zhang X. Electronic devices and myopic refraction among children aged 6-14 years in urban areas of Tianjin. China Ophthalmic Physiol Opt. 2019;39:282–93.

236. Jacobsen N, Jensen H, Goldschmidt E. Does the level of physical activity in university students influence development and progression of myopia? A 2-year prospective cohort study. Invest Ophthalmol Vis Sci. 2008;49:1322–7.
237. Rahi JS, Cumberland PM, Peckham CS. Myopia over the lifecourse: prevalence and early life influences in the 1958 British birth cohort. Ophthalmology. 2011;118:797–804.
238. Dirani M, Islam A, Baird PN. Body stature and myopia-The Genes in Myopia (GEM) twin study. Ophthalmic Epidemiol. 2008;15:135–9.
239. O'Connor AR, Stephenson TJ, Johnson A, et al. Change of refractive state and eye size in children of birth weight less than 1701 g. Br J Ophthalmol. 2006;90:456–60.

Update on Interventions to Slow Myopia Progression

2

Padmaja Sankaridurg

The awareness and importance of managing myopia progression are growing due to the burden resulting from an increasing prevalence of myopia. As outlined in Chap. 1, myopia is already seen at epidemic proportions in many East Asian and South-East Asian countries. Vision impairment may result from uncorrected or undercorrected myopia, as well as from the sight-threatening complications associated with higher levels of myopia. For an individual, the life-long nature of the condition results in a health expenditure burden that increases with higher levels of myopia and complications. In addition, myopia imposes quality of life issues with both uncorrected and corrected myopia, depending on the type of intervention. Overall, the costs to society in terms of direct health expenditure and lost productivity are significant [1].

Presently, our understanding of the mechanisms implicated in the onset and progression of myopia involves both genetic and environmental factors. Genetic involvement is evidenced by data demonstrating a greater risk of onset and progression in those with parental myopia, high heritability of refractive error in twins and linkage studies, and GWAS identifying loci associated with refractive error. Importantly, environmental exposure appears to confer significant risk, with urban-rural location, socioeconomic status, education, and certain occupations influencing risk of onset and progression [2]. With respect to environmental risk factors, early studies focused on aspects of near work whereas more recent data indicate that aspects of time outdoors may be more significant; an increased risk of myopia is evidenced in those with reduced outdoor activity [3]. While the science underpinning onset and progression of myopia is evolving, encouragingly, interest in strategies that reduce the risk of onset as well as control the progression of

P. Sankaridurg (✉)
Brien Holden Vision Institute, Sydney, Australia

School of Optometry and Vision Science, University of New South Wales, Sydney, Australia
e-mail: p.sankaridurg@bhvi.org

A. Ramasubramanian (ed.), *Pediatric Ophthalmology*, Current Practices in Ophthalmology, https://doi.org/10.1007/978-981-19-4963-0_2

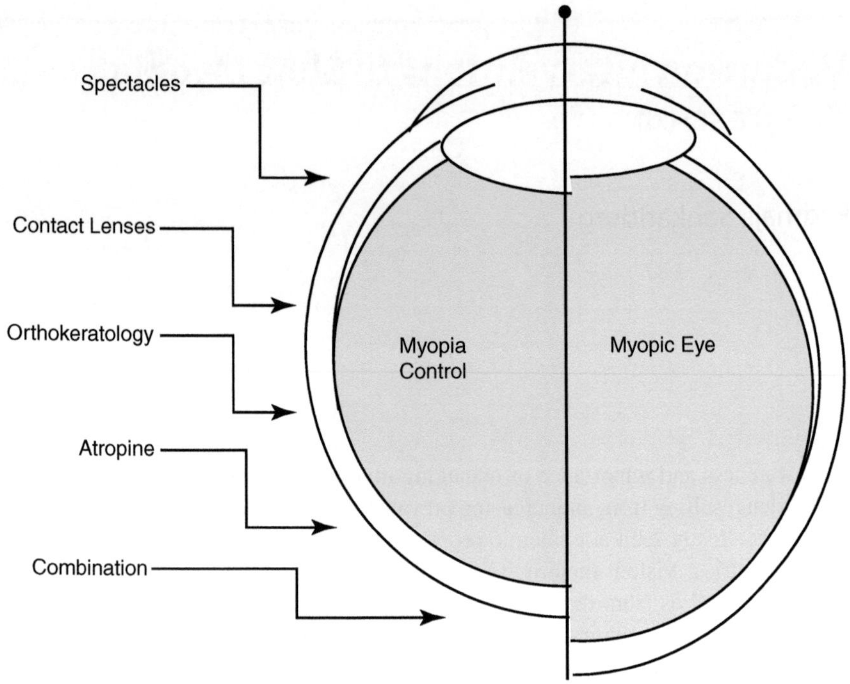

Fig. 2.1 Schematic diagram illustrating various approaches for myopia control

myopia has resulted in environmental, pharmaceutical, and optical strategies that delay and/or reduce myopia progression. The efficacy data relating to these interventions has been published extensively. In this chapter, the substantial efforts that have been directed to slowing myopia progression utilizing pharmacological and optical approaches are summarized (Fig. 2.1). Early attempts to slow myopia were focused on alleviating hyperopic blur/defocus resulting from accommodative dysfunction and include, for example, progressive addition spectacles and atropine. More recent evidence implicating the peripheral retina and defocus at the peripheral retina in the onset and progression of myopia has seen the development of a new generation of devices aimed at reducing peripheral retinal defocus, and include peripheral defocus modifying spectacles, contact lenses, and orthokeratology. Surgical methods to slow myopia involving strengthening/reinforcement of sclera, injections, and collagen cross-linking are not covered in this chapter.

2.1 Slowing Progression of Myopia: Pharmacological Measures

Pharmaceutical agents trialled thus far for slowing myopia include (a) muscarinic receptor antagonists—atropine, pirenzepine, and tropicamide (b) xanthine derivatives such as methylxanthine and caffeine, and (c) intraocular pressure-lowering agents such as timolol.

Of these, Pirenzepine—a selective M1 antimuscarinic agent—slowed myopia by up to 50% compared to a placebo control and with fewer side effects than the more widely used Atropine (less pupillary dilation than Atropine); but it is no longer pursued despite its initial success [4]. Similarly, there exists a single report with promising data for use of 1% tropicamide instilled nightly. Relaxation of the ciliary muscle was reported to be the mechanism underlying the slower progression; 29% of eyes on tropicamide progressed >0.50D compared to 63% with controls. However, the trial was nonrandomized and the cases versus controls were not matched for the commonly considered factors of age, refractive error, and duration of treatment [5].

Timolol, an ocular hypotensive agent was considered to exert a biomechanical action; by lowering intraocular pressure, the stretching of the eye would decrease and therefore reduce the risk of axial elongation [6, 7]. Although lowered progression was observed in eyes with lowered IOP from timolol, other studies found no evidence of reduced progression even though IOP was reduced [8].

7-methylxanthine used orally (400 mg) in myopic children for 24 months slowed axial elongation but not the spherical equivalent refractive error; furthermore, a shorter period of use (12 months) did not appear to confer any benefit [9]. 7-methylxanthine was regarded to exert its action by remodeling the posterior sclera by increasing the collagen concentration as well as the diameter of collagen fibrils. In primates and rabbits, 7-methylxanthine reduced axial myopia induced by hyperopic defocus. Additionally, topically instilled caffeine, another xanthine derivative reduced the likelihood of primate eyes responding to hyperopic defocus [10]. However, in recent studies conducted on chicks, 7-methylxanthine had no effect on form-deprivation myopia or on retinal dopamine system [11].

Of the pharmaceutical agents, Atropine, a nonselective muscarinic receptor antagonist remains the only agent that is widely in use. Atropine has been used for centuries for mydriasis but since the late nineteenth century, found use for slowing myopia [12]. Initially trialed at high doses of either 1.0% or 0.5% [13, 14], Atropine is quite effective in slowing myopia; however, its use especially at higher concentrations is accompanied by an increased and fixed pupillary diameter and paralysis of accommodation. Furthermore, rebound on discontinuation of Atropine was observed at high concentrations [15, 16]. In the ATOM studies, children were randomized to receive either Atropine 1% or placebo in one eye only and a significant reduction in progression was observed at the end of 2 years; however, a subsequent washout period of 1 year saw a significant rebound of myopia [15].

Consequently, lower doses of Atropine were trialed (0.1–0.01%) and found favor due to reduced risk of side effects and rebound. In a recently conducted meta-analysis, quantification of the effect size for an increase in pupillary diameter and reduced accommodative amplitude found concentrations of 0.1% Atropine and above to result in a significant effect (>10 D in accommodative amplitude and >2 mm increase in pupil size) with a much lower effect at lower doses. Efficacy was also dose-dependent; although reduction in progression was still significant, efficacy reduced with lower concentrations. Presently, concentrations ranging from 0.01% to 0.05% are increasingly considered [16, 17]. There is some controversy surrounding the use of 0.01% atropine; in both the ATOM 2 study and the more recently conducted LAMP study. Although 0.01% atropine significantly slowed myopia with respect to spherical equivalent refractive error, the change in axial elongation compared to control was not significant [16, 17]. Despite this finding, 0.01% Atropine remains the most widely used concentration. Since Atropine was widely assessed in Asian eyes, its efficacy in European eyes with lighter irides was questioned; however, recent studies demonstrated that it is equally effective in other races [18].

Despite its widespread use, the mechanism resulting in the slowing of axial elongation with Atropine remains uncertain. In early studies, Atropine was thought to act on the smooth ciliary muscle and block the accommodative function of the eye. However, sectioning of the optic nerve or lesioning of EW nucleus resulted in loss of accommodative function but did not inhibit the development of myopia; furthermore, Atropine inhibited myopia in chicks that lack muscarinic receptors. More recent studies have considered the role of Atropine on retina, choroid, and sclera. For example, the use of Atropine resulted in increased sub- and para-foveal choroidal thickness [19, 20] and Atropine was found to inhibit choroidal thinning induced by hyperopic defocus [21, 22]. The sclera as a potential site has also been explored. Synthesis of glycosaminoglycan in the scleral extracellular matrix was inhibited by atropine in chick tissue, and real-time PCR showed upregulation of the mRNA levels of M1, M3, and M4 receptors in the sclera after subconjunctival atropine treatment in addition to lens-induced myopia in mice. Despite these investigations, the mechanism underpinning slowing of eye growth with Atropine remains unclear [23].

The use of atropine requires concurrent use of an optical correction such as spectacles or contact lenses to correct for the distance refractive error. Additionally, higher concentrations of Atropine may necessitate the use of near add and/or photochromic glasses to manage near vision problems and photophobia.

2.2 Slowing Progression of Myopia: Optical Interventions

Early optical strategies for controlling myopia advocated for under correction; however, in controlled clinical trials, under correction had either no effect on progression or worsened progression. Optical interventions, i.e., spectacles, contact lenses, and orthokeratology lenses designed to slow myopia aim to reduce the hyperopic defocus/blur either at the central and/or peripheral retina.

2.2.1 Spectacle-Based Strategies

Spectacle-based strategies for slowing myopia include (1) progressive additional spectacles (PAL) [24–28], (2) peripheral asphericized progressive additional spectacles (PA-PAL) [27], (3) peripheral defocus spectacles (Peri-def) [29], (4) executive bifocal with or without prisms (exec bifocal) [30], and (5) defocus incorporated multiple segments (DIMS) or aspherical lenslet spectacles [31, 32].

The earlier spectacle based strategies for slowing myopia such as for example, bifocal spectacles and/or progressive addition spectacles were designed to reduce accommodative lag or dysfunction resulting from excessive near work; however, the performance of these designs in well-controlled clinical trials found limited efficacy. There were some exceptions; a study using executive bifocals both with and without prisms, reported myopia control effect of up to 54% with higher efficacy in the subgroup with a low lag of accommodation [30].

In recent years, mechanisms and theories related to the progression of myopia focused on the role of defocus in the peripheral retina. In experiments conducted using animal models, it was demonstrated that the peripheral visual signals could guide emmetropisation in the absence of a functioning fovea, and form-deprivation/hyperopic defocus at the peripheral retina could induce central myopic refractive error [33]. A myopic eye corrected with single vision spectacles results in hyperopic defocus at the peripheral retina due to the prolate shape of a myopic eye. This knowledge spurred the development of a new generation of spectacle lens designs designed to reduce peripheral retinal defocus. In clinical trials, early designs were observed to have limited efficacy [29]. The spectacle lens commonly incorporated a central portion/zone devoted to correcting the myopic refractive error of the eye; surrounding the central portion was a zone that was relatively more positive compared to the central zone and had a continuous power profile that increased towards the periphery of the lens [29]. More recent spectacle lens designs incorporate multiple segments/lenslets in the area surrounding the central zone rather than a continuous smooth power profile seen in the earlier designs; these segments/lenslets are relatively more positive in power. These lenses include the DIMS or defocus incorporated multiple segments (each segment in the DIMS lens is approximately 1.00 mm in diameter and +3.50D more positive than the base power) and the highly aspherical lenslets (approximately 1.2 mm in diameter, aspherical power profile) [32, 34]. In clinical studies, there was a significant treatment effect of up to 60% slowing in myopia with DIMS over a 2-year period [34]. Similarly, over 1-year period, spectacles incorporating highly aspherical lenslets were able to significantly slow myopia; 67% reduction in progression of spherical equivalent refractive error and 64% reduction of axial elongation as compared to control. In comparison, slightly reduced efficacy was observed with slightly aspherical lenslets (41% for change in spherical equivalent refractive error and 31% for change in axial length, respectively) [32].

While simple and convenient to use, due to the nature of the myopia control spectacle lens designs, there may be aspects of visual performance, that may be impacted. It should also be noted that most of the evidence is from trials considering low to moderate myopia; the efficacy of these spectacles in highly myopic eyes remains to be explored.

2.2.2 Contact Lens Based Strategies

Early studies from the 90s with rigid gas permeable lenses found slowing of myopia that was unrelated to the corneal flattening induced by the lenses [35]. However, later well-conducted clinical trials found no support for use of rigid gas permeable lenses in slowing myopia [36].

Importantly, in recent years, there has been data from many clinical trials that validate the use of multifocal or multifocal- like soft lenses to slow myopia. Such lenses are varyingly referred to in the literature as multifocal lenses, dual-focus lenses, defocus incorporated soft lenses, gradient lenses, and extended depth of focus lenses [37–46]. The optical zone of these lenses has a) portion(s) or areas that correct for the distance refractive error of the eye and, b) one or more portions that are relatively more positive than the distance power. The relatively positive portion is designed to induce myopic defocus and can be present, for example, as a concentric zone surrounding the central distance portion. Alternatively, the lens has a base power that corrects for the refractive power of the eye and rings of positive power that alternates with the base power [44]. In some designs, the relatively positive power was also present in the central optical zone [45]. Although the magnitude of the "relative positive power" that is required for myopia control is not clear, clinical studies that have used power of +2.00D and above have demonstrated success in slowing myopia. In a recent 3-year double-masked clinical trial a high add (+2.50D) multifocal lens was found to slow myopia more effectively than a medium add (+1.50D) center distance multifocal lens. (−0.60D vs −0.89D vs −1.05D for SE and 0.42 mm vs 0.58 mm vs 0.66 mm) [47].

In randomized clinical trials (1–3 years in duration), the efficacy of these lenses in slowing myopia ranged from 20% to 77%. Although myopia control strategies are commonly prescribed off-label, there are some contact lens designs that have been approved by regulatory bodies for myopia control. The MiSight contact lens has FDA approval for myopia control in children aged between 8 and 12 years; over a 3-year period, a significant reduction in progression of myopia was observed with MiSight® contact lenses compared to single vision lenses (a reduction of 59% and 52% in spherical equivalent refractive error and axial elongation with the spherical equivalent difference of approximately 0.75D) [44]. An independent, randomized clinical trial also found MiSight® contact lenses to slow spherical equivalent refractive error and axial elongation by 39% and 32% respectively as compared to single vision spectacles [48]. Additionally, MYLO contact lenses (Mark'ennovy, Spain) and NaturalVue® contact lens (Visioneering Technologies, USA) are specifically marketed to control myopia in children, and although they are referred to as extended depth of focus contact lenses, they are distinctly different in their lens design. The MYLO contact lens incorporates higher order aberrations to result in a lens power profile that is non-monotonic across the optical zone of the lens; [45] whereas the Natural Vue lens incorporates a ring of high positive power surrounding a central zone to create a pin hole effect resulting in extended depth of focus [49].

2.2.3 Orthokeratology

In recent years, overnight wear of reverse geometry rigid gas permeable lenses has achieved widespread popularity; these lenses reshape the cornea during overnight wear and enable functional vision during daytime without the need for any optical aid/correction. Additionally, in well-conducted clinical trials, these lenses were found to slow myopia [50–55]. Overnight wear of these lenses results in a reshaped corneal profile characterized by a flatter central cornea with mid-peripheral corneal steepening due to the redistribution of the corneal epithelium. The myopia control efficacy of these lenses is a result of either (a) the post ortho-k corneal profile resulting in less hyperopic defocus at the peripheral retina [50, 53–58] or (b) altered aberration profile of the eye. Greater efficacy was reported in eyes with larger pupils as a larger pupil is thought to result in a far greater reduction in myopic defocus at the far periphery. Evidence indicates that the efficacy of these lenses ranged from 30% to 63%. Orthokeratology was also found to be effective in those with high myopia and in those with moderate to high astigmatism; [59, 60] however, with high myopia, since the available OK lenses could be used to target up to −4.00D participants were required to wear single vision lenses to manage the residual refractive error [60]. However, a long-term study indicated that there may be a tapering of efficacy in later years [51]. There are reports suggesting that discontinuation of Ortho-k treatment during the progressive phase may result in an increased progression or rebound; however, the evidence is not consistent [61, 62].

2.2.4 Combination Strategies

Combination strategies in myopia management are not new, were in use over the years but were directed at improving the wearer experience rather than improving efficacy. For example, atropine use at higher concentrations necessitated the use of progressive addition lenses, and spectacles are commonly used in combination with contact lens strategies for end-of-day wear. More recently, there have been efforts to improve the efficacy of optical strategies especially Orthokeratology by using them in combination with atropine. Trials that evaluated dual therapy involving atropine (0.01–0.125%) plus Orthokeratology found improvement in efficacy over that of Orthokeratology (monotherapy) alone [63, 64]. The improvement ranged from approximately 5–50% over monotherapy alone. The mechanism underlying the improved efficacy with combination strategies is not fully clear, but the hypotheses considered include (a) a larger pupil resulting from atropine use that promotes myopic defocus from Orthokeratology; (b) Atropine and Orthokeratology act via different pathways and therefore provide an additive effect, and (c) the larger pupil promotes violet light exposure that is thought to slow progression.

The data is promising and provides another avenue to pursue for fast progressors and in those where the risk of side effects with atropine precludes the use of higher doses. However, combination therapies involve additional effort for both the practitioner and the patient and dealing with multiple systems may affect compliance.

2.3 Preventing the Onset of Myopia

Presently, strategies to reduce the onset of myopia are few and are almost entirely directed to environmental strategies such as improved time outdoors. An outdoor time of approximately 10–14 h per week reduced the risk of onset despite the presence of risk factors such as high amounts of near work or parental myopia [65]. A recently conducted meta-analysis found an inverse relation with increased time outdoors with a lowered risk of incident myopia; whilst an increase of about 80 min per day of time outdoors reduced the risk of onset of myopia by about 50%, whereas 60 min conferred a reduced risk of about 45% [66]. The reason underlying the protective effect of time outdoors is not entirely clear. With improved light luminance, spectral composition of light release of dopamine, and improved depth of focus among some of the many factors hypothesized to play a role. Additionally, it is not known if certain times of the day are more effective than other times (e.g., noon versus morning) and if time outdoors delivered continuously versus in multiple blocks matters. There is some research that indicates that outdoor time delivered over multiple breaks may be as useful as a continuous period [67].

In a single study, 0.025% Atropine was effective in preventing the onset of myopia in pre-myopes; [68] the use of low-dose Atropine to prevent myopia is also being explored in ATOM 3 study but the results are yet to be published.

2.4 Long-Term Efficacy, Rebound, and Side Effects

Over the past two decades, there have been significant developments in treatments for slowing myopia; although many of these treatments continue to be off-label (especially with multifocal soft contact lenses and atropine) in the recent years, FDA and CE certification was obtained for certain products. While this is promising for the future of myopia control strategies and their further integration into mainstream practice, improvements to maximize efficacy and minimization of associated side effects will improve uptake and success in myopia control. Presently the data on long-term efficacy is equivocal and needs further work; while some trials indicated maximal efficacy in the initial months of treatment followed by tapering efficacy [51], other trials demonstrated a consistent and stable efficacy from year to year [44]. Multiple factors may be involved and the efficacy data is confounded by age, compliance, drop-outs and discontinuations, and lack of long-term studies.

Rebound—the faster rate of progression of myopia immediately upon discontinuation of the myopia control strategies—is an issue as it leads to an increased progression. Further, it also reverses or minimizes the efforts and gains involved in managing progression—time, effort of individuals, practitioners and carers, quality of life and costs. While it is well established that Atropine is associated with rebound, the mechanisms underlying rebound remain unclear. Fortunately, rebound appears to be minimized or insignificant at lower Atropine concentrations [16]. Furthermore, there now exist clinical paradigms to reduce the risk of rebound on discontinuation [69, 70]. Continuing the treatment until late adolescence/early adulthood and/or tapering the concentration/frequency stepwise and monitoring progression is recommended to reduce the risk of rebound. Similarly, there is concern on whether rebound occurs with optical strategies; however the evidence is equivocal. In a study involving contralateral wear of orthokeratology versus rigid gas permeables, eyes that switched from orthokeratology to rigid gas permeables increased in eye length compared to the rate of change observed for an equivalent period in the GP wearing eyes [71]; however, there was no rebound in eyes that switched from progressive addition spectacles or myopia control lenses to single vision lenses [72, 73].

The ocular side effects of atropine include an increased pupillary diameter leading to symptoms of photophobia and glare, paralysis of accommodation resulting in loss of near vision, increased redness, dryness, and incidents of allergic reactions [74]. The use of multifocal spectacles and contact lenses may result in unwanted visual effects that may vary depending on the type of lens design. For example, the use of progressive addition spectacles may result in swim and distortion in the peripheral field, whereas with multifocal type contact lenses there may be haze and ghosting of images [75]. Although some of the vision-related complaints may be resolved with appropriate adjustments, they may possibly lead to a decrease in the efficacy. Additionally, with contact lenses and orthokeratology, there is the risk of complications such as microbial keratitis and infiltrates, although these are seen infrequently. With soft lenses, the risk is minimized with the use of daily wear and daily disposables and importantly, the risk of these events with lens wear is said to be no different from that observed in adult wearers [76].

2.5 Poor or Slow Responders to Myopia Control

With atropine treatment, poor or slow response was linked to the concentration of Atropine. Even with the highest concentration of 1% atropine, approximately 12% of children progressed by >0.5D/yr. These children tended to be younger, and more likely to have parental myopia and greater spherical equivalent refractive error at baseline [77]. With 0.05% atropine, approximately 17–28% of children progressed >0.5D at 1 year. Whereas with 0.01% Atropine, more than 50% of children progressed by at least 0.5D after 1 year, and about 13% by at least 1D [78–80]. At the end of 2 years, approximately 9%, 7%, and 19% had progressed by more than 2D with 0.05%, 0.025% and 0.01% Atropine respectively [80].

With MiSight® contact lenses, after 3 years of lens wear, 18% of eyes progressed by more than 1.0D [44]. With optical interventions, there have been reports of poor compliance equating to lower efficacy. With strategies where there was more than one dose available, greater efficacy was observed with higher doses [40, 45, 47].

2.6 Clinical Management of Myope

2.6.1 Risk Factors for Progression

Although any myopic eye is likely to benefit from a reduced progression, those at higher risk of progression may require more aggressive treatment strategies and/or more frequent examinations to ensure that their progression is appropriately controlled. In an already myopic eye, an individual's risk status for progression can be assessed by using some established criteria for progression. Age of detection of myopia was found to be a useful predictor, with those detected at a younger age more likely to reach higher levels of myopia later in life. It is likely that genetic factors such as parental myopia and environmental factors such as early schooling play a role in early onset myopia. However, irrespective of the underlying mechanisms, annual progression of myopia is greater in younger children [81].

Ethnicity is also useful to determine the risk of progression, with children of Asian ethnicity showing a faster annual progression compared to white European children [82]. Additionally, females progressed faster [83]. Similarly, parental myopia was found to influence progression—those with both parents being myopic had a faster progression rate compared to no parents being myopic [84].

Although peripheral retinal hyperopia was linked to greater progression in earlier studies, it was weakly linked. However, recent data indicates that eyes with asymmetry in peripheral refractive error may be at less risk of progression. (https://iovs.arvojournals.org/article.aspx?articleid=2691262). Although esophoria and accommodative lag and dysfunction were thought to influence progression, several studies showed no relation between myopia progression and accommodative lag [85, 86]. Syndromic associations such as retinal degenerations and dystrophies are likely associated with greater progression; however, the role of myopia control strategies in slowing myopia in such cases remains unexplored.

Although several lifestyle related factors such as near work distance, screen time, and near have been considered, their association with the progression of myopia is equivocal. Increased near workload with a shorter reading distance was a risk factor for progression [87]. Young school-age children, university graduates, and occupations requiring close and near work activities such as microscopists were at higher risk of progression [88, 89].

Interestingly, sleeping late was found to be a risk factor for progression in a large cohort of children, independent of age, gender, and urban-rural location [90].

2.6.2 Examining the Eye

A risk assessment should be followed by an assessment of visual acuity, binocular vision status, anterior eye health, cycloplegic refraction, and a posterior segment evaluation. In addition, depending on the type of myopia control strategy and the need, assessments, such as corneal topography, pupil diameter, and peripheral refraction, may be warranted. Of the various assessments, a cycloplegic assessment of the refractive error is important as it has been well established that non-cycloplegia may result in overestimation of myopia, especially in young children. Additionally, where available, the use of optical biometers to measure and monitor eye length is useful. Measurements with the newer generation of optical biometers are more accurate and repeatable than refractive error assessments and therefore quite useful in monitoring progression. It is important to check the eye thoroughly with lid eversion and palpebral conjunctival examination for conditions such as allergic conjunctivitis and vernal conjunctivitis. The conditions are more frequently seen in children and may influence/impact treatment with contact lenses, orthokeratology, and/or atropine.

2.6.3 Choosing a Treatment Plan, Realistic Goal Setting, and Follow-Up

Table 2.1 summarizes the various strategies and their efficacy in slowing myopia. The choice of a treatment strategy is influenced by many factors and extends beyond simply considering the efficacy of the strategy. Some of these many factors include age, onset of myopia, progression, motivation, affordability, treatment availability, lifestyle, and cultural factors. Once an appropriate strategy is chosen, it is important for the practitioner to educate the carers and/or the individual that although myopia control treatments slow progression, it is expected that there will be some progression of myopia. Percentile charts and myopia calculators may be useful to demonstrate the risk of progression with and without myopia control strategies. Thereafter, depending on the type of strategy chosen, the potential risks and benefits, and the need for any adjunct strategies should be discussed. For example, with atropine therapy, depending on the chosen concentration there may be a need for progressive addition spectacles and/or photochromic lenses to manage symptoms related to near vision and photophobia. With optical strategies, the visual performance may not be fully optimal due to, for example, multifocality of contact lenses or peripheral effects from spectacle lens-based strategies.

Once treatment has commenced, the individual should be examined within the first few weeks to ensure that they are comfortable with the chosen strategy and to ensure that their initial expectations were met. A follow-up at 3–6 monthly schedule is recommended during the initial year. The progress in the first year may be used as a guide to determine follow-up schedule for later years.

If there is a need to discontinue, age and rate of progression should be considered to determine alternative corrective or treatment modalities. There are no clear guidelines, but it is thought that minimal change in refractive error over 1.5 years to 2 years may indicate a stable refractive error. However, age is an important determinant. A minimal change in a young adult is more likely to be indicative of a stable refractive error, whereas in children caution needs to be exercised when making such a determination. With optical strategies, switching to a suitable corrective strategy appears to be the preferred approach, whereas with pharmaceutical strategies, a more conservative "tapering" approach rather than an abrupt cessation is recommended. Tapering can be done by decreasing the frequency and/or concentration. Additionally, close monitoring after cessation is recommended to determine if there is any acceleration or increase in progression [70].

Table 2.1 Interventions to slow Myopia

	Contact lenses (Soft)	Spectacles	Orthokeratology	Atropine	Combination (Atropine plus Ortho-k)
Lens design(s)	• Central zone corrects for distance ref. error; periphery plus (a treatment zone) commonly +2.00D or greater) • Non-monotonic power profile across optic zone • Alternating concentric rings of distance and relatively positive zone • Clear center distance surrounded by a zone of rapidly rising positive power • Central and peripheral plus	• Progressive addition lenses • Executive bifocals with and without prisms • Clear center distance with relatively positive power in the periphery • Clear center distance, multiple segments of relatively positive power in the mid periphery • Clear center distance, multiple rings of aspherical lenslets	Reverse geometry lens designs—Multiple	Not applicable; frequently used concentrations of 0.01–0.05%	Orthokeratology combined with atropine
Suggested frequency of use	Daily	Daily	Daily	One drop per day before bedtime	Daily
Slowing of myopia compared to control (single vision or placebo)	21–72% for Sph Eqv ref error.	11–67% for Sph Eqv ref error.	30–63% for axial length	27–67% for Sph Eqv ref error. (0.01–0.05%)	5–50% improved benefit compared to Ortho-K alone
Side effects/ complications	May result in subjective visual complaints—ghosting, haloes Risk of complications due to contact lens wear such as infiltrates, microbial keratitis	May result in subjective visual complaints—swim, peripheral distortion, ghosting, and/or poor performance	May result in subjective visual complaints—ghosting, haloes due to shaped cornea Risk of complications due to contact lens wear such as infiltrates, microbial keratitis	Glare, sensitivity to light, and near vision problems Allergic reactions Cumulative and increased light exposure-unknown effects	All side effects associated with Ortho-k and atropine apply

2.7 Summary

There is compelling evidence for optical and pharmaceutical strategies to slow myopia progression; a substantial and clinically meaningful slowing of myopia is observed with atropine, multifocal contact lenses, myopia control spectacles, and orthokeratology. The decreased risk of complications in later life as well as a decrease in burden afforded by slower progression suggests that any myope should be advocated and treated with an appropriate myopia control strategy.

Key Points

1. The goal of myopia control approaches is to reduce the risk of the eye reaching higher levels of myopia.
2. Myopia progression can be slowed using optical (spectacles, contact lenses, and orthokeratology) and pharmaceutical approaches (atropine). There is variation between approaches in terms of efficacy, safety profile, and ease of use.
3. All approaches have a role to play in myopia management based on presenting age of the individual, age at which myopia was detected, progression, motivation, affordability, treatment availability, lifestyle, and other factors.

References

1. Sankaridurg P, et al. IMI impact of myopia. Invest Ophthalmol Vis Sci. 2021;62(5):2–2.
2. Baird PN, et al. Myopia. Nat Rev Dis Primers. 2020;6(1):99.
3. Rose KA, et al. Outdoor activity reduces the prevalence of myopia in children. Ophthalmology. 2008;115(8):1279–85.
4. Siatkowski RM, et al. Two-year multicenter, randomized, double-masked, placebo-controlled, parallel safety and efficacy study of 2% pirenzepine ophthalmic gel in children with myopia. J AAPOS. 2008;12(4):332–9.
5. Abraham SV. Control of myopia with tropicamide. A progress report. Ophthalmology. 1966;3:10–22.
6. Goldschmidt E. Myopia in humans: can progression be arrested? Ciba Found Symp. 1990;155:222–9. discussion 230-4
7. Quinn GE, et al. Association of intraocular pressure and myopia in children. Ophthalmology. 1995;102(2):180–5.
8. Jensen H. Myopia progression in young school children. A prospective study of myopia progression and the effect of a trial with bifocal lenses and beta blocker eye drops. Acta Ophthalmol Suppl (1985). 1991;200:1–79.
9. Trier K, et al. Systemic 7-methylxanthine in retarding axial eye growth and myopia progression: a 36-month pilot study. J Ocul Biol Dis Infor. 2008;1(2–4):85–93.
10. Smith EL 3rd, et al. Topically instilled caffeine selectively alters emmetropizing responses in infant rhesus monkeys. Exp Eye Res. 2021;203:108438.
11. Liu H, ct al. Effects of 7-methylxanthine on deprivation myopia and retinal dopamine release in chickens. Ophthalmic Res. 2020;63(3):347–57.
12. Bedrossian RH. The effect of atropine on myopia. Ophthalmology. 1979;86(5):713–9.

13. Brodstein RS, et al. The treatment of myopia with atropine and bifocals. A long-term prospective study. Ophthalmology. 1984;91(11):1373–9.
14. Gruber E. Treatment of myopia with atropine and bifocals. Ophthalmology. 1985;92(7):985.
15. Tong L, et al. Atropine for the treatment of childhood myopia: effect on myopia progression after cessation of atropine. Ophthalmology. 2009;116(3):572–9.
16. Chia A, et al. Atropine for the treatment of childhood myopia: safety and efficacy of 0.5%, 0.1%, and 0.01% doses (atropine for the treatment of myopia 2). Ophthalmology. 2012;119(2):347–54.
17. Yam JC, et al. Low-concentration atropine for myopia progression (LAMP) study: a randomized, double-blinded, placebo-controlled trial of 0.05%, 0.025%, and 0.01% atropine eye drops in myopia control. Ophthalmology. 2019;126(1):113–24.
18. Polling JR, et al. A 3-year follow-up study of atropine treatment for progressive myopia in Europeans. Eye (Lond). 2020;34(11):2020–8.
19. Sander BP, Collins MJ, Read SA. The effect of topical adrenergic and anticholinergic agents on the choroidal thickness of young healthy adults. Exp Eye Res. 2014;128:181–9.
20. Zhang Z, et al. The effect of topical atropine on the choroidal thickness of healthy children. Sci Rep. 2016;6(1):1–8.
21. Chiang ST-H, Phillips JR. Effect of atropine eye drops on choroidal thinning induced by hyperopic retinal defocus. J Ophthalmol. 2018;2018:8528315.
22. Nickla DL, Zhu X, Wallman J. Effects of muscarinic agents on chick choroids in intact eyes and eyecups: evidence for a muscarinic mechanism in choroidal thinning. Ophthalmic Physiol Opt. 2013;33(3):245–56.
23. Lind GJ, et al. Muscarinic acetylcholine receptor antagonists inhibit chick scleral chondrocytes. Invest Ophthalmol Vis Sci. 1998;39(12):2217–31.
24. Leung J, Brown B. Progression of myopia in Hong Kong Chinese schoolchildren is slowed by wearing progressive lenses. Optom Vis Sci. 1999;76(6):346–54.
25. Gwiazda J, et al. A randomized clinical trial of progressive addition lenses versus single vision lenses on the progression of myopia in children. Invest Ophthalmol Vis Sci. 2003;44(4):1492–500.
26. Correction of Myopia Evaluation Trial 2 Study Group for the Pediatric Eye Disease Investigator Group. Progressive-addition lenses versus single-vision lenses for slowing progression of myopia in children with high accommodative lag and near esophoria. Invest Ophthalmol Vis Sci. 2011;52(5):2749.
27. Hasebe S, Jun J, Varnas SR. Myopia control with positively aspherized progressive addition lenses: a 2-year, multicenter, randomized, controlled trial. Invest Ophthalmol Vis Sci. 2014;55(11):7177–88.
28. Berntsen DA, et al. Peripheral defocus and myopia progression in myopic children randomly assigned to wear single vision and progressive addition Lenses. Invest Ophthalmol Vis Sci. 2013;54(8):5761–70.
29. Sankaridurg P, et al. Spectacle lenses designed to reduce progression of myopia: 12-month results. Optom Vis Sci. 2010;87(9):631.
30. Cheng D, et al. Effect of bifocal and prismatic bifocal spectacles on myopia progression in children: three-year results of a randomized clinical trial. JAMA ophthalmol. 2014;132(3):258–64.
31. Lam CSY, et al. Defocus incorporated multiple segments (DIMS) spectacle lenses slow myopia progression: a 2-year randomised clinical trial. Br J Ophthalmol. 2020;104(3):363–8.
32. Bao J, et al. One-year myopia control efficacy of spectacle lenses with aspherical lenslets. Br J Ophthalmol. 2021;106(8):1171–6.
33. Smith EL 3rd, Hung LF, Huang J. Relative peripheral hyperopic defocus alters central refractive development in infant monkeys. Vis Res. 2009;49(19):2386–92.
34. Lam CSY, et al. Defocus incorporated multiple segments (DIMS) spectacle lenses slow myopia progression: a 2-year randomised clinical trial. Br J Ophthalmol. 2019;104(3):363–8.
35. Perrigin J, et al. Silicone-acrylate contact lenses for myopia control: 3-year results. Optom Vis Sci. 1990;67(10):764–9.

36. Katz J, et al. A randomized trial of rigid gas permeable contact lenses to reduce progression of children's myopia. Am J Ophthalmol. 2003;136(1):82–90.
37. Anstice NS, Phillips JR. Effect of dual-focus soft contact lens wear on axial myopia progression in children. Ophthalmology. 2011;118(6):1152–61.
38. Walline JJ, et al. Multifocal contact lens myopia control. Optometry & Vision Science. 2013;90(11):1207–14.
39. Fujikado T, et al. Effect of low-addition soft contact lenses with decentered optical design on myopia progression in children: a pilot study. Clin Ophthalmol. 2014;8:1947.
40. Lam CSY, et al. Defocus incorporated soft contact (DISC) lens slows myopia progression in Hong Kong Chinese schoolchildren: a 2-year randomised clinical trial. Br J Ophthalmol. 2014;98(1):40–5.
41. Aller TA, Liu M, Wildsoet CF. Myopia control with bifocal contact lenses: a randomized clinical trial. Optom Vis Sci. 2016;93(4):344–52.
42. Sankaridurg P, et al. Novel contact lenses designed to slow progress of myopia: 12 month results. Invest Ophthalmol Vis Sci. 2017;58(8):2391.
43. Ruiz-Pomeda A, et al. MiSight assessment study Spain (MASS). A 2-year randomized clinical trial. Graefe's Arch Clin Exp Ophthalmol. 2018;256(5):1011–21.
44. Chamberlain P, et al. A 3-year randomized clinical trial of MiSight lenses for myopia control. Optom Vis Sci. 2019;96(8):556–67.
45. Sankaridurg P, et al. Myopia control with novel central and peripheral plus contact lenses and extended depth of focus contact lenses: 2 year results from a randomised clinical trial. Ophthalmic Physiol Opt. 2019;39(4):294–307.
46. Aller TA, Wildsoet C. Results of a one-year prospective clinical trial (CONTROL) of the use of bifocal soft contact lenses to control myopia progression. Ophthalmic Physiol Opt. 2006;26(Suppl 1):1–67.
47. Walline JJ, et al. Effect of high add power, medium add power, or single-vision contact lenses on myopia progression in children: the BLINK randomized clinical trial. JAMA. 2020;324(6):571–80.
48. Ruiz-Pomeda A, et al. MiSight assessment study Spain (MASS). A 2-year randomized clinical trial. Graefes Arch Clin Exp Ophthalmol. 2018;256(5):1011–21.
49. Cooper J, et al. Case series analysis of myopic progression control with a unique extended depth of focus multifocal contact lens. Eye Contact Lens. 2018;44(5):e16–24.
50. Cho P, Cheung S-W. Retardation of myopia in orthokeratology (ROMIO) study: a 2-year randomized clinical trial. Invest Ophthalmol Vis Sci. 2012;53(11):7077–85.
51. Hiraoka T, et al. Long-term effect of overnight orthokeratology on axial length elongation in childhood myopia: a 5-year follow-up study. Invest Ophthalmol Vis Sci. 2012;53(7):3913–9.
52. Santodomingo-Rubido J, et al. Myopia control with orthokeratology contact lenses in Spain: refractive and biometric changes. Invest Ophthalmol Vis Sci. 2012;53(8):5060–5.
53. Cho P, Cheung SW, Edwards M. The longitudinal orthokeratology research in children (LORIC) in Hong Kong: a pilot study on refractive changes and myopic control. Curr Eye Res. 2005;30(1):71–80.
54. Walline JJ, Jones LA, Sinnott LT. Corneal reshaping and myopia progression. Br J Ophthalmol. 2009;93(9):1181–5.
55. Chen C, Cheung SW, Cho P. Myopia control using toric orthokeratology (TO-SEE study) myopia control using toric orthokeratology. Invest Ophthalmol Vis Sci. 2013;54(10):6510–7.
56. Kakita T, Hiraoka T, Oshika T. Influence of overnight orthokeratology on axial elongation in childhood myopia. Invest Ophthalmol Vis Sci. 2011;52(5):2170–4.
57. Hiraoka T, et al. Long-term effect of overnight orthokeratology on axial length elongation in childhood myopia: a 5-year follow-up StudyLong-term effect of orthokeratology on axial length. Invest Ophthalmol Vis Sci. 2012;53(7):3913–9.
58. Santodomingo-Rubido J, et al. Myopia control with orthokeratology contact lenses in Spain: refractive and biometric changes orthokeratology in myopia progression control. Invest Ophthalmol Vis Sci. 2012;53(8):5060–5.

59. Chen C, Cheung SW, Cho P. Myopia control using toric orthokeratology (TO-SEE study). Invest Ophthalmol Vis Sci. 2013;54(10):6510–7.
60. Charm J, Cho P. High myopia-partial reduction ortho-k: a 2-year randomized study. Optom Vis Sci. 2013;90(6):530–9.
61. Cho P, Cheung SW. Discontinuation of orthokeratology on eyeball elongation (DOEE). Cont Lens Anterior Eye. 2017;40(2):82–7.
62. González-Méijome JM, et al. Stabilization in early adult-onset myopia with corneal refractive therapy. Cont Lens Anterior Eye. 2016;39(1):72–7.
63. Kinoshita N, et al. Additive effects of orthokeratology and atropine 0.01% ophthalmic solution in slowing axial elongation in children with myopia: first year results. Jpn J Ophthalmol. 2018;62(5):544–53.
64. Tan Q, et al. Combined atropine with orthokeratology for myopia control: study design and preliminary results. Curr Eye Res. 2019;44(6):671–8.
65. Jones LA, et al. Parental history of myopia, sports and outdoor activities, and future myopia. Invest Ophthalmol Vis Sci. 2007;48(8):3524–32.
66. Xiong S, et al. Time spent in outdoor activities in relation to myopia prevention and control: a meta-analysis and systematic review. Acta Ophthalmol. 2017;95(6):551–66.
67. Wu PC, et al. Outdoor activity during class recess reduces myopia onset and progression in school children. Ophthalmology. 2013;120(5):1080–5.
68. Fang PC, et al. Prevention of myopia onset with 0.025% atropine in premyopic children. J Ocul Pharmacol Ther. 2010;26(4):341–5.
69. Chia A, Lu QS, Tan D. Five-year clinical trial on atropine for the treatment of myopia 2: myopia control with atropine 0.01% eyedrops. Ophthalmology. 2016;123(2):391–9.
70. Wu PC, et al. Update in myopia and treatment strategy of atropine use in myopia control. Eye (Lond). 2019;33(1):3–13.
71. Swarbrick HA, et al. Myopia control during orthokeratology lens wear in children using a novel study design. Ophthalmology. 2015;122(3):620–30.
72. Ruiz-Pomeda A, et al. Rebound effect in the misight assessment study Spain (Mass). Curr Eye Res. 2021;46(8):1223–6.
73. Berntsen DA, et al. A randomized trial using progressive addition lenses to evaluate theories of myopia progression in children with a high lag of accommodation. Invest Ophthalmol Vis Sci. 2012;53(2):640–9.
74. Myles W, Dunlop C, McFadden SA. The effect of long-term low-dose atropine on refractive progression in myopic Australian school children. J Clin Med. 2021;10(7):1444.
75. Wildsoet CF, et al. IMI - interventions myopia institute: interventions for controlling myopia onset and progression report. Invest Ophthalmol Vis Sci. 2019;60(3):M106–m131.
76. Bullimore MA. The safety of soft contact lenses in children. Optom Vis Sci. 2017;94(6):638–46.
77. Loh KL, et al. Risk factors for progressive myopia in the atropine therapy for myopia study. Am J Ophthalmol. 2015;159(5):945–9.
78. Wei S, et al. Safety and efficacy of low-dose atropine eyedrops for the treatment of myopia progression in Chinese children: a randomized clinical trial. JAMA Ophthalmol. 2020;138(11):1178–84.
79. Lee JJ, et al. Prevention of myopia progression with 0.05% atropine solution. J Ocul Pharmacol Ther. 2006;22(1):41–6.
80. Yam JC, et al. Two-year clinical trial of the low-concentration atropine for myopia progression (LAMP) study: phase 2 report. Ophthalmology. 2020;127(7):910–9.
81. Sankaridurg PR, Holden BA. Practical applications to modify and control the development of ametropia. Eye (Lond). 2014;28(2):134–41.
82. Donovan L, et al. Myopia progression rates in urban children wearing single-vision spectacles. Optom Vis Sci. 2012;89(1):27–32.
83. Liao CC, et al. Refractive error change and its association with ocular and general parameters in junior high school students in Taiwan. Jpn J Ophthalmol. 2014;58(4):375–80.

84. Kurtz D, et al. Role of parental myopia in the progression of myopia and its interaction with treatment in COMET children. Invest Ophthalmol Vis Sci. 2007;48(2):562–70.
85. Koomson NY, et al. Relationship between reduced accommodative lag and myopia progression. Optom Vis Sci. 2016;93(7):683–91.
86. Berntsen DA, et al. Accommodative lag and juvenile-onset myopia progression in children wearing refractive correction. Vis Res. 2011;51(9):1039–46.
87. Huang PC, et al. Protective behaviours of near work and time outdoors in myopia prevalence and progression in myopic children: a 2-year prospective population study. Br J Ophthalmol. 2020;104(7):956–61.
88. Ting PW, et al. Prevalence of myopia in a group of Hong Kong microscopists. Optom Vis Sci. 2004;81(2):88–93.
89. McBrien NA, Adams DW. A longitudinal investigation of adult-onset and adult-progression of myopia in an occupational group. Refractive and biometric findings. Invest Ophthalmol Vis Sci. 1997;38(2):321–33.
90. Liu XN, et al. Sleeping late is a risk factor for myopia development amongst school-aged children in China. Sci Rep. 2020;10(1):–17194.

Current Management of Amblyopia

3

Lan Chang

Amblyopia is decreased vision due to abnormal visual development of the brain. Amblyopia is a common disorder with a prevalence of approximately 2%. There are many causes of amblyopia, including refractive error, strabismus, or visual deprivation (such as congenital ptosis or congenital cataract). Treatments of amblyopia need to address the underlying cause of vision loss and it is often coupled with penalization of the better-seeing eye. Treatments are most effective in young children, and amblyopic visual loss may become permanent if not treated early on. More recently, there has been evidence that some amblyopes can improve vision later in life.

3.1 Etiology

David Hubel and Torsten Wiesel were awarded the Nobel Prize for Physiology or Medicine in 1981 for their groundbreaking research on the visual system and visual processing. From them, we understand that there is a "critical period" early in life for the development of the visual cortex.

Good vision occurs when a sharp image is detected by the retina, and it is then transmitted to the visual cortex. Vision develops as the child uses the eye and matures the visual cortex. When strabismus (misalignment of the eyes), anisometropia (significant refractive difference between the eyes), media opacity (blocking of the visual axis due to corneal scarring, cataract, or vitreous hemorrhage), or occlusion (such as ptosis or obstructing eyelid lesion) occurs, one or both eye(s) can be disadvantaged during visual development.

Strabismic Amblyopia—Eye misalignment or strabismus accounts for approximately half of the cases of amblyopia. Visual development of one eye is favored due to constant, non-alternating, or unequally alternating tropias.

L. Chang (✉)
Pediatric Ophthalmology and Adult Strabismus, Eye Associates of New Mexico, Albuquerque, NM, USA

A. Ramasubramanian (ed.), *Pediatric Ophthalmology*, Current Practices in Ophthalmology, https://doi.org/10.1007/978-981-19-4963-0_3

Refractive Amblyopia—Anisometropic amblyopia develops when unequal refractive error causes defocusing of the image on one retina, leading to unilateral amblyopia. Bilateral refractive amblyopia can occur in the setting of high refractive error leading to bilateral reduction in visual acuity.

Visual Deprivation Amblyopia—This result from complete or partial obstruction of visual axis. Causes of this type of amblyopia include congenital or early-onset cataract, corneal opacities, intraocular inflammation, vitreous hemorrhage, and ptosis. Amblyopic visual loss from a unilateral obstruction of the visual axis tends to be more severe than that produced by bilateral deprivation of similar degree.

Occlusion or Reverse Amblyopia—This was previously observed after intense patching or atropine treatment of the nonamblyopic eye. With current regimen of lower doses of patching and atropine, reverse amblyopia is rarely observed. Also, visual acuity will return to baseline simply with cessation of patching or atropine.

Other Associations—Children with developmental delay or who are born prematurely are more likely to develop amblyopia than healthy children [1]. While amblyopia is not a directly heritable condition, several amblyopic risk factors such as strabismus and significant refractive error have genetic bases [2].

3.2 Areas of Visual Perception Affected

Acuity or sharpness of vision is just one aspect of vision affected by amblyopia. Amblyopes also experience reduced contrast sensitivity, decreased stereopsis, and visual confusion. Amblyopia has been associated with a higher incidence of reading difficulties; however, it can improve as amblyopia is treated [3]. Amblyopic children read more slowly due to fixation instability and increased frequency of saccades compared with controls [3]. Slower reading can impact a child's academic achievement; as we understand more about amblyopia, perhaps greater emphasis can be made to treat amblyopia starting at a younger age.

Development of binocular vision occurs early in life, amblyopia treatment in young children may improve binocularity as well as acuity. In anisometropic amblyopia patients treated successfully, their binocularity scores improved to normal [4].

Risk of visual impairment is substantial in those with amblyopia. A study showed that the lifelong risk of visual impairment in the fellow eye is approximately doubled for patients with amblyopia [5]. In a large population-based study analyzing the Rotterdam Study data, period of binocular visual impairment in an individual's lifetime is nearly doubled by the presence of amblyopia (0.7 years in nonamblyopic individuals to 1.3 years in amblyopic individuals) [6].

3.3 Identifying Amblyopia

Since the efficacy of treatment is age-sensitive, screening modalities would be very useful in identifying amblyopia suspects at a young age. Screening for amblyopia or its risk factors is recommended for all children between the ages of 3–5 years.

Subjective visual acuity screening in children must be performed with the age-appropriate optotype. In addition, a line of optotypes is preferred over single optotypes. The amblyopic eye can achieve higher acuity when tested with single isolated letters than lines of letters. When testing vision in young children who are unable to read a line of letters, crowding bars should be added around individual letters to avoid overestimating visual acuity. In the primary care setting, patients can be evaluated for red reflex quality, lid abnormality, pupil irregularity, ability to fix and follow, corneal light reflex, and abnormal cover testing. Instrument-based screenings can be helpful in screening in very young children and those with developmental delay. Most common instrument-based screening devices are based on photoscreening methods; newer technology uses binocular retinal birefringence scanning to detect microstrabismus associated with amblyopia. Using this newer technology, blinq.™ pediatric vision scanner, achieved a sensitivity and specificity of 96% for the detection of amblyopia or strabismus [4].

To accurately access the refractive error in children, adequate cycloplegia is necessary. This is typically accomplished using cyclopentolate 1% solution in term infants over 6 months old, and combination drop of cyclopentolate 0.2% and phenylephrine 1% in younger infants. In children with darker irises, repeat administration of cycloplegic drops may be necessary. Spray form of the cycloplegic drop may also facilitate instillation of the cycloplegic agent in children.

Unilateral amblyopia can be defined by a two-line interocular difference in best-corrected visual acuity, 20/32 or worse in the worse eye, and at least one of the following unilateral amblyopia risk factors: presence or history of strabismus, significant anisometropia, or evidence of past or present visual axis obstruction [7]. Bilateral amblyopia can be defined as decreased best-corrected visual acuity (worse than 20/50 in children under 4 years or worse than 20/40 in children 4 years and older), bilateral significant ametropia, and bilateral evidence of visual axis obstruction (Table 3.1) [7].

Table 3.1 Diagnostic criteria for amblyopia

Assessment	Finding
Unilateral amblyopia	
Response to monocular occlusion	Asymmetric objection
Fixation preference	Failure to initiate or maintain fixation
Preferential looking	Interocular difference[a] of two or more octaves
Best-corrected visual acuity	Interocular difference of two or more lines
Bilateral amblyopia	
Best-corrected visual acuity	Age 3–≤4 years: Visual acuity worse than 20/50 Age 4–≤5 years: Visual acuity worse than 20/40 Age > 5: Visual acuity worse than 20/30

In addition to visual acuity deficits, an amblyogenic factor needs to be present for the diagnosis of amblyopia

Adapted from Wallace DK, Repka MX, Lee KA, et al. on behalf of the American Academy of Pediatric Ophthalmology/Strabismus Preferred Practice Pattern Pediatric Ophthalmology Panel. Amblyopia Preferred Practice Pattern®. Ophthalmology. 2018;125(1): PP105-P14

[a]A 2-octave difference is a 4-card difference in the full set of Teller Acuity Cards

3.4 Treatment Goals

There are three primary strategies to treat amblyopia. The first is to correct any cause of visual deprivation. The second is to correct refractive errors. The third is to encourage use of the amblyopic eye by occluding or blurring the better-seeing eye. While treatment goal is to obtain equal visual acuity in both eyes, this may not always be attainable. Detailed discussion with the patient and family should take into consideration: the child's age, starting visual acuity, adherence and response to prior treatment, and the child's overall physical, social, and psychological development.

3.5 Treatment Options

Optical Correction: The initial step in the treatment of children with amblyopia is to correct significant refractive errors. Eyeglasses are generally well-tolerated by children, especially when it leads to improvement in visual function. Well-fitting and durable glasses for children are particularly important for active young children.

Patching: Patching should be considered for children who do not improve with eyeglasses alone or who experience incomplete improvement. An opaque adhesive patch directly over the fellow eye is the preferred method for patching. Prescribed eyeglasses are to be worn over the patch. Using a cloth patch mounted on the eyeglasses frame is less preferred because children may peek around the cloth patch.

The Pediatric Eye Disease Investigator Group (PEDIG) conducted many randomized clinical trials for Amblyopia Treatment Study (ATS) from 2002 to 2016. In summary, for severe amblyopia (20/100 to 20/400 starting vision) in children under 7 years of age, 6 h of daily patching is recommended. For children with moderate amblyopia (20/40–20/80 starting vision), initial patching of 2 h daily is recommended.

Pharmacological Treatment: Cycloplegic drop can be used to effect optical penalization of the nonamblyopic eye for children who do not improve with eyeglasses alone. This treatment works best when the nonamblyopic eye is hyperopic. Most often, atropine 1% is used. It has been shown to be an effective method of treatment for mild to moderate amblyopia in children 3–15 years of age. It is also useful in the presence of latent nystagmus, occlusion failure, or for maintenance treatment. PEDIG clinical trials have demonstrated daily atropine to be as effective as patching for initial treatment of moderate amblyopia (starting visual acuity of 20/40–20/100) in children aged 7–12 years [8]. Later, atropine 1% given on two consecutive days per week (weekend atropine) was shown to be equally efficacious as once daily atropine 1% for moderate amblyopia.

With regards to the concern that cycloplegia will impede a child's ability to perform schoolwork, only a minority of children (12%) could not read grade-appropriate print after cycloplegia and required reading glasses [8].

Optical Treatment: Blurring the distance correction of the fellow eye by adding 1.00 to 3.00 diopters of plus sphere has been used to treat amblyopia. This has not been evaluated in randomized clinical trials.

Bangerter Filters: It has been shown that a translucent filter can be placed on the eyeglasses lens of the fellow eye to treat mild to moderate amblyopia. Bangerter filter has been used mostly as maintenance treatment after initial treatment with either patching or atropine.

Surgery: In order to address the cause of amblyopia, surgery may be indicated in situation such as cataract, nonclearing vitreous opacity, corneal opacities, or blepharoptosis. While strabismus surgery may help in amblyopia management in some cases, usually amblyopia treatment is still necessary [9]. In a small number of cases, photorefractive keratectomy has been performed for children with anisometropic amblyopia who are unable to tolerate traditional therapy of glasses/contact lenses and occlusion therapy [10].

Other Alternative Therapies: Binocular therapy involves presenting high-contrast images to the amblyopic eye and low-contrast images to the fellow eye simultaneously through a video game such as "falling blocks" while wearing special glasses. It is thought that dichoptic contrast balancing and binocular therapies reduce suppression of the amblyopic eye thereby improving visual acuity and binocular function [11].

Using liquid crystal display eyeglasses, which can be programmed to intermittently occlude the fellow eye, may improve compliance with amblyopia treatment [12]. The Amblyz™ liquid crystal intermittent occlusion glasses alternate between opaque and transparent phases at 30-s intervals, effectively providing occlusion of one eye 50% of the time. Widespread availability of such technology has yet to be seen.

A recent review of binocular treatment of amblyopia by Pineles et al. concluded that binocular therapy cannot be recommended as a replacement for standard amblyopia therapy (patching or atropine) currently [11]. Further research and development of more engaging therapies and advanced technologies will likely change the future of amblyopia treatment. A recently published pilot study showed high efficacy and adherence of dichoptic treatment that can be applied to streamed content chosen by the patient/guardian [13].

3.6 When to Extend Treatment?

The Pediatric Eye Disease Investigator Group (PEDIG) conducted a pilot study involving 10–17-year olds with amblyopia and found improvement in visual acuity of two or more lines in 27% of subjects, a similar number in the 10–13 and 14–17 subgroups [14]. In the ATS3 clinical trial involving 7–17-year-old children, analyses achieved statistical significance in 7–<13-year olds with moderate and severe amblyopia, recommending optical correction/occlusion/atropine use compared with optical correction alone [15]. For teenagers between 13 and 17 years of age, analyses suggest better results with optical correction/occlusion combination treatment compared with optical correction alone; however, statistical significance was not reached [15]. In the 13–17 years group, responder rate was 47% in patients not previously treated compared with 16% in those previously treated [15].

Improvement of vision in the amblyopic eye during adulthood has been observed. In Rahi et al., they saw an improvement of vision in the amblyopic eye when adults in the United Kingdom lost function of their good eye [16]. The improvement was greater when amblyopia was less severe.

3.7 Follow-up Examinations

Once amblyopia has been diagnosed, treatment options should be discussed with the parent/guardian/child. The time-sensitive nature of amblyopia treatment should be emphasized. The importance of adherence to treatment and regular follow-ups needs to be discussed with the family. For older children, active engagement of the patient in the treatment plan will also improve outcomes (Table 3.2).

3.8 When to Taper/Stop Treatment?

We are still learning about what contributes to the great variability in treatment response, regardless of age [17]. Even with cessation of amblyopia treatment after improvement plateaus, the patient should be monitored for possible regression and subsequent need for reinstituting amblyopia treatment. Levartovsky et al. showed

Table 3.2 Recommendations for adjusting treatment in amblyopia

Indication to change treatment	Action on treatment
Visual acuity is not improved after 3 months	Maintain or increase patching or atropine, or consider alternative therapy
Severe skin irritation develops with patching	Try a well-designed cloth patch on glasses or other alternative therapy
Visual acuity is not improved with occlusion	Taper or terminate treatment
Treatment is futile (e.g., organic lesion)	Taper or terminate treatment. Still emphasize monocular protection with glasses
Strabismus and/or diplopia develop	Temporarily stop treatment and monitor
Visual acuity decreases in the fellow eye by two or more lines	Temporarily stop treatment, review diagnosis, and monitor. Consider treating the previously amblyopic eye
Visual acuity is stabilized at normal or near normal over a period of 4 or more months confirmed on two or more visits	Taper or terminate therapy

Note: These recommendations are generated by consensus based on professional experience and clinical impressions

Adapted from Wallace DK, Repka MX, Lee KA, et al. on behalf of the American Academy of Pediatric Ophthalmology/Strabismus Preferred Practice Pattern Pediatric Ophthalmology Panel. Amblyopia Preferred Practice Pattern®. Ophthalmology. 2018;125(1): PP105–P14 that following cessation of amblyopia treatment at 9 years of age, 51% of patients with ≤1.50 diopters of anisometropia and 75% of patients with ≥1.75 diopters of anisometropia experienced regression [18].

Once a child achieves maximal expected improvement, amblyopia treatment can be maintained with lower dose occlusion, full- or part-time optical treatment, Bangerter filters, or part-time cycloplegic treatment. If the visual acuity in the amblyopic eye remains stable on maintenance therapy for at least 4 months, the treatment may be stopped and a follow-up appointment scheduled to monitor for recurrent amblyopia.

3.9 Amblyopia and Risk to Fellow Eye

Children with unilateral vision impairment due to amblyopia are at high risk of losing vision in the better eye due to disease or injury (1 in 1000) [5]. The importance of proper protective eyewear full time should be encouraged in all children with vision of 20/50 or worse. In the setting of most ball and contact sports, children need to wear proper impact-resistant goggles and face protection.

3.10 Amblyopia as a Public Health Focus

Treating amblyopia during childhood is also valuable in preventing binocular visual impairment later in life [16]. In the United Kingdom study of unilateral amblyopia patients, worse vision loss in the nonamblyopic eye was also associated with higher risk of death [16]. In the same study, half of those employed were unable to continue their work due to decreased vision [16]. Authors estimate the lifetime risk of serious vision loss for individuals with amblyopia being at least 1.2–3.3% [16].

Key Points

1. Earlier and more profound visual deprivation lead to more dense amblyopia.
2. While treatment later in childhood may have some effect in improving vision, early and consistent treatments are recommended for the best outcome. Monitoring should continue after treatment to avoid regression.
3. Commitment and collaboration of the child/parent/caregiver/physician team is essential to reversing amblyopia, as compliance with treatment and follow-ups are critical.
4. Suitable treatment options for amblyopia may include optical correction, patching, atropine drops, optical treatment, Bangerter filters, and/or surgery to treat the cause of amblyopia.

References

1. van Hof-Van DJ, Leunen A E-v, et al. Effects of very low birth weight (VLBW) on visual development during the first year after term. Early Hum Dev. 1989;3-4:255–66.
2. Levi D. Rethinking amblyopia. Vis Res. 2020;176:118–29.
3. Kelly KR, Jost RM, et al. Amblyopic children read more slowly than controls under natural, binocular reading conditions. J AAPOS. 2015;19(6):515–20.
4. Loudon SE, Rook CA, et al. Rapid, high-accuracy detection of strabismus and amblyopia using the pediatric vision scanner. Invest Ophthalmol Vis Sci. 2011;52(8):5043–8.
5. Tommila V, Tarkkanen A. Incidence of loss of vision in the healthy eye in amblyopia. Br J Ophthalmol. 1981;65(8):575–7.
6. van Leeuwen R, Eijkemans MJC, et al. Risk of bilateral visual impairment in individuals with amblyopia: the Rotterdam study. Br J Ophthalmol. 2007;91(11):1450–1.
7. Friedman DS, Repka MX, et al. Prevalence of amblyopia and strabismus in white and African American children aged 6 through 71 months: the Baltimore pediatric eye disease study. Ophthalmology. 2009;116(11):2128–34.
8. PEDIG. Patching vs atropine to treat amblyopia in children aged 7 to 12 years. Arch Ophthalmol. 2008;126(12):1634–42.
9. Lam GC, Repka MX. Timing of amblyopia therapy relative to strabismus surgery. Ophthalmology. 1993;100(12):1751–6.
10. Paysse EA, Coats DK, et al. Long-term outcomes of photorefractive keratectomy for anisometropic amblyopia in children. Ophthalmology. 2006;113(2):169–76.
11. Pineles SL, Aakalu VK, et al. Binocular treatment of amblyopia: a Report by the American Academy of Ophthalmology. Ophthalmology. 2020;127(2):261–72.
12. Wang J, Neely DE, et al. A pilot randomized clinical trial of intermittent occlusion therapy liquid crystal glasses versus traditional patching for treatment of moderate unilateral amblyopia. J AAPOS. 2016;20(4):326–31.
13. Xiao S, Gaier ED, et al. Digital therapeutic improves visual acuity and encourages high adherence in amblyopic children in open-label pilot study. J AAPOS. 2021;25(2):87–9.
14. PEDIG. A prospective, pilot study of treatment of amblyopia in children 10 to < 18 years old. Am J Ophthalmol. 2004;137:581–3.
15. PEDIG. Randomized trial of treatment of amblyopia in children aged 7 to 17 years. Arch Ophthalmol. 2005;123(4):437–47.
16. Rahi J, Logan S, et al. Risk, causes and outcomes of visual impairment after loss of vision in the non-amblyopic eye: a population-based study. Lancet. 2002;360(9333):597–602.
17. Holmes JM, Levi DM. Treatment of amblyopia as a function of age. Vis Neurosci. 2018;35:E015.
18. Levartovsky S, Olive M, et al. Long-term effect of hypermetropic anisometropia on the visual acuity of treated amblyopic eyes. Br J Ophthalmol. 1998;55–58:82(1).

Pediatric Refractive Surgery

4

Kamran Ahmed

The field of refractive surgery has historically been a science of modifying refractive error in adult patients for the purpose of improving uncorrected visual acuity (UCVA). More recently within pediatric ophthalmology, refractive surgery has emerged as a beneficial tool to address refractive errors and their associated comorbidities such as amblyopia and strabismus in special needs children intolerant of spectacles or contact lenses. Like any technology, the indications for use continue to evolve and expand as the safety, ease, and efficacy of the procedures are repeatedly demonstrated. At present, these procedures are mostly reserved for children with neurobehavioral disorders. Such children are physically incapable of properly wearing spectacles or are perturbed by the stimulation of wearing spectacles on their face even in the presence of disabling refractive errors which cause them to live in a world of blur. Contact lenses can be considered for a minority of these patients but require highly motivated and vigilant caretakers to ensure regular contact lens hygiene and prevent complications. This is usually impractical for such children who have multiple systemic comorbidities which are time-consuming for the caretaker to manage, or their behavioral disorder precludes cooperation with contact lens placement and removal.

K. Ahmed (✉)
Phoenix Children's Hospital, Phoenix, AZ, USA

Department of Child Health, University of Arizona College of Medicine-Phoenix, Phoenix, USA

Department of Medicine, Creighton University School of Medicine, Phoenix, USA

Department of Ophthalmology, Mayo Clinic Alix School of Medicine, Phoenix, USA

A. Ramasubramanian (ed.), *Pediatric Ophthalmology*, Current Practices in Ophthalmology, https://doi.org/10.1007/978-981-19-4963-0_4

The field of pediatrics in general is a risk-averse field, as it should be, because treatments are applied to children who lack the ability for autonomous medical decision-making. Therefore, new technologies within pediatric ophthalmology must undergo great scrutiny before achieving widespread acceptance. This chapter will provide an overview of the past, present, and future developments within the exciting and burgeoning field of pediatric refractive surgery.

4.1 Classification and History of Pediatric Refractive Surgery

Correction of ametropia can occur at multiple planes: spectacle, contact lens, corneal, anterior chamber, posterior chamber, and lens. Pediatric refractive surgery involves modification of the last four planes in this list when the first two options are not feasible.

The earliest reported cases of pediatric refractive surgery include clear lens excision with resultant aphakia for high myopia dating back to the late nineteenth century. This procedure involved dissection of the crystalline lens, allowing the liberated lens material to swell within the anterior chamber, and then removing the intumescent lens material via needling. Treated patients included children as young as 8-years old [1].

Angle-supported anterior chamber phakic IOLs (pIOLs) were first implanted in the 1950s, again to correct myopia [2]. Also, during this time, the iris-enclavated IOL was initially used for the correction of aphakia after intracapsular cataract extraction. In 1986, the first iris-enclavated IOL implantation for myopic correction of a phakic eye was performed [3]. The first published report of iris-enclavated IOL implantation in pediatric patients as young as 12-years old was published in 1998 [4]. Posterior chamber pIOL implantation began in the 1980s with the introduction of a silicone pIOL with a "mushroom" configuration. This lens had an optic which projected anteriorly through the pupil and haptics behind the iris [5]. Technological advancements eventually lead to the development of two new posterior chamber pIOLs: the implantable collamer lens (ICL) by STAAR Surgical and the phakic refractive lens (PRL) by Carl Zeiss Meditec. The earliest published report of implantation of posterior chamber pIOLs in children was in 1999 utilizing the ICL. This study included four children ranging from ages 3 to 16-years old with a mean refractive error of −12.8 D [6].

Over 8.5 million people in the United States underwent keratorefractive surgery from 1995 to 2010 and by 2015 over 13 million LASIK procedures had been performed in the United States [7]. The earliest published report of excimer laser photorefractive keratectomy in pediatric patients was in 1995. This was a small case series of 9 patients ranging from ages 10- to 15-years old with refractive errors from −17.75 D to +8.25 D [8]. Since that time, many reports of successful excimer laser corneal surgery in children have been published in the literature with low rates of complications [9–20]. The largest study reported outcomes in 405 ametropic children with 96% of myopic and 91% of hyperopic eyes corrected to within ±1 D of their target value. Of eyes treated with intraoperative mitomycin-C, 91% had no corneal haze, and no child with postoperative haze lost best-corrected visual acuity (BCVA). The retreatment rate was 1.5% of treated eyes [10].

4.2 The Need for Pediatric Refractive Surgery

Myopia is a growing epidemic and the most common visually significant refractive error, with a rising prevalence of 25–40% in Western countries [21, 22]. In the United States, the prevalence of myopia doubled in a 30-year period ending in 2004, and pathologic myopia (over 8.0 D) rose eightfold [23]. There are over 80 million reported myopic children worldwide, and myopia is among the five conditions that have been identified as immediate priorities by the World Health Organization (WHO) in its Global Initiative for the Elimination of Avoidable Blindness [24]. Myopia of prematurity has become an increasingly recognized entity and according to WHO, every year an estimated 15 million babies are born preterm (before 37 completed weeks of gestation), and this number is rising [25].

Naturally occurring astigmatism is common with a prevalence of 14.9% in children using a cutoff value >0.5 D. Children in South-East Asia have the lowest prevalence at 9.8%, while children in the Americas have the highest at 27.2% [26]. The degree of astigmatism is higher in premature infants and has an inverse relationship with birth weight and gestational age [27, 28]. Astigmatism has been shown to reduce visual acuity by 0.31 logMAR per diopter of myopic astigmatism and 0.23 logMAR per diopter of hyperopic astigmatism [29]. That is equivalent to reducing the visual acuity from 20/20 to 20/40 for 1.0 D of uncorrected myopic astigmatism and from 20/20 to 20/35 for 1.0 D of uncorrected hyperopic astigmatism.

Hyperopia has a bimodal distribution with the majority of full-term infants exhibiting physiologic hyperopia between 0.25 D and 4.00 D. Prevalence of hyperopia $\geq$ +2.0 D decreases as age increases down to 1% at age 15 with an average prevalence of about 5% in children of all ages [26, 30–32]. Prevalence then rises again in adulthood affecting about 10% of the population age 40 and above [22]. Anisometropic hyperopia and astigmatism tend to be more amblyogenic than myopia [18]. Uncorrected high hyperopia is also associated with accommodative esotropia or exotropia [33].

Although there is a significant need for ametropic correction among children, there is a subpopulation of children who cannot tolerate correction at the spectacle or contact lens planes. These children have poor spectacle compliance which can be defined as wearing glasses for 25% or less of their waking time. Spectacles are also frequently dislodged particularly in children with poor head control, or children may develop a habit of viewing around the spectacle frames. Spectacle noncompliance arises for a variety of reasons including high power lens distortions, prismatic effects, narrowed field of view, social stigma, aniseikonia, anisovergence, asthenopia, neurobehavioral disorders, craniofacial, or ear abnormalities. The most common neurobehavioral disorders are cerebral palsy, autism, Down syndrome, Angelman syndrome, seizure disorders, idiopathic developmental delay/mental retardation, and progressive childhood encephalopathies. Uncorrected ametropia exacerbates the neurobehavioral disorder giving rise to visual autism which is described as heightened social isolation due to living in a cocoon of blur. Contact lenses are usually even more problematic in this group of patients. They can be expensive, difficult to insert and remove in children, increase the risk of corneal infection, and are frequently lost [18, 19, 34].

Many studies have shown dramatic improvements in uncorrected visual acuity in children undergoing refractive surgery with low rates of complications. A multitude of other benefits for children with neurobehavioral disorders undergoing refractive surgery are improvements in communication, socialization, motor skills, adaptive behaviors, visual perception, and cognitive function [35]. Refractive surgery is highly valued by parents of children with large refractive errors and spectacle non-compliance, and bilateral LASEK for these children ranked among the most cost-effective procedures in ophthalmology [36].

4.3 Unique Aspects of Refractive Surgery for the Pediatric Patient

The preoperative evaluation of the pediatric patient prior to refractive surgery has unique differences from the adult patient, but also similarities including a full ocular history and examination, motility assessment, cycloplegic refraction (manifest usually obtained in adults but difficult to obtain in children), and ocular biometry.

The history should include the reason for the child's aversion to spectacles and the lack of feasibility of contact lenses. It is important to know if a child with a neurobehavioral disorder has a sensory aversion to objects near their face. This is a common aversion within this group of patients and can make tasks such as wearing spectacles, haircuts, dental exams, or even wearing a hat challenging. If such a sensory aversion exists, then parents need to be informed about the challenges of postoperative management which will arise due to the need for eye drops, eye shields, and multiple examinations of the eyes. This gives parents time to arrange for assistance by other family members or social services during the postoperative period. Discussion should also include the possible use of arm restraints so that the child does not cause self-inflicted trauma to the surgical site. Arm restraints should be used sparingly when the parent cannot be with the child so as to avoid persistent elbow stiffness. Other less restrictive methods to protect the surgical site include distraction, repositioning, swaddling, and pain management.

The patient's target refraction is determined by considering the current cycloplegic refraction and the patient's age. Unlike in adults for whom emmetropia is the usual target, younger children need a more hyperopic target to account for the eye growth and myopic shift that will occur over the ensuing years. The practice of targeting a hyperopic refraction in pediatric refractive surgery is similar to that in pediatric cataract surgery but with the advantage of preserved lens accommodation depending upon the method of refractive surgery. The caveat however is that spectacle compliance will not be possible postoperatively, since this was the reason for undergoing refractive surgery. Evaluation of ocular motility and alignment is a regular practice for pediatric ophthalmologists and plays a role in the assessment for refractive surgery as well. For example, multiple studies have demonstrated effective treatment of accommodative esotropia with the use of refractive surgery to correct the hyperopia [34, 37–39]. In contrast to this, one must also consider the loss of correction of small heterotropias by the prismatic effects of spectacles if the patient undergoes refractive surgery. In general, hyperopic lenses provide a partial prismatic correction of any horizontal or vertical tropia, because the base of the prism is always pointing in the appropriate direction as long as the optical centers of the lenses are correctly placed.

The presence of amblyopia which may be a contraindication to refractive surgery for an adult is frequently an indication of refractive surgery in the pediatric patient who requires a sharp, focused image on the retina for the amblyopia to improve [11, 13, 14, 40]. In addition to strabismus and amblyopia, common comorbidities with high ametropia also include optic neuropathies, foveopathies, and nystagmus. The presence of these comorbidities does not mean that the ametropia is not important and does not warrant correction [18]. Rather, the visual function should be optimized to the maximum potential of the child, sometimes requiring both refractive and eye muscle surgery.

When possible, preoperative biometric evaluation is performed in the clinic. However, children, particularly those with neurobehavioral disorders or cerebral palsy, are unable to remain stationary and fixate on diagnostic imaging such as specular microscopy or IOL biometry. In this case, an examination under anesthesia (EUA) is required, and biometry is obtained with ultrasound for measurement of axial length, anterior chamber depth (ACD), and lens thickness. Central corneal thickness is measured with a handheld pachymeter and horizontal white-to-white (WTW) with industrial-grade digital calipers with precision to the hundredth of a millimeter. The EUA also provides an opportunity for a complete exam of all ocular structures, because many of these children can be difficult to thoroughly examine in the clinic. Children undergoing refractive surgery have at least two full EUAs and two cycloplegic refractions before finally undergoing surgery. During the EUA, the eyes should be evaluated for contraindications to keratorefractive surgery, such as severe dry eye, exposure keratopathy, ocular surface cicatrization, keratoectasias, corneal dystrophies, uveitis, and uncontrolled glaucoma. The absence of sufficient support structures for pIOL implantation or refractive lens exchange (RLE), such as ectopia lentis or a hypoplastic iris, should be noted. The posterior segment is examined with a 360° scleral depressed exam to evaluate for risk factors for retinal detachment such as lattice degeneration which may benefit from prophylactic laser barrier retinopexy prior to refractive surgery. At the completion of the EUA with cycloplegic refraction and biometric data in hand, one can decide upon the best refractive surgery option for the patient and discuss this with the parents. The ACD and magnitude of ametropia frequently drive the decision-making, because pIOLs have minimum ACD requirements (Fig. 4.1). Children can have a wide range of ACD, and those with a history of prematurity and in particular retinopathy of prematurity tend to have reduced ACD [27, 41]. Other factors to consider include adequate corneal thickness for excimer laser ablation and sufficient horizontal WTW, which serves as a proxy to iridociliary sulcus diameter, for ICL implantation.

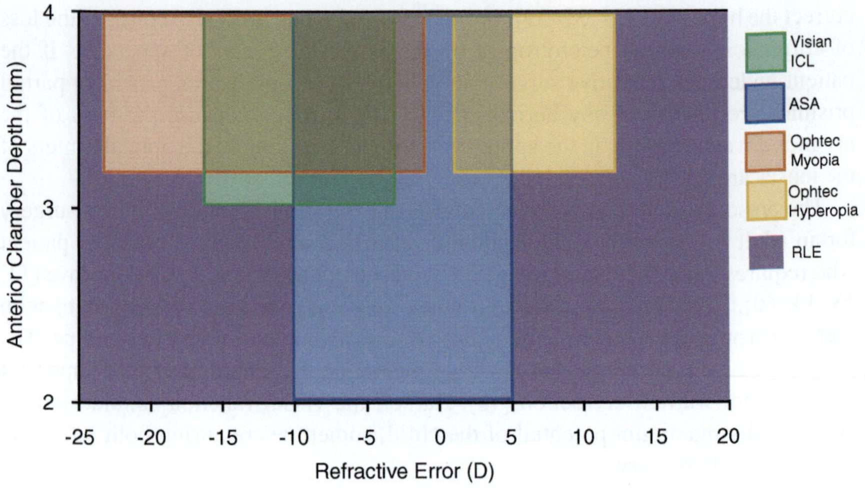

Fig. 4.1 This chart shows the available refractive surgery options based on the sphere of the refractive error on the *X*-axis and anterior chamber depth on the *Y*-axis. The Visian ICL (green) comes in powers from −3.00 D to −16.00 D. The ICL requires an anterior chamber depth (ACD) of at least 3.0 mm and a horizontal white-to-white (WTW) diameter between 10.7 and 13.1 mm. Advanced surface ablation (blue) can reliably correct refractive errors from −10.00 D to +5.00 D without an ACD limitation. The Ophtec myopia lens (orange) and hyperopia lens (yellow) are available in powers from −1.00 D to −23.5 D for myopia and + 1.0 D to +12.0 D for hyperopia, respectively. The Ophtec lenses require an ACD of at least 3.2 mm. Refractive lens exchange (purple) can correct very large refractive errors beyond the limits of the previous options or when there is insufficient ACD

4.4 Excimer Laser

Excimer lasers allow for precise reshaping of the corneal surface down to the submicron range, especially with the use of modern scanning lasers [42]. This powerful tool allows for the correction of myopia, hyperopia, and astigmatism (Fig. 4.2) using advanced surface ablation (ASA) and anterior corneal opacities using phototherapeutic keratectomy. ASA is a broad term covering photorefractive keratectomy (PRK), LASEK, and Epi-LASEK, which are methods to reshape the corneal stroma without the creation of a stromal flap as performed in LASIK. Although there have been successful reports of pediatric LASIK [20, 37–39], it is preferable in the author's opinion to use ASA in children. This is because children are at greater risk for traumatic flap dislocation which can be visually devastating to the eye. Other advantages for children are that ASA may have a lower long-term risk of ectasia and when properly performed leaves the eye appearing as though a procedure was never done, even with a close examination at the slit lamp [43, 44].

In addition to the general preoperative evaluation discussed previously, evaluating for keratoectasia is important since such a condition would be a contraindication to ASA. Patients are asked about chronic eye rubbing and atopy which are risk factors for keratoconus [45]. Children with Down syndrome are at greater risk for developing keratoconus, and ASA in these patients should be approached with caution or avoided [46].

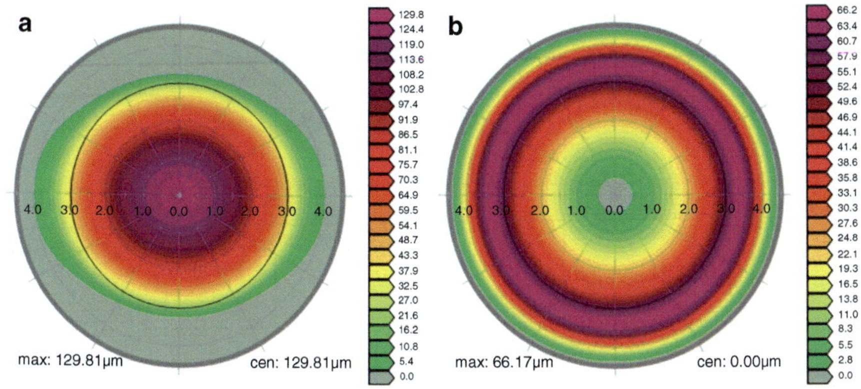

Fig. 4.2 Wavefront-optimized ablation profiles for a compound myopic astigmatism treatment (**a**) and simple hyperopic treatment (**b**) in two separate pediatric patients. Color-coding toward the pink side of the spectrum indicates greater ablation depth (values in microns), while the green side indicates less ablation depth. The numbers arranged horizontally across the ablation profile indicate optical zones of the cornea in millimeters. The numbers at the bottom of the profile indicate maximum and central ablation depth. The patient in (**a**) had refraction of −8.25 + 2.25 × 90 with a correction of −9.25 + 2.25 × 90 for a target of +1.00 D. Notice there is more ablation in the center of the cornea with less ablation in the periphery in order to flatten the central cornea for a myopic correction. Also notice that the ablation profile is ovalized in order to create steepening along the horizontal meridian to correct for astigmatism. The patient in (**b**) had a refraction of +5.00 with a correction of +4.00 for a target of +1.00 D. Notice that the highest amount of ablation is between the 3.0 and 4.0 mm optical zones with no ablation in the center in order to steepen the central cornea for a hyperopic correction. The ablation profile is spherical, because there is no astigmatic correction

Although older children may be able to undergo corneal ablation awake in the clinic [12], most children require brief general anesthesia in the operating room [9–11, 16–18, 47–49]. Excimer lasers are large machines and in operating rooms where space is limited, an organized and efficient setup is critical for performing this procedure safely and with rapid turnover (Fig. 4.3). Another advantage of ASA over LASIK is that it does not require the additional set up of a femtosecond laser or microkeratome in usually an already crowded operating room. For general anesthesia, patients are premedicated with nasal midazolam if needed. Standard induction is performed with sevoflurane, oxygen, and nitrous gas mixture. A laryngeal mask airway is placed, and the extension tube is oriented toward the feet so as not to obstruct the laser. Positioning of the patient becomes critical, since the patient is unconscious. The iris plane should be parallel with the floor. The head and neck should be vertically aligned beneath the laser, so that treatment of astigmatism will be on the correct axis. Propofol supplementation is provided as needed, and intravenous morphine or ketorolac are given at the end of the procedure to help with initial postoperative pain. Elbow restraints can be placed before emergence from anesthesia. General anesthesia also allows for ASA to be performed in patients with nystagmus or other conditions with fixation impersistence.

The procedure itself follows the same steps as adult ASA. A conservative residual stromal bed of 400 microns is set as a limit in children similar to that in adults

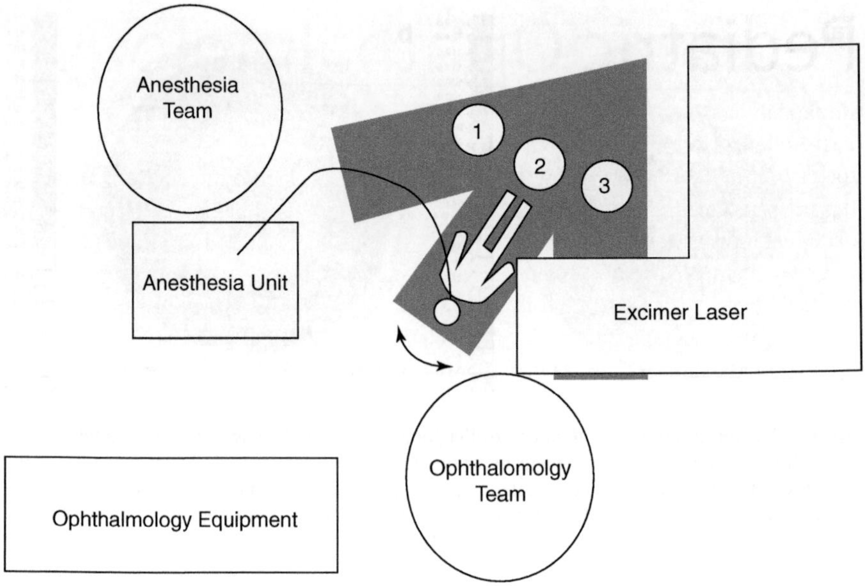

Fig. 4.3 Operating room layout for photorefractive keratectomy (PRK) under general anesthesia. The swiveling patient bed (grey) can rotate the patient to position 1 for induction and emergence from anesthesia, position 2 for exam under anesthesia by the ophthalmology team, and position 3 for excimer laser treatment. The ventilatory tubing should have sufficient length for the full excursion of the patient to position 3. The laryngeal mask airway should be oriented toward the patient's feet once exiting the mouth in order to avoid interference with the eye-tracking system of the excimer laser

[50]. After ablation, the stromal bed is treated with mitomycin-C to reduce corneal haze [51]. A bandage contact lens is placed, and the patient is started on topical tobradex, fluorometholone, and ketorolac. Goggles are then placed over the eyes. Patients are seen on postoperative day 1 to ensure the bandage contact lens is still in place and to review postoperative instructions. Vitamin C supplementation is encouraged to further reduce the risk of postoperative corneal haze. On postoperative day 5, the corneal epithelium should be healed, and the bandage contact lens can be removed. Then the patient is continued only on fluorometholone for 6 months. The postoperative refraction is checked at the 1-month visit and at subsequent visits to determine the effectiveness of treatment and regression. Visual acuity is not always obtainable, particularly in delayed children, and therefore the patient's cycloplegic refraction, visual behavior, and pattern visual evoked potential become the indicators of successful treatment.

Long-term, there is evidence of refractive regression in children, especially with higher degrees of corneal ablation [9, 11, 52, 53]. This practically limits the amount of treatment at the primary ablation to −10 D of myopia and +5 D of hyperopia (Fig. 4.1). Treatment of high degrees of astigmatism, in particular when combined with hyperopic ablations, seems to create even greater refractive regression [53]. Regression leads to under correction of the refractive error over time, which sometimes requires retreatment if the patient has sufficient corneal thickness.

4.5 Phakic Intraocular Lens (pIOL)

The two pIOLs which have most widely been implanted in children are the Visian implantable collamer lens (ICL) made by STAAR Surgical and the iris-enclavated Artisan lens made by Ophtec. The ICL is placed in the posterior chamber between the crystalline lens and iris, while the Artisan lens clips onto the anterior surface of the iris thus residing in the anterior chamber (Fig. 4.4). Phakic IOLs have shown excellent refractive outcomes in children with minimal regression, because they do not have the problem of tissue remodeling, which drives refractive regression after corneal ablation [6, 17, 40, 54–57]. However, the feasibility of pIOLs is limited by the need for sufficient anterior chamber depth (ACD). The ICL requires an ACD of 3.0 mm, and the Artisan lens requires 3.2 mm. In children who tend to have smaller eyes than adults, the ACD plays an important role in choosing a refractive surgery option (Fig. 4.1). Additionally, the ICL requires a horizontal white-to-white (WTW) of 10.7–13.1 mm. Implantation of a pIOL in the setting of insufficient ACD can result in angle-closure glaucoma, accelerated corneal endothelial cell loss, subclinical inflammation, pigmentary dispersion, and cataractogenesis [58]. This is why it is critical for the pediatric refractive surgeon to perform multiple checks of the patient's ACD, WTW, and corneal endothelial health prior to implantation to ensure that the appropriately sized ICL is used.

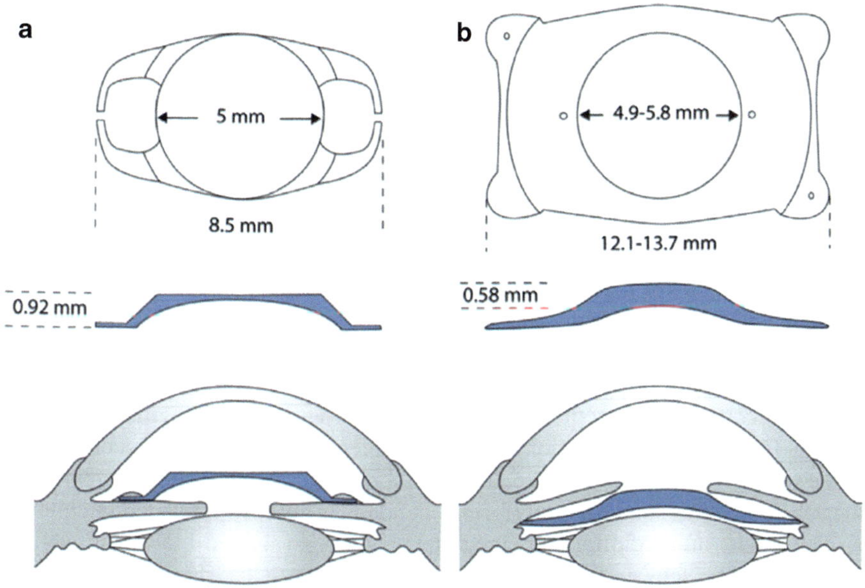

Fig. 4.4 Dimensions and anatomic position of the Ophtec-Artisan (**a**) and Visian ICL (**b**) phakic intraocular lens (pIOL) in the anterior segment. (Reprinted with permission from Faron N, Hoekel J, Tychsen L. Visual acuity, refractive error, and regression outcomes in 169 children with high myopia who were implanted with Ophtec-Artisan or Visian phakic IOLs. *J Am Assoc Pediatric Ophthalmol Strabismus*. 2021;25:27.e1–27.e8)

The ICL can correct myopia from −3.0 to −16.0 D. There is also a toric ICL (TICL) used for the correction of cylinder from 1.0 to 4.0 D at the spectacle plane. It is a single-piece lens with an overall length ranging from 12.1 to 13.7 mm. Different sizes are used due to anatomical variation in iridociliary sulcus diameter, which can be directly measured with ultrasound biomicroscopy, though in children the horizontal WTW is used as a proxy. All ICLs can be implanted through a 3.2 mm corneal incision. It is made from a copolymer of hydroxyethyl methacrylate and porcine-collagen and has nearly 100% transmittance of visible light, making it nearly imperceptible after implantation [59, 60].

In a 2016 study of 23 special needs children implanted with an ICL, 88% were corrected to within ±1.0 D of goal refraction. Eighty-five percent of children with a neurobehavioral disorder were reported to have enhanced visual awareness, attentiveness, or social interactions after ICL implantation. At an average of 9 months follow-up, average shift of spherical refractive error was +0.59 D, which was non-significant. Endothelial cell density had an average 1% decline in 10 eyes able to undergo measurement. Two children (8%) required an unplanned return to the operating room on the first postoperative day to relieve pupillary block caused by non-patent iridotomy. The authors explain this occurred in the first two children implanted in their series who both had Nd:YAG laser iridotomies. Thereafter, laser iridotomy was abandoned in favor of scissor iridectomy at the time of ICL implantation. Afterward, no further complications were encountered. Other recommendations by the authors for adapting ICL surgery for special needs children include administration of IV acetazolamide during surgery to prevent postoperative ocular hypertension due to retained viscoelastic, use of a bridle suture to stabilize eye position while the patient is under general anesthesia, and closure of all corneal incisions with absorbable suture [54].

The Artisan lens can correct −1.0 to −23.5 D of myopia and +1.0 to +12.0 D of hyperopia. Toric lenses are also available correcting 1.0 to 7.5 D of cylinder. Currently, in the US, only the myopic lens has been approved and is available in powers −5.0 to −20.0 D. There is also an Artisan aphakia lens currently undergoing a multicenter clinical trial for patients aged 2–21-years old. Its power ranges from +10.0 to +30.0 D, and it requires a minimum ACD of 3.2 mm [61]. The Artisan lens is made from polymethyl methacrylate and comes in optic sizes of 5.0 mm and 6.0 mm in diameter. Typically, the 5.0 mm diameter optic is used in children, which requires a corneal incision of 5.2 mm for insertion. The overall length of the lens is 8.5 mm [62, 63]. De-enclavation of the Artisan lens from the iris can occur usually in the setting of trauma. Therefore, in the author's opinion, retropupillary fixation of the aphakic lens as sometimes performed in adults is not recommended in children.

The largest study of pIOL implantation in children evaluated 115 eyes implanted with the Artisan lens and 154 eyes implanted with the ICL. These children had a history of high myopia and spectacle-aversion. Average age at surgery was 9.9 years, and mean follow-up was 3.9 years. Spherical correction averaged 12.3 D, and 92% of eyes were corrected to within ±0.5 D of goal refraction. There were significant gains in uncorrected distance visual acuity, corrected distance visual acuity, and binocular fusion. The reason for postoperative improvement in corrected distance visual acuity is due to the relative image magnification achieved after reducing the amount of myopic lens power needed at the spectacle plane. Of the 169 children in the study, 81% were noted to have enhanced visual awareness, attentiveness, or social interactions. Of the eyes implanted with the Artisan lens, 8% required surgical repositioning/re-enclavation for traumatic dislocation. Three percent of the children implanted with either pIOL required return to the operating room in the days following surgery because of iridotomy closure causing pupillary block. The authors note the two major advantages of pIOL implantation for high myopia in this study were the marked low rate of refractive regression and no removal of corneal tissue, both of which are considerable drawbacks of excimer laser ablation for high levels of refractive error [55].

4.6 Refractive Lens Exchange (RLE)

RLE is a procedure in which lensectomy of the natural, crystalline lens with simultaneous implantation of an artificial intraocular lens (IOL) is performed for the treatment of refractive error. In eyes with a long axial length and/or steep keratometry values, aphakia may yield the desired refractive target. In this case, lensectomy without IOL implantation is performed, and the procedure is called clear lens extraction (CLE). These procedures are usually a secondary option in pediatric refractive surgery, because they result in loss of accommodation. Typically, in adults, RLE is performed around the age of presbyopia onset, so the loss of accommodation has minimal significance [64]. However, in children, who can have an amplitude of accommodation greater than 16.0 D [65, 66], the loss of accommodation is a major drawback to consider before removing the natural lens. RLE/CLE is used when other options are not possible due to insufficient space for a pIOL or too large of a refractive error for ASA or a pIOL (Fig. 4.1).

An exam under anesthesia is performed a few months before the planned procedure in order to obtain accurate biometry and perform a thorough scleral depressed exam of the peripheral retina. If there are risk factors for retinal detachment, such as axial length exceeding 29 mm, lattice degeneration, or asymptomatic retinal tears, then a barrier diode laser may be prophylactically applied. However, the use of barrier diode laser for retinal detachment prophylaxis is debated [67, 68]. Standard lensectomy with posterior capsulectomy and anterior vitrectomy is performed as in the manner of pediatric cataract surgery. The primary posterior capsulectomy and anterior vitrectomy are important to prevent posterior capsule or anterior hyaloid opacification, which can have an incidence as high as 50% [52]. Families should also be informed that the capsulectomy may need to be repeated in the future. Older children who can cooperate with an Nd:YAG capsulotomy in clinic may have the posterior capsule left intact at the time of surgery but should be closely monitored for the development of posterior capsule opacification.

If an IOL needs to be implanted to achieve the refractive target, then consider implantation of an acrylic, foldable 3-piece IOL in the iridociliary sulcus with posterior optic capture. This allows for implantation through a small incision with excellent long-term centration of the lens and facilitates future IOL exchange if needed. Multifocal lenses may be beneficial to counteract the loss of accommodation for older children outside of the amblyogenic age. These children should have normal pupillary movement and the ability to maintain stable centration of the multifocal IOL [69].

In a study of unilateral lens extraction for high anisometropic myopia in a pediatric population, 86% of eyes were corrected within ±3 D of goal refraction. Myopia correction averaged 17.3 D, and myopic regression averaged 0.43 D per year [70]. In another study of clear lens extraction and refractive lens exchange for high bilateral myopia in children with neurobehavioral disorders, 81% were corrected to within ±2 D of goal refraction. Uncorrected acuity improved an average of 2 log units in all 26 eyes, with commensurate gains in behavior and environmental visual interaction in 88% of children. Myopic regression averaged 0.16 D per year. Focal retinal detachment occurred in one eye with a history of cicatricial retinopathy of prematurity and trauma and was successfully repaired but resulted in loss of visual acuity [52].

The most vision-threatening complication of RLE is retinal detachment because unlike other refractive surgery options, the procedure necessitates surgery within the vitreous chamber. Myopic eyes are at higher risk of retinal detachment, and lens extraction increases this risk. In adults, the reported incidence of retinal detachment after RLE ranges from 0.37% to 8.1% [71, 72]. In the two pediatric studies mentioned above, the authors estimate the incidence to be about 3% at an average follow-up of 4.5 years [52, 70]. It is prudent to note that other serious complications may only appear after prolonged follow-up.

4.7 Future Technologies

Pediatric refractive surgery is a rapidly advancing field with new technologies continually emerging in the areas of preoperative evaluation, treatment interventions, and postoperative care.

Iris anatomy and limbal vessel registration obtained during preoperative biometry create a map of the ocular surface which can then be overlayed onto the surgeon's view in the microscope. The axis of astigmatism can then be precisely treated without the confounding effect of globe cyclotorsion when the patient is in the supine position. For children who can cooperate with preoperative biometry, this will greatly assist in the treatment of astigmatism, because children usually cannot tolerate preoperative toric marking. Intraoperative anterior segment optical coherence tomography allows for a very accurate evaluation of pIOL position and vaulting. This is critical for ensuring long-term anterior segment health in children.

In the realm of keratorefractive surgery, treatment of higher order aberrations is becoming increasingly important in improving contrast sensitivity along with visual acuity. Advancements in this area include wavefront-optimized, wavefront-guided, and topography-guided treatments. Wavefront-optimized treatments are already being applied to pediatric patients. Wavefront and topography-guided treatments will be more available to pediatric patients as the preoperative diagnostic equipment becomes more facile for use in children and for exams under anesthesia. A drawback of these customized ablations is that they remove more corneal tissue than traditional ablations. Bioptics is another methodology already being used in pediatrics and involves a combination of keratorefractive and pIOL/IOL procedures to customize refractive error treatment. Small incision lenticule extraction (SMILE) provides an advantage in pediatric patients in that there is minimal disruption of corneal epithelium while still reshaping corneal stroma. This may reduce the risk of infection and would effectively remove the need for postoperative bandage contact lens management as currently performed with PRK. Surgical management of astigmatism, particularly hyperopic astigmatism, is currently a challenge in pediatric refractive surgery. The use of femtosecond laser nonpenetrating limbal relaxing incisions appears promising in children because the treatments are highly precise and should result in minimal pain, postoperative recovery time, and infection risk as there is no epithelial incision. These limbal relaxing incisions also do not remove a significant amount of tissue and are repeatable.

Phakic IOLs with a central opening will obviate the need for a peripheral iridotomy at the time of surgery. This will be safer for children who tend to have more inflammation and scarring postoperatively and thus are at greater risk for closure of the iridotomy.

In postoperative management of children, simplicity is key. Combination drops which mix antibiotic, steroid, and NSAID can help reduce the eyedrop burden on caregivers of children with neurobehavioral disorders. In a similar approach, punctal steroid implants and intracameral antibiotic given at the end of surgery may abolish the need for postoperative drop regimens altogether.

As the safety of these procedures improves and repeatedly manifests itself, the indications for pediatric refractive surgery will expand, like any medical technology. The surgeon's enthusiasm for achieving better results with cutting-edge technology must be continually tempered by the concern for the long-term visual health of young patients. Pediatric refractive surgery can make meaningful and lasting impacts in the lives of children when surgeons combine the knowledge and skills of refractive surgery and pediatric ophthalmology.

Key Points

1. Pediatric refractive surgery addresses refractive errors and their associated comorbidities such as amblyopia and strabismus in special needs children intolerant of spectacles or contact lenses.
2. Contrary to adults, amblyopia is frequently an indication for pediatric refractive surgery.
3. Pediatric refractive surgery involves modification of ametropia at the corneal, anterior chamber, posterior chamber, and lens planes.
4. The most common modalities used for pediatric refractive surgery today are advanced surface ablation, phakic intraocular lenses, and refractive lens exchange.
5. Children with neurobehavioral disorders undergoing refractive surgery have improvements in visual acuity, communication, socialization, motor skills, adaptive behaviors, visual perception, and cognitive function.

References

1. Schmidt D, Grzybowski A. Vincenz Fukala (1847–1911) and the early history of clear-lens operations in high myopia. Saudi J Ophthalmol. 2013;27:41–6.
2. Strampelli B. Tolerance of acrylic lenses in the anterior chamber in aphakia and refraction disorders. Ann Di Ottalmologia E Clin Ocul. 1954;80:75–82.
3. Fechner PU, Worst JGF. A new concave intraocular lens for the correction of myopia. European J Implant Refract Surg. 1989;1:41–3.
4. Fechner PU, Singh D, Wulff K. Iris-claw lens in phakic eyes to correct hyperopia: preliminary study. J Cataract Refract Surg. 1998;24:48–56.
5. Simsek S, Demirok A, Yasar T, Yilmaz O. The correction of high myopia by posterior chamber lens implantation into phakic eyes. East J Med. 1998;3:54–7.
6. Lesueur LC, Arne JL. Phakic posterior chamber lens implantation in children with high myopia. J Cataract Refract Surg. 1999;25:1571–5.
7. Chuck RS, Jacobs DS, Lee JK, et al. Refractive Errors & Refractive Surgery Preferred Practice Pattern®. Ophthalmology. 2018;125:P1–P104.
8. Singh D. Photorefractive keratectomy in pediatric patients. J Cataract Refract Surg. 1995;21:630–2.
9. Faron N, Tychsen L, Hoekel J. Excimer laser refractive surgery for astigmatism in children and adolescents. J AAPOS. 2014 18(4):e28-e29.
10. Faron N, Hoekel J, Tychsen L. Excimer laser refractive surgery outcomes in 405 children and adolescents. J AAPOS. 2015;19(4):e22.
11. Tychsen L, Packwood E, Berdy G. Correction of large amblyopiogenic refractive errors in children using the excimer laser. J AAPOS. 2005;9:224–33.
12. Phillips CB, Prager TC, McClellan G, Mintz-Hittner HA. Laser in situ keratomileusis for treated anisometropic amblyopia in awake, autofixating pediatric and adolescent patients. J Cartaract Refract Surg. 2004;30:2522–8.
13. Autrata R, Rehurek J. Laser-assisted subepithelial keratectomy and photorefractive keratectomy versus conventional treatment of myopic anisometropic amblyopia in children. J Cartaract Refract Surg. 2004;30:74–84.
14. Paysse EA, Coats DK, Hussein MAW, et al. Long-term outcomes of photorefractive keratectomy for anisometropic amblyopia in children. Ophthalmology. 2006;113:169–76.
15. Song J, Al-Ghamdi I, Awad A. Pediatric refractive surgery in evolution. Middle East Afr J Ophthalmol. 2012;19:22–3.
16. Paysse EA, Tychsen L, Stahl E. Pediatric refractive surgery: corneal and intraocular techniques and beyond. J AAPOS. 2012;16:291–7.
17. Tychsen L. Refractive surgery for children: excimer laser, phakic intraocular lens, and clear lens extraction. Curr Opin Ophthalmol. 2008;19:342–8.
18. Tychsen L. Refractive surgery for children: laser, implants, current results and future directions. Expert Rev Ophthalmol. 2008;3(6):635–43.
19. Daoud YJ, Hutchinson A, Wallace DK, et al. Refractive surgery in children: treatment options, outcomes, and controversies. Am J Ophthalmol. 2009;147:573–582.e2.
20. Agarwal A, Agarwal T, Siraj AA, et al. Results of pediatric laser in situ keratomileusis. J Cartaract Refract Surg. 2000;26:684–9.
21. McCarty CA, Livingston PM, Taylor HR. Prevalence of myopia in adults: implications for refractive surgeons. J Refract Surg (Thorofare, NJ : 1995). 1997, 13:229–34.
22. Kempen JH, Mitchell P, Lee KE, et al. The prevalence of refractive errors among adults in the United States, Western Europe, and Australia. Arch Ophthalmol. 2004;122:495–505.
23. Vitale S, Sperduto RD, Ferris FL. Increased prevalence of myopia in the United States between 1971-1972 and 1999-2004. Arch Ophthalmol. 2009;127:1632–9.
24. Siatkowski RM, Cotter SA, Crockett RS, et al. Two-year multicenter, randomized, double-masked, placebo-controlled, parallel safety and efficacy study of 2%pirenzepineophthalmicgelinchildrenwithmyopia. J AAPOS. 2008;12:332–9.

25. OECD, WHO. Preterm birth and low birth weight. 2020.
26. Hashemi H, Fotouhi A, Yekta A, et al. Global and regional estimates of prevalence of refractive errors: systematic review and meta-analysis. J Curr Ophthalmol. 2018;30:3–22.
27. Cook A, White S, Batterbury M, Clark D. Ocular growth and refractive error development in premature infants with or without retinopathy of prematurity. Invest Ophthalmol Vis Sci. 2008;49:5199–207.
28. Friling R, Weinberger D, Kremer I, et al. Keratometry measurements in preterm and full term newborn infants. Br J Ophthalmol. 2004;88:8–10.
29. Singh A, Pesala V, Garg P, Bharadwaj SR. Relation between uncorrected astigmatism and visual acuity in Pseudophakia. Optometry Vision Sci. 2013;90:378–84.
30. Castagno VD, Fassa AG, Carret MLV, et al. Hyperopia: a meta-analysis of prevalence and a review of associated factors among school-aged children. BMC Ophthalmol. 2014;14:163.
31. Varghese RM, Sreenivas V, Puliyel JM, Varughese S. Rcfractive status at birth: its relation to newborn physical parameters at birth and gestational age. PLoS One. 2009;4:e4469.
32. Semeraro F, Forbice E, Nascimbeni G, et al. Ocular refraction at birth and its development during the first year of life in a large cohort of babies in a single Center in Northern Italy. Front Pediatr. 2020;7:539.
33. Kassem IS, Rubin SE, Kodsi SR. Exotropia in children with high hyperopia. J AAPOS. 2012;16:437–40.
34. Fecarotta CM, Kim M, Wasserman BN. Refractive surgery in children. Curr Opin Ophthalmol. 2010;21:350–5.
35. Paysse EA, Gonzalez-Diaz M, Wang D, et al. Developmental improvement in children with neurobehavioral disorders following photorefractive keratectomy for high refractive errors. J AAPOS. 2011;15:e6.
36. Ghasia F, Tychsen L. Utility values for surgical treatment of high refractive errors in children. J AAPOS. 2007;11:89.
37. Phillips CB, Prager TC, McClellan G, Mintz-Hittner HA. Laser in situ keratomileusis for high hyperopia in awake, autofixating pediatric and adolescent patients with fully or partially accommodative esotropia. J Cataract Refract Surg. 2004;30:2124–9.
38. Polat S, Can Ç, İlhan B, et al. Laser in situ Keratomileusis for treatment of fully or partially refractive accommodative Esotropia. Eur J Ophthalmol. 2009;19:733–7.
39. Magli A, Iovine A, Gagliardi V, et al. LASIK and PRK in refractive accommodative Esotropia: a retrospective study on 20 adolescent and adult patients. Eur J Ophthalmol. 2008;19:188–95.
40. Lesueur LC, Arne JL. Phakic intraocular lens to correct high myopic amblyopia in children. J Refract Surg Thorofare N J. 1995;2002(18):519–23.
41. Garcia-Valenzuela E, Kaufman LM. High myopia associated with retinopathy of prematurity is primarily lenticular. J AAPOS. 2005;9:121–8.
42. Thompson V, Seiler T, Hardten DR. Photorefractive keratectomy. In: Azar D, editor. Refractive surgery. 3rd ed. Philadelphia, PA: Elsevier; 2019. p. 280–90.
43. Moisseiev E, Sela T, Minkev L, Varssano D. Increased preference of surface ablation over laser in situ keratomileusis between 2008–2011 is correlated to risk of ecatasia. Clin Ophthalmol. 2013;7:93–8.
44. O'Brart DPS, Shalchi Z, McDonald RJ, et al. Twenty-year follow-up of a randomized prospective clinical trial of Excimer laser photorefractive keratectomy. Am J Ophthalmol. 2014;158:651–663.e1.
45. Najmi H, Mobarki Y, Mania K, et al. The correlation between keratoconus and eye rubbing: a review. Int J Ophthalmol. 2019;12:1775–81.
46. Kristianslund O, Drolsum L. Prevalence of keratoconus in persons with down syndrome: a review. BMJ Open Ophthalmol. 2021;6:e000754.
47. Paysse EA, Hussein MAW, Koch DD, et al. Successful implementation of a protocol for photorefractive keratectomy in children requiring anesthesia. J Cartaract Refract Surg. 2003;29:1744–7.
48. Stahl ED. Pediatric refractive surgery. Curr Opin Ophthalmol. 2017;28:305–9.

49. Tychsen L. Refractive surgery for special needs children. Arch Ophthalmol (Chicago, Ill : 1960). 2009;127:810–3.
50. Bamashmus MA, Saleh MF, Awadalla MA. Reasons for not performing keratorefractive surgery in patients seeking refractive surgery in a hospital-based cohort in "Yemen". Middle East Afr J Ophthalmol. 2010;17:349–53.
51. Sy ME, Zhang L, Yeroushalmi A, et al. Effect of mitomycin-C on the variance in refractive outcomes after photorefractive keratectomy. J Cataract Refract Surg. 2014;40:1980–4.
52. Tychsen L, Packwood E, Hoekel J, Lueder G. Refractive surgery for high bilateral myopia in children with neurobehavioral disorders: 1. Clear lens extraction and refractive lens exchange. J AAPOS. 2006;10:357–63.
53. Ahmed K, Faron N, Hoekel J, Tychsen L. Excimer laser keratectomy for hyperopia in special needs children: longer term outcomes. J AAPOS. 2021;25:e32.
54. Tychsen L, Faron N, Hoekel J. Phakic intraocular collamer lens (visian ICL) implantation for correction of myopia in spectacle-aversive special needs children. Am J Ophthalmol. 2017;175:77–86.
55. Faron N, Hoekel J, Tychsen L. Visual acuity, refractive error, and regression outcomes in 169 children with high myopia who were implanted with ophtec-Artisan or Visian phakic IOLs. J AAPOS. 2021;25:27.e1–8.
56. Tychsen L, Hoekel J, Ghasia F, Yoon-Huang G. Phakic intraocular lens correction of high ametropia in children with neurobehavioral disorders. J AAPOS. 2008;12:282–9.
57. Pirouzian A, Bansal P, O'Halloran H. Phakic IOL in children. Ophthalmology. 2007;114:194–5.
58. Arne J-L. Posterior chamber phakic intraocular lens. In: Azar D, editor. Refractive surgery. 3rd ed. Amsterdam: Elsevier; 2019. p. 412–20.
59. STAAR Surgical Visian ICL® (Implantable Collamer Lens) For Myopia Brochure 2018.
60. STAAR Surgical Visian® TORIC ICL (Implantable Collamer® Lens) for Myopia Brochure. 2018.
61. Artisan Aphakia Lens for the Correction of Aphakia in Children - Full Text View. ClinicalTrials.gov. https://clinicaltrials.gov/ct2/show/NCT01547442; Accessed 26 June 2021.
62. Ophtec. Artisan Myopia Model 206; 2021 . https://www.ophtec.com/products/refractive-surgery/p-iols/artisan-myopia-model-206#downloads. Accessed 20 June 2021.
63. Ophtec. The ARTISAN® Phakic IOL Clinical Study and Post-Approval Study (PAS) I & II Results 2019.
64. Alio JL, Grzybowski A, Kanclerz P. Refractive lens exchange. In: Azar D, editor. Refractive surgery. 3rd ed. Elsevier; 2019. p. 400–6.
65. Rosenfield M, Benzoni JA. Amplitude of accommodation in children between 5 and 10 years of age | IOVS | ARVO journals. Invest Ophthalmol Vis Sci. 2007;48:975.
66. Sterner B, Gellerstedt M, Sjöström A. The amplitude of accommodation in 6–10-year-old children – not as good as expected! Ophthal Physl Opt. 2004;24:246–51.
67. Wilkinson CP. Evidence-based analysis of prophylactic treatment of asymptomatic retinal breaks and lattice degeneration. Ophthalmology. 2000;107:12–5.
68. Folk JC, Bennett SR, Klugman MR, et al. Prophylactic treatment to the fellow eye of patients with phakic lattice retinal detachment: analysis of failures and risks of treatment. Retin. 1990;10:165–9.
69. Hunter DG. Multifocal intraocular lenses in children. Ophthalmology. 2001;108:1373–4.
70. Ali A, Packwood E, Lueder G, Tychsen L. Unilateral lens extraction for high anisometropic myopia in children and adolescents. J AAPOS. 2007;11:153–8.
71. Colin J, Robinet A, Cochener B. Retinal detachment after clear lens extraction for high myopia seven-year follow-up. Ophthalmology. 1999;106:2281–5.
72. Westin O, Koskela T, Behndig A. Epidemiology and outcomes in refractive lens exchange surgery. Acta Ophthalmol. 2015;93:41–5.

Advances in the Management of Retinopathy of Prematurity

5

Deeksha Katoch, Ashish Markan, and Mangat Ram Dogra

5.1 Introduction

Retinopathy of prematurity (ROP) is a retinal disorder characterized by abnormal neovascular proliferation that occurs secondary to arrest of the physiologic retinal vascularization. ROP accounts for nearly 40% of childhood blindness and is estimated to affect three-fourth of premature infants born with a birth weight of less than 1250 grams (g) [1]. The epidemiology of ROP is described in three epidemics [2]. Unrestricted use of oxygen led to the first epidemic of ROP in the USA and the UK between 1940 and 1960. Restriction of oxygen usage curtailed the first epidemic albeit with some increase in pulmonary complications and mortality. The second epidemic was again seen in developed countries due to increased survival of preterm babies with very low birth weights. The burden of ROP in current times is limited to the low- and middle-income countries and is postulated to be similar to the situation in the developed countries in the first epidemic. Out of the estimated 15 million preterm infants born worldwide every year, nearly 3.8 million are born in low- and middle-income countries [3]. High rates of preterm births, suboptimal neonatal care, low screening coverage, and paucity of trained ophthalmologists have caused ROP to become an emerging public health problem in these nations. Studies in Asian Indian infants have shown that ROP can occur in heavier and more mature infants with birth weight >1250 g [4, 5]. In India, for example, as per WHO (2010) out of the 3.5 million preterm births, about 6,00,000 babies are born at gestational age (GA) <32 weeks. Out of these, approximately 2,00,000 babies are at the risk of developing ROP every year. Even if 10% of them develop treatable disease, roughly 20,000 newborns will require ROP management every year in India alone [6, 7].

D. Katoch (✉) · A. Markan · M. R. Dogra
Advanced Eye Centre, Postgraduate Institute of Medical Education and Research, PGIMER, Chandigarh, India
e-mail: drdeekshakatoch@yahoo.in

A. Ramasubramanian (ed.), *Pediatric Ophthalmology*, Current Practices in Ophthalmology, https://doi.org/10.1007/978-981-19-4963-0_5

Amid the growing number of infants requiring ROP screening and treatment, there have been evolutionary changes in disease classification, disease documentation, and treatment which will be discussed in this chapter.

5.2 Classification

ROP is classified using the International Classification of ROP (ICROP) into zones (I–III) for disease location, stage 1–5 for disease severity, and clock hours 1–12 for disease extent. Dilatation and tortuosity of the posterior retinal vessels are noted as the presence or absence of plus disease. The ICROP classification was revised in 1987 and again in 2005 to include the terms "pre-plus" and "Aggressive Posterior ROP" (APROP). Appearance of posterior retinal vessels which was less than the definition of plus was categorized as pre-plus, warranting closer observation for progression to plus and treatment requiring disease [8]. APROP was classified as a severe, rapidly progressive disease characterized by location in zone I or posterior zone II, prominence of plus, flat neovascularization, circumferential shunt vessels, and vascular loops. APROP can progress directly to retinal detachment without passing through the typical intervening stages if left untreated [8].

ICROP was recently updated in 2021 (ICROP 3) with the following salient new additions [9].

(a) Definition of "posterior zone II" as an intermediate zone that begins at the margin of zone I and zone II and extends into zone II for 2 disc diameters.
(b) Description of a "Notch" as an incursion of the ROP lesion for 1 or 2 clock hours into a more posterior zone. In the presence of a posterior notch, the zone for eyes is labeled by the most posterior zone of retinal vascularization.
(c) Aggressive ROP—ICROP 3 recognized that APROP may occur beyond the posterior retina and in larger preterm infants, particularly in regions of the world with limited resources. Therefore, replacement of the term APROP with Aggressive ROP (A-ROP) has been recommended.
(d) Subclassifications of stage 5 as 5A when the optic disc is visible by ophthalmoscopy, 5B—when the optic disc is not visible because of retrolental fibrovascular tissue or closed-funnel detachment, 5C—presence of anterior segment changes such as anterior chamber shallowing, iridocorneolenticular adhesions, and corneal opacification.
(e) Regression: Signs of regression include reduction of plus, advancement of vascularization into the peripheral avascular retina, involution of tunica vasculosa lentis, better pupillary dilation, greater media clarity, and resolution of intraretinal hemorrhages.
(f) Reactivation: Appearance of recurrent vascular dilation, tortuosity, or both, similar to acute-phase pre-plus or plus disease. Documentation of reactivation should specify the presence and location(s) of new ROP features, using the modifier *reactivated*. For example, the presence of a ridge during reactivation would be noted as "reactivated stage 2."
(g) Long term Sequelae: Include late retinal detachments, Persistent Avascular Retina, Macular anomalies, Retinal vascular changes, and glaucoma.

5.2.1 Risk Factors

ROP is a multifactorial disease. Identification of the risk factors can aid neonatologists as well as ophthalmologists to perform careful risk stratification for screening and take necessary measures to prevent disease progression. Among the several risk factors linked to ROP, low birth weight, prematurity, and postnatal oxygen exposure are well known to confer independent risk. Apart from this, prolonged mechanical ventilation, APGAR score, anemia, sepsis, pulmonary complications, use of surfactant, multiple blood transfusions, necrotizing enterocolitis, intraventricular hemorrhage (IVH), thrombocytopenia, and cardiac disease are some of the other risk factors for development of ROP in preterm infants [10].

5.2.2 Screening Guidelines

Screening guidelines vary across different demographic regions based on different risk profiles and quality of neonatal care. The American Academy of Pediatrics (AAP), American Association for Pediatric Ophthalmology and Strabismus (AAPOS), and the American Academy of Ophthalmology (AAO) recommend a retinal screening examination for infants with a birth weight of ≤1500 g or gestational age of ≤30 weeks. Infants between 1500 and 2000 gm and GA >30 weeks with risk factors such as prolonged oxygen supplementation are also eligible for screening [11]. The United Kingdom guidelines recommend screening all preterm infants with GA < 32 weeks and birth weight <1501 gm [12].

Development of severe ROP in more mature and heavier infants in developing countries who may be missed if western guidelines are used for screening has been reported previously [4]. This has necessitated a need to alter screening guidelines based on country-specific incidence and disease distribution [4]. The current Indian ROP guidelines as an example recommend screening of all children born with GA <34 weeks and/or BW <2000 g. Those born at >34 weeks GA to be screened in presence of risk factors (prolonged oxygen requirement, respiratory distress syndrome, chronic lung disease, blood transfusions, sepsis, apneas, poor postnatal weight gain, cardiorespiratory support, IVH). Screening should be performed before the baby is discharged from NICU/SNCU, or by 30 days of life, whichever is earlier [7]. Babies with GA <28 weeks and birth weight <1200 grams should be screened by 2–3 weeks of chronological age.

5.2.3 Imaging for ROP

Indirect ophthalmoscopy with scleral depression by an experienced ophthalmologist is considered the gold standard for ROP screening. The difficulty with this approach is the paucity of trained ophthalmologists, lack of objectivity, and an associated learning curve. All these factors have translated into remote telemedicine screening by nonphysicians such as trained ophthalmic technicians and nurses [13, 14]. Digital retinal imaging devices have now been validated for objective disease documentation, parental counseling, and telemedicine-based screening in remote areas where no ROP specialists are available [13–15].

Fundus photography in premature babies presents unique challenges due to the absence of fixation and voluntary cooperation from the infant. Imaging systems for ROP also need to be portable to allow transport across different NICUs, have a wide field of view, be able to image eyes and fundi of different colors, and allow easy export of files in standardized medical image formats for telemedicine.

The most commonly used fundus camera for ROP screening and also proven useful for telemedicine is the RetCam (Natus Medical Systems, Inc., Pleasanton, CA, US). It is a contact, wide-angle, mydriatic, hand-held imaging device that can capture upto 130^0 of the retina [16]. The RetCam Shuttle is the compact, easily portable, and lighter version of the RetCam. RetCam 3 version of this system has a Fluorescein Angiography feature to delineate retinal vascular details.

Trinetra Neo (Forus health, Bangalore, India) is a novel low-cost, handheld, light-weight, and portable fundus camera which provides approximately 120° field of view. It uses a light-emitting diode (LED) illumination and a liquid lens-based focusing system. It has been found to be safe for ocular use [17, 18]. This camera has the potential to be used in low-resource countries allowing better telemedicine care (Fig. 5.1).

The ICON (Phoenix Clinical, Inc., Pleasanton, CA, US) is also a mydriatic, contact, handheld camera with reported improved resolution and color profile for capturing images in dark fundi; Fluorescein Angiography is also available with this device. The Panocam (Visunex Medical Systems, Inc., Fremont, CA, US) is a wireless, contact, handheld camera system with a 130° field of view.

Noncontact fundus cameras have also been used for capturing ROP images and detecting treatment/referral warranted ROP. The disadvantage of noncontact systems are difficulties in infant positioning, motion artifacts, and inability to capture the retinal periphery in majority. Nidek NM200-D is a portable, posterior pole retinal camera with a 30° field of view [17]. Skalet et al. have shown the feasibility of this fundus camera to screen for ROP in remote areas and identify referral warranted ROP (RW-ROP). Pictor is an FDA-approved narrow-angle retinal camera with a field of view of 45°. Plus and pre-plus disease can be documented with high sensitivity and specificity using this modality for ROP screening [19].

Optos 200Tx is an ultrawide field noncontact fundus camera which allows fundus imaging upto 200°. Mao et al. have shown feasibility to perform ultrawide imaging using Optos 200Tx by placing the baby in the "flying baby" position [20]. It involves placing one arm to support the chin/chest and the other hand supporting the head. Eyelid speculum is used to keep the eyelids open and stabilize the eye movements. The ultrawide field images show areas of non-perfusion, demarcation line and ridge, presence of neovascularization and hemorrhages. This allowed the physician to clearly identify the stage and zone of the disease.

Smartphone-based fundus imaging (SBFI) has also been used for documentation of ROP [21, 22]. With the help of different condensing lenses and specialized lens holders, smartphones can be used as cost-effective, handy, and noncontact devices to capture reasonable quality retinal images.

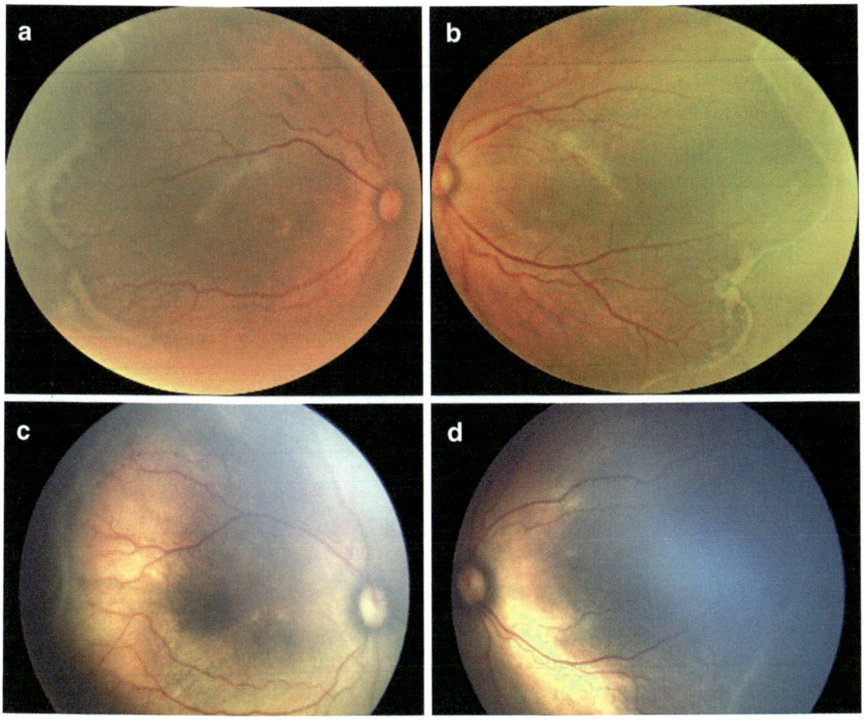

Fig. 5.1 Comparison of wide-field fundus photographs using the Trinetra neo fundus camera (top panel) showing stage 3 Retinopathy of prematurity (ROP) (**a**) in the right eye and stage 2 ROP in the left eye (**b**) in zone II in a preterm infant. Bottom panel shows fundus photographs using the Retcam 3 depicting stage 2 ROP in zone II in right (**c**) and left eye (**d**)

5.3 Optical Coherence Tomography (OCT)

With the introduction of portable Spectral domain OCT (SD-OCT) and age-adjusted scanning protocols, it is now possible to perform OCT in preterm infants [23]. Subclinical findings are being detected on OCT in both APROP and other stages of ROP which are difficult to pick up on indirect ophthalmoscopy. Presence of isolated extraretinal lesions [24] which correspond to popcorn retinopathy, and shown to be precursors to stage 3 disease have also been detected close to the optic disc on OCT in APROP [25]. Epiretinal membranes causing alterations in foveal contour in preterm infants have been detected on SD-OCT [26]. Presence of hyporeflective cystoid spaces predominantly in the inner nuclear layer in preterm infants has been described as macular edema of prematurity (MEOP). MEOP is usually bilateral and is known to be a transient event which resolves spontaneously [27]. Two patterns of MEOP have been described: one with a dome-shaped fovea and the other with a normal foveal morphology [28]. These cystic changes are independent of the stage of ROP. Long-term effects of MEOP on foveal development and photoreceptor function are still unknown. Visual function testing is needed to determine if these cysts have any adverse effect on normal foveal development.

Tilting the handheld probe can allow the physician to screen the retinal periphery and detect stage 3 disease in zone 2. OCT can also be useful in determining the extent of foveal involvement in stage 4 disease. Studies have shown the presence of foveal architecture abnormalities thus explaining poor visual outcomes despite a successfully attached retina [29].

Subfoveal choroidal thickness can also be measured using SD-OCT devices in premature infants. Mean choroidal thickness in premature infants range from 324 ± 79 um to 356.9 ± 75.8 um [30, 31]. Erol et al. have shown a decrease in choroidal thickness with increasing stages of ROP and attributed it to increased oxidative stress at worse stages of ROP [31].

Novel information provided by OCT in ROP will help in better understanding of disease pathophysiology and may provide answers to the possible implications of ROP in foveal and visual development. Furthermore, OCT may provide new quantifiable references for future treatments.

5.4 OCT Angiography (OCT-A)

There are currently no commercially available handheld OCT-A devices to perform OCT-A in preterm infants. Vinekar et al. reported OCT-A findings in APROP using Optovue [32]. Campbell et al. were able to successfully visualize microvascular changes in various stages of ROP using a handheld prototype OCT-A device [33]. The study demonstrated attenuated flow signal in areas of atrophic retina, increased signal transmission in areas of laser scars, and lack of flow in overlying preretinal fibrous proliferation. Kothari et al. have shown the feasibility of arm-mounted OCT-A to detect changes in FAZ in extremely low birth weight babies and allow a better understanding of foveal development in premature babies [34]. OCT-A studies have shown a better foveal development in previously anti-VEGF treated eyes compared to laser treatment [35]. Mataftsi et al. have shown a significantly smaller FAZ and a lower vessel density in spontaneously regressed ROP compared to preterm babies with no ROP and age-matched normal controls [36].

5.5 Fundus Fluorescein Angiography (FFA)

FFA has been a useful adjunct to clinical examination in pediatric retinal vascular diseases. Widefield FFA helps to document and analyze subtle peripheral vascular changes that can be missed on clinical examination (Fig. 5.2). Retcam 3 and Optos

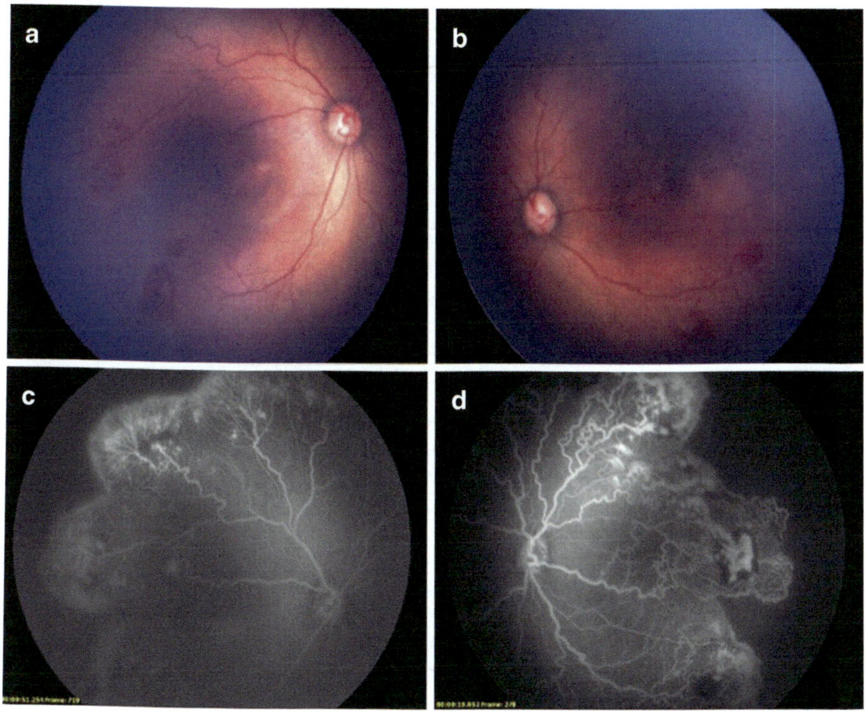

Fig. 5.2 Wide-field retcam fundus photographs in a preterm infant born at 28 weeks of gestation with a birth weight of 1000 grams showing flat neovascularization or hemorrhage in posterior zone II with pre-plus. (**a**, **b**). Fluorescein angiography confirms and also demonstrates the extent of neovascularization at the vascular avascular junction (**c**, **d**)

200Tx have been successfully used to record widefield angiograms in infants [20, 37]. FFA has helped identify vascular abnormalities such as areas of non-perfusion, extent of neovascularization, avascular loops, residual skip areas, and status of macular perfusion in APROP [20, 37].

Anti-VEGF therapy is preferred over laser in infants with severe vaso-obliteration and vascularization limited to posterior zone I (Fig. 5.3). Fluorescein angiography helps to clearly delineate persistent avascular retina following treatment with Anti-VEGF agents and helps guide the need for retreatment and follow-up.

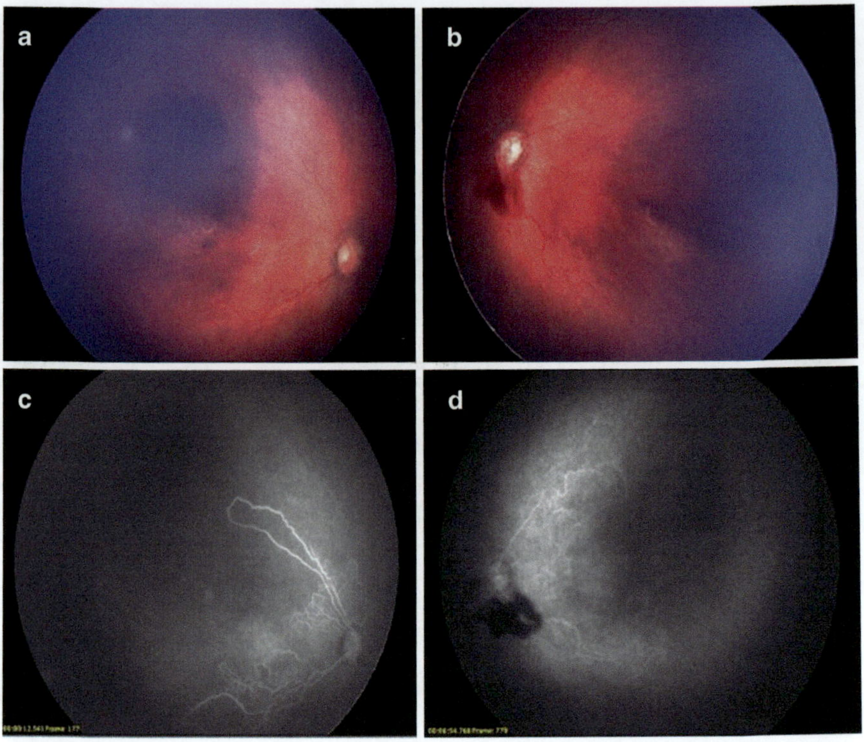

Fig. 5.3 Retcam fundus photography showing posterior zone I APROP with loops and shunts in posterior zone I (**a, b**) along with a preretinal bleed over the optic disc (**b**). Fluorescein angiography confirms non-perfusion of the macula in both eyes (**c, d**). This infant was treated with Anti-VEGF therapy to provide an opportunity to allow vascularization to progress beyond macula

5.6 Telemedicine in ROP

Amid the growing numbers of infants requiring screening and significant workforce limitation, the role of telemedicine-based screening has expanded in the field of ROP. Telemedicine allows non-ophthalmologists to capture and then transfer images online to a remotely located ROP specialist. The specialist examines the images and provides opinion regarding treatment or follow-up. Infants requiring urgent intervention can be called for management to the referral center.

Photo-ROP trial compared telemedicine with bed-side binocular indirect ophthalmoscopy and found them to be equally effective [38]. e-ROP study showed that training and certifying nonphysician graders to read and interpret ROP images under the supervision of a reading center director was reliable in detecting potentially serious ROP with good intragrader and intergrader consistency [39]. The Stanford University Network for Diagnosis of ROP (SUNDROP) is a telemedicine screening program based on a hub and spoke model [40]. The central hub (remote screener) at the university collects digital images generated by Retcam (Clarity Medical Systems) from six peripheral NICUs. The screener looks for all referral warranted and treatment warranted disease. The screening program has a sensitivity of 100% and specificity over 99.5% with good negative and positive predictive values. A similar telescreening program which has successfully completed over 46,000 imaging sessions and over 1000 treatment procedures is the "Karnataka Internet Assisted Diagnosis of Retinopathy of Prematurity" (KIDROP). Technicians are trained to color code the images as red (Type 1 ROP), orange (Type 2 ROP), and green (normal or mature retina). Images are uploaded on a secure tele-ROP platform and are finally analyzed by the ROP experts. Red flagged images are given a priority so that diagnosis can be provided the same day and parents are referred for time management [41]. Use of imaging, grading, and computer-based image analysis can improve accuracy and consistency of diagnosis of plus disease compared to indirect ophthalmoscopy-based diagnosis.

5.7 Management

5.7.1 Laser Therapy

Laser photocoagulation of the peripheral avascular retina is considered the gold standard for the treatment of ROP. Topical anesthesia with 5% proparacaine or general anesthesia can be utilized to perform the laser procedure. The Early Treatment of Retinopathy of Prematurity (ETROP) showed both anatomical and functional benefits of treating the avascular retina with diode laser photocoagulation at an earlier than threshold stage when compared to cryoablation. Laser photocoagulation was recommended for type 1 ROP defined as a) presence of any ROP stage with plus or stage 3 without plus in zone I or b) stage 2 or 3 with plus in zone II [42]. Laser therapy converts the peripheral hypoxic retina into anoxic retina thereby reducing the stimulus for neovascularization and disease progression. More recently, laser photocoagulation using the frequency doubled Nd:YAG (532 nm green) laser has been shown to be as effective as the 810 nm wavelength. Sanghi et al. have reported comparable efficacy with both infrared diode and frequency doubled Nd: YAG laser [43]. This study also showed the feasibility to perform frequency doubled Nd: YAG laser in eyes with tunica vasculosa lentis and preretinal hemorrhage without any accentuated risk of inducing cataract, anterior segment ischemia, or hyphema. Other reported advantages with Nd: YAG laser include higher "defocus threshold" resulting in lesser spots being wasted, lesser pain and more confluent spots being achieved as compared to infrared diode laser.

Conventionally laser burns are applied to the avascular retina upto the ora serrata in a near confluent manner. Despite this, the ETROP reported a 15.7% risk of progression to stage 4 or 5. Subtle modifications in the technique have been reported to be useful for severe stage 3 ROP. Ells et al. have shown rapid regression of the disease with posterior laser treatment in severe stage 3 zone II disease with no increased safety concerns [44]. The study proposed the role of primary "posterior to ridge" laser for eyes with thick stage 3 in four or more confluent temporal clock hours, plus disease in temporal two quadrants, subretinal fluid associated with the ridge, minimal temporal traction and minimum 3000 um distance between the ridge and the fovea.

Yetik et al. have advocated the role of limited laser treatment (covering the demarcation line with 5–6 rows of laser spots 360°) in zone 2 type 1 prethreshold cases [45]. This prevents ablation of a large amount of peripheral retina. Limited laser treatment is based on a newly proposed hypothesis by the author that ROP is a disease initially confined to the vitreoretinal interface and results from aberrant growth of normal retinal vessels into the vitreous gel. Ambiguity of the premature vitreoretinal interface with immature ILM causes misretinalization of retinal vasculogenesis. Limited laser treatment around the demarcation line/ridge can cease the vascular growth into the vitreous gel thus allowing ILM and vitreoretinal interface to mature more and allowing the disease to regress.

5.7.2 Surgical Management

Management of progressive stage 4 and stage 5 ROP involve surgical intervention in the form of scleral buckling or vitrectomy. The primary aim of surgery is to relieve tractional forces from the ridge to ora serrata, ridge to lens, and ridge to ridge. Whereas scleral buckling may be possible for stage 4 A or 4B ROP, the need for removal of the scleral buckle to allow growth of the eyeball necessitates a second surgery before the first year of life. Introduction of microincision vitrectomy surgery (MIVS) has not only improved functional and structural outcomes but also reduced surgical times and surgical trauma [46]. Several advancements in the MIVS including the use of smaller gauges (23, 25, and 27 gauge), high cut rates upto 10,000 cuts per minute, valved cannulas, improved illumination, and availability of specialized instruments allows improved access to the tight retinal folds (Fig. 5.4). Lens sparing vitrectomy involves making sclerotomy ports 1–1.5 mm from the limbus through the pars plicata or the iris root. Lensectomy with vitrectomy is primarily employed in cases with stage 5 ROP, associated retrolental fibroplasia, or stage 4B ROP where the traction or the ridge extends anteriorly upto the lens capsule.

The primary aim of stage 5 ROP surgery is to remove the fibrous stalk from the disc which holds the retina along the central axis, allowing the posterior funnel to open up. This is followed by careful dissection of peripheral tough present between the peripheral avascular retina and the ridge [46].

Surgical outcomes for stage 4 disease with 25 gauge vitrectomy (81–100%) are much better than 20 gauge vitrectomy (62–92%) [47–50]. There are limited reports of MIVS in stage 5 disease. Reported surgical success with 23/25 gauge MIVS systems ranges from 33 to 45.4% in stage 5 disease as compared to 13–42% with 20 gauge vitrectomy systems [46, 51].

Factors associated with favorable outcomes include stage 4 disease, previous laser treatment, LSV, and surgery with 25 G MIVS compared to 23 G [46]. Formation of inadvertent intraoperative retinal breaks is associated with poor anatomical outcomes in ROP surgery and should be avoided by careful and meticulous dissection.

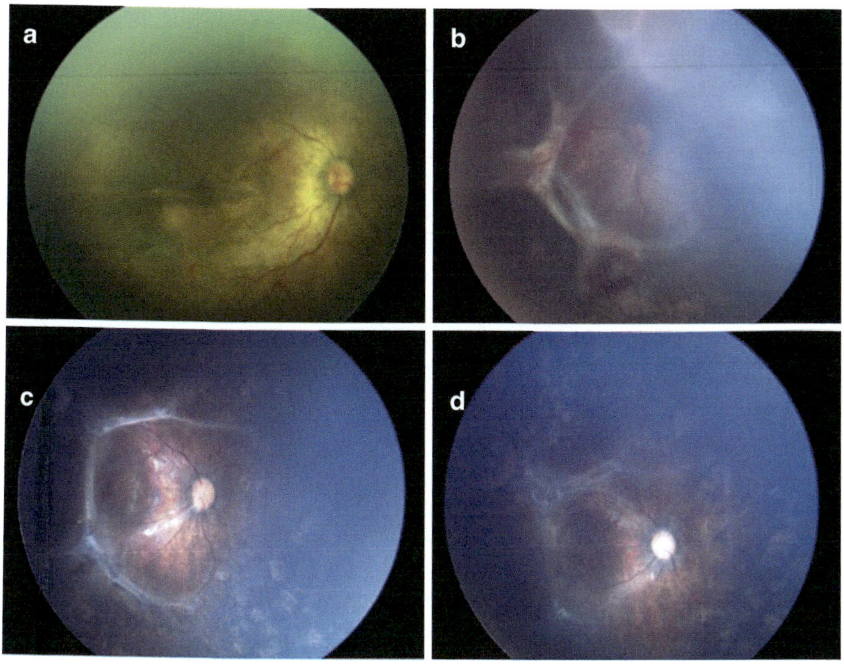

Fig. 5.4 Retcam fundus photographs showing the presence of Aggressive posterior ROP in the right eye of a preterm infant (**a**) which showed progression to a stage 4A tractional retinal detachment despite confluent laser photocoagulation (**b**). The same eye following 25-gauge microincision lens sparing vitrectomy 1 week (**c**) and 2 months (**d**) postoperatively with complete flattening of the ridge

5.7.3 Anti-VEGF Treatment

Vascular endothelial growth factor (VEGF) is important for angiogenesis in fetal life and is also regarded as a key mediator in the pathogenesis of abnormal neovascularization in ROP. Cryotherapy and laser ablation, which are standard of care for ROP, help decrease the VEGF levels by converting hypoxic peripheral avascular retina into anoxic retina. Through effective therapy, studies have shown poor structural and functional outcomes with both laser and cryoablative therapy in eyes with zone 1 disease and APROP [52]. Apart from this, both these are associated with ocular complications like high myopia and peripheral field loss. In such a scenario, anti-VEGF injections have emerged as a promising therapy for the management of ROP, especially for disease in zone 1. Currently, various anti-VEGFs like bevacizumab, ranibizumab, aflibercept, pegaptanib, and conbercept have been evaluated in ROP treatment [53].

The BEAT-ROP study was the first prospective randomized study to show the efficacy of 0.625 mg bevacizumab in the treatment of stage 3 ROP with plus disease in zone 1 or posterior zone II [54]. Fewer recurrences (22% in laser vs 4% in the bevacizumab group) were reported at 54 weeks postmenstrual age and the results were statistically significant for zone I eyes but not for eyes in zone II. At 2.5 years the Anti-VEGF treated eyes in the BEAT-ROP study showed lower degrees of myopia compared to the laser-treated eyes [55].

One of the major concerns with intravitreal therapy with anti-VEGF agents is the long-term systemic side effects [53]. Studies have shown a reduction in serum VEGF levels with the presence of anti-VEGF agents in systemic circulation following anti-VEGF injection in the vitreous cavity. VEGF is known to regulate the growth of various other organs like the brain, kidney, liver, hematopoietic system, lungs, and bones. Being a bigger and heavier molecule, vitreous and serum half-life of bevacizumab is much higher than ranibizumab (vitreous half-life: 5.6–6.7 days versus 3.2 days; serum half-life: 20 days versus 2 h respectively). Aflibercept has an intermediate value between the two (vitreous half-life: 4.8 days; serum half-life: 11.4 ± 4.8 days) [53].

As a result, long-term systemic effects of Anti-VEGF injections on organ growth and function including neurodevelopment cannot be overlooked and need to be studied in detail.

PEDIG group studied variable doses of bevacizumab (0.25 mg, 0.125 mg, 0.063 mg, and 0.031 mg) in the treatment of type 1 ROP and concluded that even the lowest dose of bevacizumab (0.031 mg) which was 5% of dose used by BEAT-ROP study was effective after 4 weeks in 9 out of 10 eyes [56]. Ranibizumab after its intravitreal administration in premature infants has been shown to have less prolonged (7 days) systemic suppression of VEGF compared to bevacizumab. Recent studies have evaluated the effect of decreasing the dosage of ranibizumab on the disease outcome and associated systemic adverse events [53].

RAINBOW, an open-label randomized controlled trial studied the efficacy of ranibizumab 0.1 mg or 0.2 mg versus laser in very low birth weight infants (<1500 g) with ROP in zone I and II. The study reported overall treatment success to be 80% (0.1 mg) and 88% (0.2 mg) compared to 66% with laser photocoagulation alone [57]. The study showed no clear evidence of systemic VEGF suppression following intravitreal ranibizumab therapy. Ranibizumab also showed an acceptable short-term safety profile with systemic side effects equally distributed in all three treatment arms (0.1 mg ranibizumab, 0.2 mg ranibizumab, and laser arm). Systemic events were reported to be likely related to preterm birth and not dependent upon therapy.

Contrary to the above trials, some investigators have shown deleterious effects on neurocognitive development in preterm infants treated with anti-VEGF injections including a lower motor score, poor early cognitive function, and high mortality in preterm infants treated with anti-VEGF injection. However, in all such studies, the role of other confounding factors like lower birth weight, prematurity itself, prolonged ventilation, and prolonged oxygen supplementation in the anti-VEGF group could not be ruled out [58]. Though there are reports regarding thromboembolic events, respiratory failure, hepatic dysfunction, and nephropathy post-injection, their association with the anti-VEGF drug itself has not been convincingly proven. Long-term studies are required to look into the ocular and systemic side effects associated with anti-VEGF agents.

5.7.4 Artificial Intelligence (AI) and Deep Learning in ROP

With the increasing trend of telemedicine in ROP, there is a paradigm shift in computer-based image analysis (CBIA) in ROP. Before the advent of deep learning, traditional machine-based learning involved tedious steps of defining the disease features of specific interest followed by feature extraction using explicit algorithms and training a classifier, and lastly testing system performance on previously unseen dataset. The performance of the system is likely to be affected by any of the above steps. Earlier CBIA systems used manual or semi-automated approaches to look at vessel diameter and tortuosity using fundus photographs for ROP diagnosis. These systems lacked adequate diagnostic performance due to inaccuracy of vessel segmentation or time-consuming manual inputs to delineate posterior pole vessels [59].

In the last few years, there has been a shift from machine-based learning to deep convolutional neural networks (CNNs), also known as deep learning. Deep learning classifiers do not need external training and learn without being told what to focus on. CNN-based systems perform similar to human graders in determining cases of ROP [59].

DeepROP is an automated ROP screening application which can successfully detect the presence or absence of ROP features (Id-Net) and can additionally grade the severity of the disease (Gr-Net) [60]. i-ROP-deep learning system (i-ROP-DL) is another CNN-based system which can classify plus disease by accurate vessel segmentation [61]. As both DeepROP and i-ROP-DL use publicly available ImageNet databases for training, they demonstrate strong agreement with expert opinion. The ROP vascular severity score (score derived from i-ROP-DL for ROP screening) can be used to monitor disease progression, and regression following treatment and differentiate the pace of disease in APROP.

AI seems to be an upcoming technology expected to solve some of the problems related to ROP screening. Its implementation into routine ROP care seems to be a distant reality. To implement the use of AI for ROP diagnosis in the practical world, concerted efforts targeted at developing standards for data acquisition, true external validation, and demonstration of feasibility should be made. There are several unaddressed technical, ethical, clinical, financial, and regulatory considerations which need to be understood before it can be brought into clinical practice.

5.7.5 Medicolegal Aspects in ROP

Malpractice claims in ROP are a result of errors that result in failure to screen the infant in a timely manner, leading to failure/delays in intervention and/or referral [62]. Medicolegal risks can be avoided by understanding the complex interplay between the parents of the infant, the NICU, various caregivers, social workers, office staff, and screening physicians. Some key aspects to keep in mind include (a) engaging the family in the ROP screening process by providing clear written and verbal communication regarding timely follow-up, potentially blinding complications of ROP, and the importance of timely treatment. Performing the first screening before discharge is likely to result in better follow-ups. (b) Coordination among the various stakeholders (pediatricians, gynecologists, nurses, and ophthalmologists) is another key element to ensure no infant escapes the screening program. Lastly, ophthalmologists should remain updated with current screening guidelines in their demographic region and follow-up protocols.

Key Points

1. This chapter briefly summarizes the current disease burden of ROP, the latest screening guidelines, and recent advances in the management of ROP.
2. Fundus imaging, FFA, OCT, and OCT-A have proven a useful adjunct to clinical examination using binocular indirect ophthalmoscopy (BIO). Novel information provided by these modalities will help in better understanding of disease pathophysiology and improving our understanding of foveal and visual development and its maturation.
3. Telemedicine offers a viable, validated, and objective alternative to screening using BIO and is a boon for places with shortage of trained ophthalmologists.
4. Anti-VEGF injections have been a useful addition in the treatment of severe zone I ROP, though long-term safety and timeline for long term follow ups in view of a persistent avascular retina induced by the treatment are yet to be addressed, and laser photocoagulation still remains a highly effective therapy for most ROP cases
5. Artificial intelligence and automated detection of ROP seem to hold promise for ROP detection and its clinical utility needs further study...

References

1. Carroll L, Owen LA. Current evidence and outcomes for retinopathy of prematurity prevention: insight into novel maternal and placental contributions. Explor Med. 2020;1:4–26.
2. Gilbert C. Retinopathy of prematurity: a global perspective of the epidemics, population of babies at risk and implications for control. Early Hum Dev. 2008;84:77–82.
3. Blencowe H, Lawn JE, Vazquez T, et al. Preterm-associated visual impairment and estimates of retinopathy of prematurity at regional and global levels for 2010. Pediatr Res. 2013 Dec;74(Suppl 1):35–49.
4. Vinekar A, Dogra MR, Sangtam T, et al. Retinopathy of prematurity in Asian Indian babies weighing greater than 1250 grams at birth: ten year data from a tertiary care center in a developing country. Indian J Ophthalmol. 2007;55(5):331–6.
5. Jalali S, Matalia J, Hussain A, et al. Modification of screening criteria for retinopathy of prematurity in India and other middle-income countries. Am J Ophthalmol. 2006;141(5):966–8.
6. Blencowe H, Cousens S, Oestergaard MZ, et al. National, regional, and worldwide estimates of preterm birth rates in the year 2010 with time trends since 1990 for selected countries: a systematic analysis and implications. Lancet Lond Engl. 2012;379(9832):2162–72.

7. Honavar SG. Do we need India-specific retinopathy of prematurity screening guidelines? Indian J Ophthalmol. 2019;67(6):711–6.
8. International Committee for the Classification of Retinopathy of Prematurity. The international classification of retinopathy of prematurity revisited. Arch Ophthalmol. 2005;123(7):991–9.
9. Chiang MF, Quinn GE, Fielder AR, Ostmo SR, Paul Chan RV, Berrocal A, et al. International classification of retinopathy of prematurity, third edition. Ophthalmology. 2021;S0161-6420(21):00416–4. https://doi.org/10.1016/j.ophtha.2021.05.031.
10. Kim SJ, Port AD, Swan R, et al. Retinopathy of prematurity: a review of risk factors and their clinical significance. Surv Ophthalmol. 2018;63(5):618–37.
11. Fierson WM. American academy of pediatrics section on Ophthalmology; American academy of ophthalmology; American association for pediatric ophthalmology and strabismus; American association of certified orthoptists. Screening Examination of Premature Infants for Retinopathy of Prematurity. Pediatrics. 2018;142(6):e20183061. https://doi.org/10.1542/peds.2018-3061.
12. Wilkinson AR, Haines L, Head K, et al. Guideline Development Group of the Royal College of Paediatrics and Child Health, Royal College of Ophthalmologists, et al. UK retinopathy of prematurity guideline. Eye Lond Engl. 2009;23(11):2137–9.
13. Richter GM, Sun G, Lee TC, et al. Speed of telemedicine vs ophthalmoscopy for retinopathy of prematurity diagnosis. Am J Ophthalmol. 2009;148(1):136–142.e2.
14. Athikarisamy SE, Lam GC, Ross S, et al. Comparison of wide field imaging by nurses with indirect ophthalmoscopy by ophthalmologists for retinopathy of prematurity: a diagnostic accuracy study. BMJ Open. 2020;10(8):e036483.
15. Richter GM, Williams SL, Starren J, et al. Telemedicine for retinopathy of prematurity diagnosis. Surv Ophthalmol. 2009;54(6):671–85.
16. Salcone EM, Johnston S, VanderVeen D. Review of the use of digital imaging in retinopathy of prematurity screening. Semin Ophthalmol. 2010;25(5–6):214–7.
17. Skalet AH, Quinn GE, Ying G-S, et al. Telemedicine screening for retinopathy of prematurity in developing countries using digital retinal images: a feasibility project. J AAPOS. 2008;12(3):252–8.
18. Vinekar A, Rao SV, Murthy S, Jayadev C, Dogra MR, Verma A, Shetty B. A novel, low-cost, wide-field, infant retinal camera, "neo": technical and safety report for the use on premature infants. Transl Vis Sci Technol. 2019;8(2):2. https://doi.org/10.1167/tvst.8.2.2.
19. Prakalapakorn SG, Wallace DK, Freedman SF. Retinal imaging in premature infants using the Pictor noncontact digital camera. J AAPOS. 2014;18(4):321–6.
20. Mao J, Shao Y, Lao J, et al. Ultra-wide-field imaging and intravenous fundus fluorescein angiography in infants with retinopathy of prematurity. Retina (Phila Pa.). 2020;40(12):2357–65.
21. Goyal A, Gopalakrishnan M, Anantharaman G, et al. Smartphone guided wide-field imaging for retinopathy of prematurity in neonatal intensive care unit – a smart ROP (SROP) initiative. Indian J Ophthalmol. 2019;67(6):840–5.
22. Wintergerst MWM, Petrak M, Li JQ, et al. Non-contact smartphone-based fundus imaging compared to conventional fundus imaging: a low-cost alternative for retinopathy of prematurity screening and documentation. Sci Rep. 2019;9(1):19711.
23. Maldonado RS, Toth CA. Optical coherence tomography in retinopathy of prematurity. Clin Perinatol. 2013;40(2):271–96.
24. Wallace DK, Kylstra JA, Greenman DB, et al. Significance of isolated neovascular tufts ("popcorn") in retinopathy of prematurity. J AAPOS. 1998;2(1):52–6.
25. Chavala SH, Farsiu S, Maldonado R, et al. Insights into advanced retinopathy of prematurity using handheld spectral domain optical coherence tomography imaging. Ophthalmology. 2009;116(12):2448–56.
26. Lee AC, Maldonado RS, Sarin N, et al. Macular features from spectral-domain optical coherence tomography as an adjunct to indirect ophthalmoscopy in retinopathy of prematurity. Retina (Phila Pa). 2011;31(8):1470–82.

27. Maldonado RS, O'Connell R, Ascher SB, et al. Spectral-domain optical coherence tomographic assessment of severity of cystoid macular edema in retinopathy of prematurity. Arch Ophthalmol 1912. 2012;130(5):569–578.
28. Vinekar A, Avadhani K, Sivakumar M, et al. Understanding clinically undetected macular changes in early retinopathy of prematurity on spectral domain optical coherence tomography. Invest Ophthalmol Vis Sci. 2011;52(8):5183–8.
29. Joshi MM, Trese MT, Capone A. Optical coherence tomography findings in stage 4A retinopathy of prematurity: a theory for visual variability. Ophthalmology. 2006;113(4):657–60.
30. Moreno TA, O'Connell RV, Chiu SJ, et al. Choroid development and feasibility of choroidal imaging in the preterm and term infants utilizing SD-OCT. Invest Ophthalmol Vis Sci. 2013;54(6):4140–7.
31. Erol MK, Coban DT, Ozdemir O, et al. Choroidal thickness in infants with retinopathy of prematurity. Retina (Phila Pa). 2016;36(6):1191–8.
32. Vinekar A, Chidambara L, Jayadev C, et al. Monitoring neovascularization in aggressive posterior retinopathy of prematurity using optical coherence tomography angiography. J AAPOS. 2016;20(3):271–4.
33. Campbell JP, Nudleman E, Yang J, et al. Handheld optical coherence tomography angiography and ultra-wide-field optical coherence tomography in retinopathy of prematurity. JAMA Ophthalmol. 2017;135(9):977–81.
34. Kothari N, Chu A, Huang JM, et al. Arm-mounted optical coherence tomography angiography in extremely low birth weight neonates with retinopathy of prematurity. Am J Ophthalmol Case Rep. 2020;18:100624.
35. Zhao J, Wu Z, Lam W, et al. Comparison of OCT angiography in children with a history of intravitreal injection of ranibizumab versus laser photocoagulation for retinopathy of prematurity. Br J Ophthalmol. 2020;104(11):1556–60.
36. Mataftsi A, Dermenoudi M, Dastiridou A, et al. Optical coherence tomography angiography in children with spontaneously regressed retinopathy of prematurity. Eye. 2021;35(5):1411–7.
37. Klufas MA, Patel SN, Ryan MC, et al. Influence of fluorescein angiography on the diagnosis and Management of Retinopathy of prematurity. Ophthalmology. 2015;122(8):1601–8.
38. Photographic Screening for Retinopathy of Prematurity (Photo-ROP) Cooperative Group. The photographic screening for retinopathy of prematurity study (photo-ROP). Primary outcomes. Retina (Phila Pa.). 2008;28(3 Suppl):S47–54.
39. Daniel E, Quinn GE, Hildebrand PL, et al. Validated system for centralized grading of retinopathy of prematurity: telemedicine approaches to evaluating acute-phase retinopathy of prematurity (e-ROP) study. JAMA Ophthalmol. 2015;133(6):675–82.
40. Murakami Y, Jain A, Silva RA, et al. Stanford University network for diagnosis of retinopathy of prematurity (SUNDROP): 12-month experience with telemedicine screening. Br J Ophthalmol. 2008;92(11):1456–60.
41. Vinekar A, Gilbert C, Dogra M, et al. The KIDROP model of combining strategies for providing retinopathy of prematurity screening in underserved areas in India using wide-field imaging, tele-medicine, non-physician graders and smart phone reporting. Indian J Ophthalmol. 2014;62(1):41–9.
42. Good WV. Early treatment for retinopathy of prematurity cooperative group. Final results of the early treatment for retinopathy of prematurity (ETROP) randomized trial. Trans Am Ophthalmol Soc. 2004;102:233–48.
43. Sanghi G, Dogra MR, Vinekar A, et al. Frequency-doubled Nd:YAG (532 nm green) versus diode laser (810 nm) in treatment of retinopathy of prematurity. Br J Ophthalmol. 2010;94(9):1264–5.
44. Ells AL, Gole GA, Lloyd Hildebrand P, et al. Posterior to the ridge laser treatment for severe stage 3 retinopathy of prematurity. Eye. 2013;27(4):525–30.
45. Yetik H. Limited laser treatment for retinopathy of prematurity: a new hypothesis for pathogenesis of ROP based on ambiguity of vitreoretinal interface, immaturity of internal limiting membrane and mis-retinalization. New Front Ophthalmol. 2016;2

46. Sen P, Bhende P, Sharma T, et al. Surgical outcomes of microincision vitrectomy surgery in eyes with retinal detachment secondary to retinopathy of prematurity in Indian population. Indian J Ophthalmol. 2019;67(6):889–95.
47. Gonzales CR, Boshra J, Schwartz SD. 25-gauge pars plicata vitrectomy for stage 4 and 5 retinopathy of prematurity. Retina (Phila Pa.). 2006;26(7 Suppl):S42–6.
48. Shah PK, Narendran V, Kalpana N. Safety and efficacy of simultaneous bilateral 25-gauge lens-sparing vitrectomy for vascularly active stage 4 retinopathy of prematurity. Eye (Lond Engl). 2015;29(8):1046–50.
49. Choi J, Kim JH, Kim S-J, et al. Long-term results of lens-sparing vitrectomy for stages 4B and 5 retinopathy of prematurity. Korean J Ophthalmol. 2011;25(5):305–10.
50. Hubbard GB, Cherwick DH, Burian G. Lens-sparing vitrectomy for stage 4 retinopathy of prematurity. Ophthalmology. 2004;111(12):2274–7.
51. Gadkari S, Kamdar R, Kulkarni S, et al. Vitreoretinal surgery for advanced retinopathy of prematurity: presentation and outcomes from a developing country. Can J Ophthalmol. 2015;50(1):54–60.
52. Nicoară SD, Ştefănuţ AC, Nascutzy C, et al. Regression rates following the treatment of aggressive posterior retinopathy of prematurity with bevacizumab versus laser: 8-year retrospective analysis. Med Sci Monit Int Med J Exp Clin Res. 2016;22:1192–209.
53. Enríquez AB, Avery RL, Baumal CR. Update on anti-vascular endothelial growth factor safety for retinopathy of prematurity. Asia-Pac J Ophthalmol. 2020;9(4):358–68.
54. Mintz-Hittner HA, Kennedy KA, Chuang AZ. BEAT-ROP cooperative group. Efficacy of intravitreal bevacizumab for stage 3+ retinopathy of prematurity. N Engl J Med. 2011;364(7):603–15.
55. Geloneck MM, Chuang AZ, Clark WL, Hunt MG, Norman AA, Packwood EA, Tawansy KA, Mintz-Hittner HA. BEAT-ROP cooperative group. Refractive outcomes following bevacizumab monotherapy compared with conventional laser treatment: a randomized clinical trial. JAMA Ophthalmol. 2014;132:1327–33.
56. Wallace DK, Kraker RT, Freedman SF, et al. Assessment of lower doses of Intravitreous bevacizumab for retinopathy of prematurity: a phase 1 dosing study. JAMA Ophthalmol. 2017;135(6):654–6.
57. Stahl A, Lepore D, Fielder A, et al. Ranibizumab versus laser therapy for the treatment of very low birthweight infants with retinopathy of prematurity (RAINBOW): an open-label randomised controlled trial. Lancet (Lond Engl). 2019;394(10208):1551–9.
58. Natarajan G, Shankaran S, Nolen TL, et al. Neurodevelopmental outcomes of preterm infants with retinopathy of prematurity by treatment. Pediatrics. 2019;144(2):e20183537. https://doi.org/10.1542/peds.2018-3537.
59. Gensure RH, Chiang MF, Campbell JP. Artificial intelligence for retinopathy of prematurity. Curr Opin Ophthalmol. 2020;31(5):312–7.
60. Wang J, Ju R, Chen Y, et al. Automated retinopathy of prematurity screening using deep neural networks. EBioMedicine. 2018;35:361–8.
61. Brown JM, Campbell JP, Beers A, et al. Automated diagnosis of plus disease in retinopathy of prematurity using deep convolutional neural networks. JAMA Ophthalmol. 2018;136(7):803–10.
62. Moshfeghi DM. Top five legal pitfalls in retinopathy of prematurity. Curr Opin Ophthalmol. 2018;29(3):206–9.

Periocular Infantile Hemangiomas

6

Swathi Somisetty, Lili Montoya, Harper Price, and Aparna Ramasubramanian

6.1 Introduction

Infantile hemangiomas (IH) are the most common benign vascular tumors of infancy, and they can present as small isolated lesions to large masses with segmental involvement anywhere on the body. Depending on the location and size of the IH, complications can arise ranging from ulceration to vital functional impairment to poor cosmesis upon regression. Due to the prevalence and significant ocular complications associated with periocular infantile hemangiomas, a thorough understanding of the natural history, clinical presentations, treatment, and complications will be valuable for ophthalmologists who will be encountering these cases. This chapter will review the epidemiology, pathogenesis, clinical manifestations, diagnosis, and latest updates on the management of patients with periocular IH [1].

6.2 Epidemiology

Infantile hemangiomas have an estimated incidence of about 4–5% [2]. IH are more common in females and white non-Hispanic infants [3–5]. The most significant risk factor is prematurity and low birth weight [3]. In infants weighing less than 1000 g, up to 23% have at least one IH while the incidence in full-term infants is 1–4% [3]. Other risk factors include advanced maternal age, multiple births, in vitro

Aparna Ramasubramanian, M.D. has had full access to all the data in the study and takes responsibility for the integrity of the data.

S. Somisetty · L. Montoya · H. Price · A. Ramasubramanian (✉)
Phoenix Children's Hospital, Phoenix, AZ, USA
e-mail: swathiSomisetty@creighton.edu; lmontoya@phoenixchildrens.com; hprice@phoenixchildrens.com; aramasubramanian@phoenixchildrens.com

A. Ramasubramanian (ed.), *Pediatric Ophthalmology*, Current Practices in Ophthalmology, https://doi.org/10.1007/978-981-19-4963-0_6

fertilization, amniocentesis, chorionic villus sampling, prenatal maternal vaginal bleeding, and multiple gestations [3, 6].

Twelve percent of all infantile hemangiomas occur in the periocular region [2]. Complications from periocular or orbital IH arise in about 60% of cases, leading to significant morbidity [7]. Amblyopia is a common sequelae of periorbital/orbital IH with a prevalence of 43–60% (Lyons, Chap. 20). Early recognition and treatment initiation of periorbital IH can lead to significant improvement in morbidity and patient outcomes.

6.3 Pathogenesis

The pathogenesis of infantile hemangiomas has not been fully elucidated. These vascular tumors are characterized by a proliferative phase and an involution phase, and evidence suggests that the blood vessels found in IH are unique from normal vasculature. Vasculogenesis, or formation of new primitive blood vessels from stem cell precursors, leads to the growth of these vascular tumors through clonal proliferation of vascular endothelial cells. Studies have shown that endothelial cells within proliferating and involuting hemangiomas are unique in that they have high expression of glucose transporter-1 (GLUT-1) and placenta-associated vascular antigens, and these markers can help distinguish between IH and other vascular tumors or vascular malformations. The only other vasculature known to have similar gene expression is placental chorionic villi, suggesting a connection between IH and placental pathogenesis [8, 9]. During the proliferative growth phase, vasculogenic factors are overexpressed, including fibroblast growth factor, proliferating cell nuclear antigen, vascular endothelial growth factor (VEGF), and type IV collagenase [10]. As IH transition into the involution phase, apoptosis of endothelial cells outpaces vasculogenesis, and fibrofatty tissue deposition begins to occur (Khan 2008). Histologically, fibrosis of the capillary lamina heralds the involution process, and higher numbers of mast cells are seen. Expression of tissue metalloproteinases increases, and this inhibits blood vessel formation [10]. The underlying mechanism that triggers transition from the proliferative to regression phase is unknown.

Similarities between retinopathy of prematurity and IH have also been found. “Premature infants with IH have been found to be more likely to have retinopathy of prematurity than those without IH” [11].

6.4 Clinical Presentation

The natural history of infantile hemangiomas, including periocular IH, is characterized by a proliferative growth phase during the first year of life, followed by an involution phase thereafter. About one-third of IH’s have a precursor lesion noted at birth, often a faint telangiectatic patch with a circumferential pale halo of vasoconstriction or an erythematous to violaceous patch that can be mistaken for a bruise or abrasion. Shortly after birth, the proliferative phase begins, with the fastest growth period between 5.5 and 7.5 weeks of age [12]. By 3 months of age, most hemangiomas have reached 80% of their final size and 80% of hemangiomas have completed growth by 5 months of age [2, 12]. In the remaining IHs, growth may continue through months 6–12, but the rate is slower. After about 9–12 months old, IHs begin the involution process, which can last a variable number of years. By 4 years of age, about 90% of IH involution has occurred [13]. It is important to recognize that even after complete involution, 55% of IHs leave permanent skin changes, such as telangiectasias, atrophy, or fibrofatty tissue deposition, which depending on the location, can be cosmetically undesirable [13].

Classification of infantile hemangiomas is based on the depth of skin or soft tissue involvement (superficial, deep, mixed) and extent of the lesion (localized, segmental, indeterminate). Superficial hemangiomas present as a bright red, vascular papules or plaques, without a deep subcutaneous component (Fig. 6.1a). Deep IHs are subcutaneous growths without overlying skin changes, and therefore can have a bluish hue noted beneath the skin. Mixed hemangiomas exhibit features of both deep and superficial lesions. It is important to recognize these different hemangioma subtypes when evaluating a patient because their growth pattern is slightly different. The average onset of growth for deep IH is 1 month later than superficial hemangiomas, and they also continue growing for longer [14]. Segmental and periorbital hemangiomas also exhibit prolonged growth phases and are associated with increased morbidity. Because of this, these IH subtypes typically require longer follow-up, treatment, and monitoring [11].

Periocular infantile hemangiomas can be classified based on location in relation to the orbit. IHs can be anterior to the globe with eyelid involvement, extraconal or behind the bony orbit but not involving extraocular muscles, or intraconal or within the cone of extraocular muscles. Periocular infantile hemangiomas are most often found on the upper eyelid or within the orbit. In patients with periocular IH, about 30% have hemangiomas elsewhere on the body, showcasing the importance of a full-body skin exam when the diagnosis of IH is entertained. The natural history of periocular hemangiomas coincides with visual axis development in infants thereby leading to the risk of amblyopia.

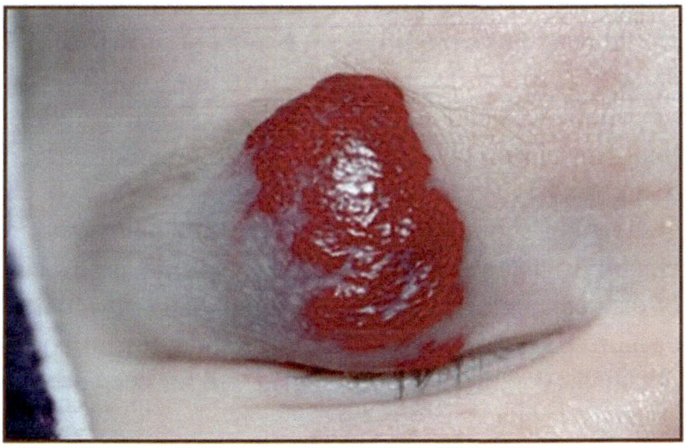

Fig. 6.1 Right upper eyelid hemangioma causing ptosis and visual obscuration

Periocular infantile hemangiomas or other large facial segmental IH can be associated with systemic disorders, including PHACE (posterior fossa anomalies, hemangioma, arterial lesions, cardiac abnormalities/aortic coarctation, eye anomalies) syndrome. It is important to be familiar with this entity because specific imaging and specialty consultation are necessary. PHACE syndrome should be considered in any patient with a large, segmental IH measuring >5 cm. The hemangioma may or may not directly involve the periocular region, but due to associations with structural eye abnormalities, ophthalmologic examination is prudent (controversial though).

Periocular IH and other possible systemic associations

- PHACE syndrome (posterior fossa anomalies, hemangioma, arterial lesions, cardiac abnormalities/aortic coarctation, eye anomalies).
- IH in PHACE are segmental and large (>5 cm).
- IH in PHACE may be periocular.
- Separate from the IH, PHACE is associated with structural eye abnormalities which include posterior segment abnormalities (major criteria for PHACE diagnosis) and anterior segment abnormalities (minor criteria for PHACE diagnosis).
- While controversial [11], states that all infants undergoing workup for PHACE should be evaluated by an ophthalmologist ([15]—states eye exam is low yield in patients with PHACE syndrome without a periocular infantile hemangioma).

6.5 Diagnosis

Infantile hemangiomas are typically diagnosed clinically, and rarely require further investigation with imaging or biopsy. Obtaining a detailed history from the family elucidating the onset of the lesion and growth history coupled with clinical appearance is often enough to make the diagnosis. However, clinical diagnosis can become challenging in certain scenarios, particularly when the lesion mimics vascular malformations, capillary malformations (like port-wine stains or nevus simplex), or other subcutaneous tumors. For instance, during the first few weeks of life, IH and port-wine stains can be challenging to differentiate, and the lesion would need to be monitored for signs of growth and thickening, as this is suggestive of IH. Deep IH can also be difficult to differentiate from other subcutaneous tumors or vascular malformations, and a high index of suspicion is needed and imaging and/or biopsy should be completed early if there is any doubt in the diagnosis.

Imaging should also be considered if there is a concern for systemic involvement. For instance, when PHACE syndrome is suspected, MRI/MRA with contrast of the head and neck should be completed to evaluate for anatomy. If there are five or more IH, a liver ultrasound to evaluate for intrahepatic hemangiomas should be obtained. Also, MRI orbit is considered for deep orbital hemangioma to evaluate the extent of lesion.

6.6 Differential Diagnosis

Below is the differential diagnosis of infantile hemangiomas, particularly of the periocular region. This is not an exhaustive list but describes the most commonly encountered alternative diagnoses.

- Capillary malformations.
  - Nevus simplex.
  - Port-wine stain.
- Other vascular tumors.
  - Venous and/or lymphatic malformations.
  - RICH (rapidly involuting congenital hemangioma).
  - NICH (non-involuting congenital hemangioma).
  - Tufted angioma.
  - Kaposiform hemangioendothelioma.
- Deep IH vs intra/periocular tumors.
  - Rhabdomyosarcoma.
  - Neuroblastoma.
  - Plexiform neurofibroma.
- Deep IH vs orbital cysts.
  - Dermoid cyst.
  - Epidermoid cyst.
  - Teratomas.
  - Choristomas.

6.7 Complications

Periocular IH are more often associated with complications compared to the overall complication rate in hemangiomas, with complications occurring 63% vs 24% of the time, respectively [2, 7].

- Amblyopia due to periocular IH can result from three different mechanisms:
  - Astigmatism or myopia can occur from compression of the eye by the mass of the hemangioma, and this can lead to asymmetric refractive error between the two eyes (anisometropia). Subsequent refractive amblyopia can develop if not corrected quickly. This is the most common cause of amblyopia in patients with periocular IH.
  - Partial or complete obstruction of the visual axis can lead to deprivation-associated amblyopia.
  - Globe displacement from the mass effect of the IH tumor or involvement of extraocular muscles can lead to strabismus (misalignment of the eyes), which can then subsequently lead to amblyopia.
  - Luckily, amblyopia occurs less commonly in the post-propranolol versus pre-propranolol era [2].

- Proptosis from the IH mass can lead to exposure keratopathy.
- Extension of IH into the retrobulbar space can lead to compressive optic neuropathy or compression of orbital structures, although this is rare.
- Nasolacrimal duct obstruction can also occur depending on the location of the mass.
- Ulceration tends to be less common in periocular IH than other sites, but can still occur.
- Permanent disfigurement or skin changes can result from IH proliferation including fibrofatty tissue residua, anetoderma, telangiectasias, skin discoloration, distortion of facial landmarks (eyelid skin, lid margin, eyelashes, eyebrows), or indentation. In one study by [2], 42% of children had residual skin changes are involution of periocular IH.
- Complications associated with periocular IH are more likely when the hemangioma is classified as deep or mixed-type, larger in size measuring >1 cm, involving the upper eyelid (particularly if causing ptosis), nasally located, segmental, intraconal, or extraconal [2].

6.8 Management

- While most infantile hemangiomas do not require treatment due to their favorable location and small size, a significant number of more complicated hemangiomas do require treatment [16]. Because periocular hemangiomas are more often associated with morbidity, a high proportion of them require treatment. In one study by [2], 89 patients with periocular IH were included and 89% of those required treatment of some kind [2]. Morbidity resulting from these more complicated hemangiomas is reduced when treatment is initiated prior to the significant growth phase, which occurs from 5.5 to 7.5 weeks of age [12].
- Comanagement and close communication between pediatric dermatologists and ophthalmologists can be helpful, especially in complex cases.
- The current mainstay of treatment is oral propranolol (Fig. 6.2a, b) and, in certain circumstances, topical timolol. Oral propranolol is effective in treating and promoting regression of IH in 97% of cases and is generally well-tolerated [7].
- The dose of oral propranolol is typically 2–3 mg/kg/day divided twice daily or three times daily. Higher doses of propranolol (3 mg/kg/day) are often needed for deep IH, including those in the periocular region. Treatment ideally should start before the rapid proliferative phase and should be continued through at least the first year of life. A propranolol wean can then begin with close monitoring for rebound growth. Occasionally, hemangiomas require treatment with oral propranolol for several years [17].
- Topical timolol has been shown to induce regression of small and superficial IH (Fig. 6.3a, b) but should be used cautiously for periocular hemangiomas. Response rates to topical timolol are slower than systemic beta-blockers and

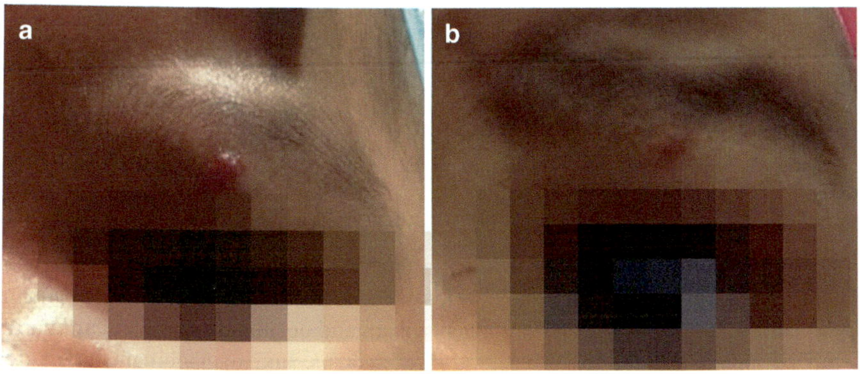

Fig. 6.2 Left upper eyelid hemangioma causing astigmatism (**a**) treated with propranolol showing a good response (**b**)

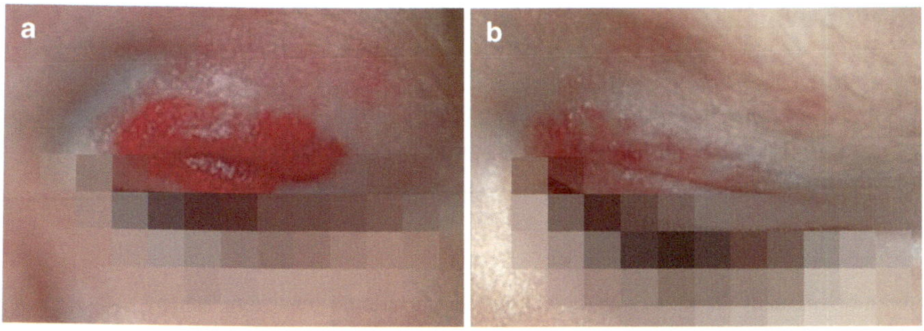

Fig. 6.3 Superficial upper eyelid hemangioma (**a**) showing a good response to topical timolol (**b**)

given the risk of vision loss, rapid onset of action with systemic medications may be necessary.

- Other treatment options available for consideration when beta-blockers are ineffective or contraindicated include corticosteroids, pulsed dye laser, or surgical debulking procedures. These therapies were utilized more often in the past before the efficacy of beta-blockers in IH regression was discovered.
- Even after management with propranolol, there may be a residual mass requiring surgical correction.
- Rarely, patients may not be able to tolerate the side effects of propranolol resulting in discontinuation of the medication. In a study by [7], propranolol adverse events occur up to 33% of the time, although the side effects were only severe enough to warrant discontinuation in 5% of patients [7]. In another study published by the American Academy of Ophthalmology in 2019 [18] only two patients out of 227 required treatment cessation because of complications from beta-blockers. Minor side effects of propranolol are more common and include sleep disturbances, acrocyanosis, diarrhea, emesis, or restlessness. Other more severe, but less common, side effects include hypoglycemia, transient bradycar-

dia, hypotension, or bronchospasm. Appropriate counseling and monitoring of infants on propranolol are crucial to reduce the likelihood of adverse events. Unfortunately, there are no consensus guidelines detailing monitoring of infants on oral propranolol for IH.

6.9 Conclusion

Periocular infantile hemangiomas are a unique subset of IH associated with increased morbidity related to vision loss. They more often necessitate treatment with beta-blockers to prevent permanent visual and cosmetic sequelae. Familiarity with periocular IH clinical presentation, diagnosis, and management is key for ophthalmologists.

Key Points

1. Hemangioma is a common benign vascular tumor seen in children and is often seen in the periocular region.
2. Amblyopia is seen in approximately half of the patients with hemangioma.
3. Propranalol is an effective treatment for hemangioma and is the first line of treatment.

Acknowledgment This research did not receive any specific grant from funding agencies in the public, commercial, or not-for-profit sectors.

References

1. Tavakoli M, Yadegari S, Mosallaei M, Aletaha M, Salour H, Lee WW. Infantile periocular hemangioma. J Ophthalmic Vis Res. 2017;12(2):205–11. https://doi.org/10.4103/jovr.jovr_66_17.
2. Zhao J, Huang AH, Rainer BM, et al. Periocular infantile hemangiomas: characteristics, ocular sequelae, and outcomes. Pediatr Dermatol. 2019;36(6):830–4. https://doi.org/10.1111/pde.13925.
3. Haggstrom AN, Drolet BA, Hemangioma Investigator Group, et al. Prospective study of infantile hemangiomas: demographic, prenatal, and perinatal characteristics. J Pediatr. 2007;150(3):291–4. https://doi.org/10.1016/j.jpeds.2006.12.003.
4. Chiller KG, Passaro D, Frieden IJ. Hemangiomas of infancy: clinical characteristics, morphologic subtypes, and their relationship to race, ethnicity, and sex. Arch Dermatol. 2002;138(12):1567–76. https://doi.org/10.1001/archderm.138.12.1567.
5. Drolet BA, Esterly NB, Frieden IJ. Hemangiomas in children. N Engl J Med. 1999;341(3):173–81. https://doi.org/10.1056/NEJM199907153410307.
6. Garzon MC, Drolet BA, Baselga E, et al. Comparison of infantile hemangiomas in preterm and term infants: a prospective study. Arch Dermatol. 2008;144(9):1231–2. https://doi.org/10.1001/archderm.144.9.1231.
7. Men CJ, Ediriwickrema LS, Paik JS, et al. Surgical intervention of periocular infantile hemangiomas in the era of β-blockers. Ophthalmic Plast Reconstr Surg. 2020;36(1):70–3. https://doi.org/10.1097/IOP.0000000000001466.

8. Leon-Villapalos J, Wolfe K, Kangesu L. GLUT-1: an extra diagnostic tool to differentiate between haemangiomas and vascular malformations. Br J Plast Surg. 2005;58(3):348–52.
9. Barnés CM, Huang S, Kaipainen A, Sanoudou D, Chen EJ, Eichler GS, Guo Y, Yu Y, Ingber DE, Mulliken JB, Beggs AH, Folkman J, Fishman SJ. Evidence by molecular profiling for a placental origin of infantile hemangioma. Proc Natl Acad Sci U S A. 2005;102(52):19097–102.
10. Takahashi K, Mulliken JB, Kozakewich HP, et al. Cellular markers that distinguish the phases of hemangioma during infancy and childhood. J Clin Invest. 1994;93:2357–64.
11. Spence-Shishido AA, Good WV, Baselga E, Frieden IJ. Hemangiomas and the eye. Clin Dermatol. 2015;33(2):170–82. https://doi.org/10.1016/j.clindermatol.2014.10.009.
12. Tollefson MM, Frieden IJ. Early growth of infantile hemangiomas: what parents' photographs tell us. Pediatrics. 2012;130(2):e314–20. https://doi.org/10.1542/peds.2011-3683.
13. Baselga E, Roe E, Coulie J, et al. Risk factors for degree and type of Sequelae after involution of untreated Hemangiomas of infancy. JAMA Dermatol. 2016;152(11):1239–43. https://doi.org/10.1001/jamadermatol.2016.2905.
14. Chang LC, Haggstrom AN, Drolet BA, et al. Growth characteristics of infantile hemangiomas: implications for management. Pediatrics. 2008;122(2):360–7. https://doi.org/10.1542/peds.2007-2767.
15. Samuelov L, Kinori M, Mancini AJ, et al. Ocular complications in PHACE syndrome: a true association or a coincidence? J Pediatr. 2019;204:214–218.e2. https://doi.org/10.1016/j.jpeds.2018.08.031.
16. Darrow DH, Greene AK, Mancini AJ, et al. Diagnosis and management of infantile hemangioma. Pediatrics. 2015;136(4):e1060–104. https://doi.org/10.1542/peds.2015-2485.
17. Krowchuk DP, Frieden IJ, Mancini AJ, et al. Clinical practice guideline for the management of infantile hemangiomas. Pediatrics. 2019;143(1):e20183475. https://doi.org/10.1542/peds.2018-3475.
18. Hutchinson AK, Kraker RT, Pineles SL, VanderVeen DK, Wilson LB, Galvin JA, Lambert SR. The Use of β-Blockers for the Treatment of Periocular Hemangiomas in Infants: A Report by the American Academy of Ophthalmology. Ophthalmology. 2019;126(1):146–155.

7 Current Management of Pediatric Uveitis

Maureen C. Farrell, Pujan R. Patel, and Meghan K. Berkenstock

7.1 Introduction to Pediatric Uveitis

The pediatric uveitides are uncommon conditions with an estimated incidence of 4.3 per 100,000 and prevalence of 27.9 per 100,000 people [1]. Non-infectious causes are the most common and account for 75–88% of pediatric uveitis cases [2]. Within the United States, non-infectious uveitis affects an estimated 22,000 children [2], three-quarters of which have inflammation limited to the anterior chamber. The most common etiologies include juvenile idiopathic arthritis (JIA), sarcoidosis, and tubulointerstitial nephritis and uveitis syndrome (TINU) [2]. While pediatric uveitides are an uncommon disease, they are often painless and chronic. Thus, children may present late with significant morbidities due to the cumulative disease burden over time, which includes the risk of amblyopia [3].

Several retrospective cohort studies have described demographics, disease course, and visual outcomes in pediatric uveitis [3, 4]. One retrospective, multicenter study consisted of 527 patients, with median age at diagnosis of 9.4 years with no gender predominance [3]. In this study, the most common causes of uveitis were idiopathic (29%), JIA (21%), and pars planitis (17%) [3]. In addition to etiology, uveitis can also be categorized based on the anatomic location of the inflammation as defined by the Standardization of Uveitis Nomenclature criteria: anterior, intermediate, posterior, or panuveitis [5]. Of these subtypes, anterior uveitis was the most common (45%) [4], and was less associated with severe visual impairment

M. C. Farrell · P. R. Patel
Drexel University College of Medicine, Philadelphia, PA, USA

M. K. Berkenstock (✉)
Division of Ocular Immunology, Wilmer Eye Institute, Baltimore, MD, USA
e-mail: mberken2@jhmi.edu

A. Ramasubramanian (ed.), *Pediatric Ophthalmology*, Current Practices in Ophthalmology, https://doi.org/10.1007/978-981-19-4963-0_7

than posterior uveitis or panuveitis [3, 6]. JIA was identified as the cause of the uveitis in nearly half of the anterior uveitis cases [3]. In comparison, pars planitis was identified in the majority (57%) of intermediate uveitis cases [3]. Posterior uveitis and panuveitis were the least common subtypes, with toxoplasmosis (35%) and other infectious etiologies (26%) comprising most of the posterior cases [3]. In contrast, autoimmune disorders were the predominant causes of the panuveitis, including Vogt Koyanagi Harada disease (VKH), Behcet's Disease (BD), and sarcoidosis [3].

When discussing treatment options, it is first critical to understand that most cases of uveitis in children are gradually progressive and chronic [3]. Common complications at the time of presentation include posterior synechiae, cataract, and band keratopathy [5]. Importantly, the development of each complication is associated with the disease duration [3]. Years of chronic, uncontrolled inflammation can lead to the formation of cataracts, ocular hypertension (OHT), glaucoma, and cystoid macular edema (CME) [3]. All of these complications carry the risk of visual impairment [3]. Thus, treatment for noninfectious uveitis is centered around the use of topical and oral corticosteroids for immediate control of the inflammation, while initiating the use of non-corticosteroid immunosuppressive agents to maintain long-term suppression of the ocular inflammation [6–9]. This avoids the systemic side effects of corticosteroids, to which children are particularly susceptible including premature closure of the long bone epiphyses, hyperglycemia, osteoporosis, and dysregulation of the developing hypothalamus-pituitary-adrenal axis [10]. Herein, we discuss each of the aforementioned uveitis and review the evidence-based guidelines for treatment specific to each condition.

7.2 Juvenile Idiopathic Arthritis-Associated Uveitis

7.2.1 Epidemiology

Juvenile idiopathic arthritis (JIA) is the most common rheumatological condition of childhood [11]. There are seven subtypes of JIA and a common complication of JIA is uveitis, which has an annual incidence between 2 and 21% and a prevalence ranging from 9 to 14% [12–14]. Risk factors for JIA-associated uveitis include female sex, oligoarticular subtype, less than 6-years old at disease onset, and serologic positivity for antinuclear antibodies and negative for rheumatoid factor [11]. However, other subtypes of JIA may also present with uveitis. This includes enthesitis-related arthritis, which is associated with HLA-B27 positivity and typically causes acute anterior uveitis [12]. This differs from the majority (67–89%) of uveitis cases in JIA, which are chronic, anterior, and bilateral [13]. The uveitis is usually diagnosed following systemic diagnosis, but up to 10% can predate joint symptoms [15]. Ocular symptoms and external signs such as pain and redness are not always present at disease onset [12]. Thus, screening eye exams are essential to identify the development of occult ocular inflammation.

7.2.2 Screening

According to the 2019 American College of Rheumatology/Arthritis Foundation guidelines, children with JIA should undergo regular ocular screening every 3–12 months [16]. The exact frequency should be based on individual-specific risk factors, including JIA subtype, ANA seropositivity, age of onset, and disease duration. For example, patients with either systemic JIA, RF-positive polyarthritis, or enthesitis-related arthritis can be categorized as low-moderate risk and only need to be screened every 6–12 months [16]. For all other JIA subtypes, the concurrent presence of ANA positivity and JIA onset at <7 years of age and disease duration ≤4 years is considered high risk and necessitates screening every 3 months [16]. If any of these three features are lacking, then the patient can be considered low-moderate risk thus requiring screening every 6–12 months [16]. Subsequent follow-up after diagnosis is based on the severity of the inflammation, response to therapy, and monitoring for the development of ocular complications [6, 16–18].

7.2.3 Treatment

Initial treatment consists of topical corticosteroids, such as prednisolone acetate 1% [19, 20]. One or two drops of prednisolone acetate 1% is an acceptable daily dose, while ≥3 drops daily have greater possible risks for complications, including cataract formation [21]. In addition, topical cycloplegics such as tropicamide or cyclopentolate 0.5–1% can be considered if there is a high grade of flare, which increases the risk of posterior synechiae formation [20]. If inflammation is not adequately controlled after 3 months of topical steroids or if more than 2 drops daily of prednisolone acetate 1% or equivalent of corticosteroid drops are required, then immunosuppressive therapy is indicated [18, 20, 21]. Among these agents, the disease modifying anti-rhrumatic drugs (DMARD), including methotrexate, are considered first-line therapies. Specifically, methotrexate can be administered orally or via subcutaneous injection. The latter allows for less gastrointestinal side effects and a higher plasma concentration through bypassing first-pass metabolism in the liver [11, 16, 19, 20]. All DMARDs require three or more months to show a therapeutic benefit, which occurs in 75% of cases [11, 19, 20, 22]. This treatment strategy is in alignment with the management of other uveitides where two immunosuppressive drugs are required in about 25% of patients [23]. Due to the potential for systemic side effects with these medications, a CBC and CMP should be repeated every 4–8 weeks initially, and then every 2–3 months to assess the development of systemic toxicities; however, more frequent monitoring may be needed if the dose exceeds 17.5 mg/m^2 [24].

If quiescence cannot be achieved at the maximum or highest tolerated dose using a single agent, a second immunosuppressive medication is required [20]. After the 2016 United States Food and Drug Administration (FDA) approval of adalimumab for the treatment of JIA-associated uveitis and with several studies showing the efficacy of infliximab, the TNF-inhibitors have been recommended by the American Uveitis Society as second-line agents [25]. The 5-year outcomes from the SYCAMORE trial, which studied the effectiveness of adalimumab in controlling JIA-associated uveitis refractory to methotrexate showed that adalimumab was well tolerated [26]. Furthermore, withdrawal after 1–2 years of treatment was not associated with disease recurrence [27]. However, a cost-effectiveness analysis of adalimumab use among patients in the SYCAMORE trial estimated that the drug would require an 84% price reduction to justify its use based on its incremental cost per quality-adjusted life year compared to methotrexate alone [26]. ADJUST is a currently enrolling clinical trial where 118 patients with adalimumab-controlled JIA-associated uveitis are to be randomized to either continue adalimumab therapy or discontinue treatment [28]. The primary endpoint will determine if the cessation of treatment is associated with uveitis recurrence at 1 year [29]. Compared to the subcutaneous, self-administration of adalimumab, infliximab is administered through intravenous infusion and is not FDA-approved for the treatment of noninfectious uveitis [19]. However, it is another off-label treatment option with the ability to increase the dose in mg/kg or decrease the infusion interval to tailor treatment based on clinical inflammation. Once quiescence is achieved, methotrexate should be continued for at least another 12–24 months in conjuction with a biologic agent [20]. However, the 2019 American College of Rheumatology/Arthritis Foundation guidelines for the treatment of JIA-Associated Uveitis conditionally recommend continued treatment for a duration of 2 years for all JIA-associated uveitis patients [16].

When treatment failure occurs with DMARDs and TNF-inhibitors, third-line agents such as abatacept and tocilizumab can be considered. The quality of evidence for these treatments is limited. In the APTITUDE phase II trial, tocilizumab failed to meet its primary endpoint of a two-step decline or absence of cells in the anterior chamber at 3 months [29]. Nevertheless, the authors noted that 33% of subjects showed response to tocilizumab, and suggested use when first-and second-line options fail [29]. Another study examined the efficacy of tocilizumab in eight patients (mean age of 23 years) with severe, long-term, uncontrolled JIA-associated uveitis. Findings included decreased uveitis activity in all patients beginning 4–5 months after beginning infusions and stable visual acuities in the subsequent study period, and reduced need for corticosteroid agents and immunosuppressants in five patients [30]. A recent case series of four patients aged 18–43 years with longstanding, complicated JIA-associated uveitis (mean disease duration of 21 years) reported that Janus Kinase inhibitors significantly reduced anterior chamber cells by ≥2 steps [31].

Of note, for all pediatric patients on immunosuppressive agents, there are several additional considerations for clinical management. In terms of prevention, patients can receive inactivated vaccines per clinical guidelines by the Center for Disease Control and Prevention [32, 33]. In addition, children and adolescents on immunosuppressive drugs should also receive the pneumococcal polysaccharide vaccine [33]. However, the use of live vaccines is contraindicated with high-dose immunosuppressants [32]. In pediatric patients who have reached puberty and are on DMARD therapy, a discussion with the patient and their caregiver is required to review the teratogenic risk of these medications and their contraindication in pregnancy. In addition, the effect of methotrexate on spermatogenesis is still not fully understood [34]. Contraception is advised while taking methotrexate and for an additional 3–6 months after discontinuation [32]. Specific to the use of TNF-α inhibitors, patients should be tested for tuberculosis infection prior to initiating treatment and yearly thereafter [35]. As previously mentioned, laboratory testing (CBC and CMP) is recommended every 3–6 months to monitor for systemic side effects [35]. Some patients may develop neutralizing antibodies to the anti-TNF-α monoclonal antibodies resulting in decreased effectiveness over time [36]. Serious infections in pediatric patients on adalimumab have been reported, but are rare with only 2.7 serious infections per 100 patient-years [37]. Finally, TNF-α inhibitors are contraindicated in patients with multiple sclerosis (MS) or other central nervous system demyelinating diseases [38].

7.2.4 Complications

It has been reported that nearly 40% of patients with JIA-associated uveitis may experience ocular complications, with the highest risk in those who develop uveitis shortly after JIA diagnosis or have positive antinuclear antibody titers [39]. Cataract and glaucoma are the most common complications, as seen in a retrospective 4-year study of JIA-associated uveitis patients where the risk of incident cataract was strongly associated with topical corticosteroid use in a dose-dependent manner [21]. Another factor associated with cataract development is the presence of posterior synechiae during initial presentation [11, 21]. Additional sight-threatening complications in JIA uveitis include band keratopathy, ocular hypertension, hypotony, optic disc edema, cystoid macular edema (Fig. 7.1), and serous retinal detachments [1, 11, 40–43].

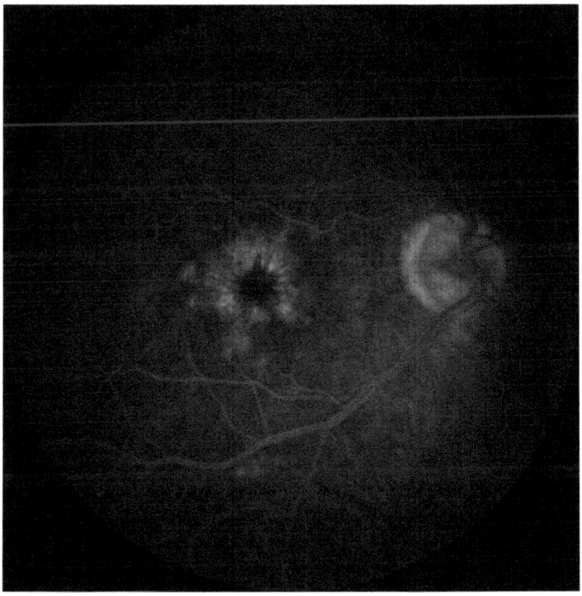

Fig. 7.1 A fluorescein angiogram of a right eye showing petaloid leakage in a patient with cystoid macular edema and uveitis

7.3 Tubulointerstital Nephritis and Uveitis (TINU) Syndrome

7.3.1 Epidemiology

Tubulointerstitial nephritis and uveitis (TINU) syndrome is a rare disease limited to the renal and ocular systems and is responsible for about 2% of uveitis cases at tertiary care centers [44]. However, this number likely underestimates the actual number of cases given renal and ocular symptoms may not present concurrently complicating the diagnosis. Risk factors for TINU include young age, female sex, and NSAID or antibiotic use [45, 46]. In addition the following risk alleles have been identified: HLA-DQA101, HLA-DRB101, HLA-DQB105 [47].

Tubulointerstitial nephritis (TIN) typically has the earlier onset in 65% of patients and is characterized by nonspecific constitutional symptoms such as fever, malaise, rash, anorexia, flank pain, arthralgia, and myalgia [44, 47]. Renal injury is usually mild, but acute kidney injury may occur [44]. Conversely, it should be noted that patients with bilateral anterior uveitis with simultaneous onset should be screened for TINU with urine beta-2 microglobulin to identify subclinical renal disease prior to progression [47]. Of note, elevated levels of beta-2 microglobulin is a nonspecific finding and can be elevated in any kidney disorder affecting the renal tubules [47].

7.3.2 Screening

All patients with TIN should be evaluated by an ophthalmologist for uveitis given the relatively high proportion of subclinical cases and potential for development after TIN onset [48]. Patients should be monitored every 3 months initially and for at least 1 year following a diagnosis of TIN [48]. The onset of uveitis may present up to 14 months after renal symptoms [44]. However, ocular symptoms precede renal symptoms in about 20% of patients and present concurrently in another 15% of patients [44]. Of note, systemic steroids for treating TIN has not been shown to decrease the incidence of uveitis, and bilateral anterior uveitis with simultaneous onset is the most common type of presentation [44, 45]. Up to half of the children with TINU do not have ocular symptoms at the time of diagnosis [48].

TINU is a diagnosis of exclusion after serologic evaluation to exclude other causes of anterior uveitis, including HLA-B27 positivity or infectious etiologies. Simplifying the diagnosis is if the acute bilateral uveitis occurs after the development of azotemia of unknown origin and generalized malaise. With this clinical presentation, urinalysis may show elevated urinary ß-2 microglobulin levels, which provides a sensitive marker for diagnostic screening [47, 49, 50]. Furthermore, the combination of elevated urinary ß-2 microglobulin and elevated serum creatinine was found to have 100% positive predictive value for detecting TINU in patients with uveitis [50]. Confirmatory diagnosis can be made by renal biopsy, which shows a predominant T cell infiltration of the renal interstitium along with some neutrophils and plasmatocytes [44].

7.3.3 Treatment

Initial treatment for anterior uveitis in TINU mirrors that of JIA-associated uveitis and consists of topical corticosteroids with refractory cases requiring initiation of oral corticosteroids and immunosuppressive agents, including methotrexate or azathioprine [44]. With aggressive treatment and maintained quiescence, the prognosis of TINU is good with the preservation of visual function [48]. Compared to adults, children are more likely to have recurrent or chronic uveitis but are less likely to develop chronic kidney disease [45]. Posterior synechiae are the most commonly reported complications in TINU [44]. Other complications include optic disc edema, CME, and chorioretinal scarring [44].

7.4 Blau-Jabs Syndrome (Juvenile Systemic Granulomatosis)

7.4.1 Epidemiology

Blau-Jabs Syndrome (BJS) is a rare autosomal dominant autoinflammatory disorder that affects the eyes, skin, and joints [51]. It has also been known as pediatric granulomatous arthritis and juvenile granulomatous systemic disorder. The classic triad of BJS is painful granulomatous arthritis, dermatitis, and uveitis. However, not all patients develop each of these manifestations [51, 52]. Polyarticular arthritis is the most common clinical feature, affecting an estimated 97% of patients and occurs in the first few years of life [37, 51]. Most often involved joints are the ankles, knees, wrists, and fingers in addition to the development of synovial cysts, tenosynovitis, or intraphalangeal contractures [51].

Dermatitis is another feature of BJS and consists of a generalized, non-confluent, erythematous or pigmented, papular rash on the trunk or extremities [51, 53]. The initial rash develops after infancy and may often show interval improvement followed by eruptions of ichthyosiform dermatosis, panniculitis, livedoid lesions, and vasculitis [51, 53]. In addition, patients may also develop additional skin features including erythema nodosum, leukocytoclastic, or plaque-like dermatitis [51].

Uveitis is the least common and the latest onset feature of BJS but is sight-threatening, bilateral, and chronic [51]. Panuveitis is the most common presentation in patients with BJS (51% of eyes) [52], followed by isolated granulomatous anterior uveitis (Fig. 7.2) [51]. Posterior segment involvement is often marked by multifocal choroidal infiltrates with sclerotic lesions peripheral to vascular arcades (Fig. 7.3) [51, 52]. Patients may develop additional ocular features and secondary inflammatory complications including coin-shaped corneal opacities, retinal vasculitis, optic nerve atophy or edema, glaucoma, exudative retinal detachments, and cataracts [51]. An estimated 50% of patients with BJS may develop other manifestations, which can include recurrent fevers, tubulointerstitial nephritis, hepatic or salivary gland inflammation, vasculitis, pulmonary fibrosis, malignant hypertension, cranial nerve palsies, or cardiac hypertrophy [51].

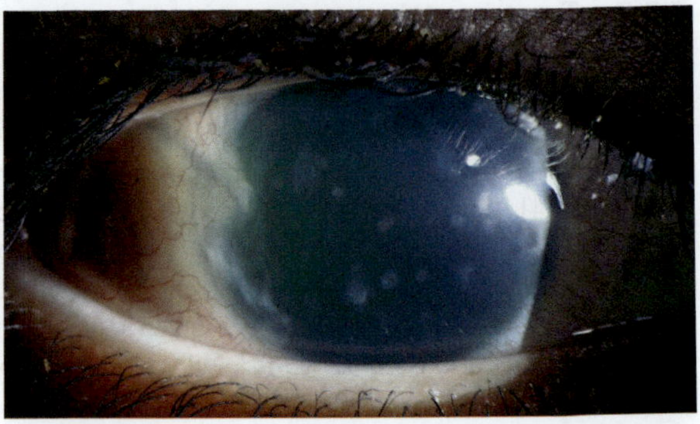

Fig. 7.2 An external photo of the right eye of a patient with Blau-Jabs Syndrome showing corneal opacities and superotemporal glaucoma drainage tube

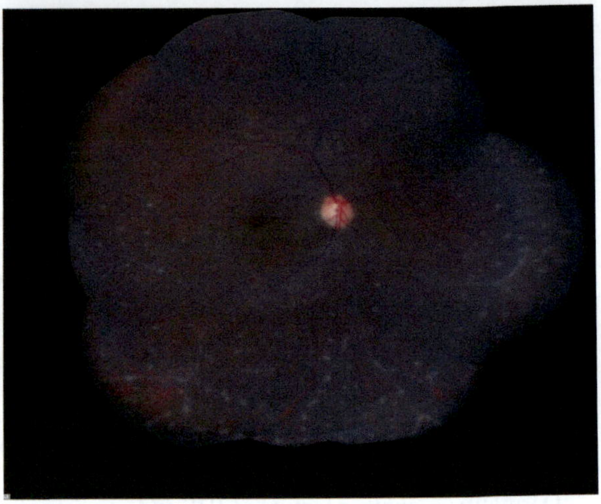

Fig. 7.3 A color fundus photo of a right eye in a patient with Blau-Jabs Syndrome showing extensive peripheral vascular sheathing

7.4.2 Screening

The diagnosis of BJS may be complicated by overlapping phenotypes with other pediatric inflammatory diseases including JIA and juvenile sarcoidosis. While most cases of JIA only involve a few joints or oligoarthritis, BJS is a polyarthritis involving five or more joints. Additionally, the anatomic location of the ocular inflammation can provide another means of differentiation, as JIA most commonly involves the anterior chamber and BJS has a predilection for retinochorioretinal involvement. Further complicating diagnosis is that cases of juvenile sarcoidosis have been shown to be caused by de novo *NOD2/CARD15* variants, which has been identified to be the affected gene in BJS and both disorders also cause granulomatous anterior uveitis [49]. In contrast to BJS, patients with juvenile sarcoidosis develop characteristic features of bilateral hilar adenopathy and non-caseating pulmonary granulomas [51]. The onset is often not until the teen years in juvenile sarcoidosis, compared to the early childhood onset of clinical features in BJS.

Based on clinical suspicion, laboratory testing should include testing to rule out infectious causes of granulomatous uveitis, such as TB and syphilis. Genetic testing for pathogenic *NOD2* variants is confirmatory.

7.4.3 Etiology

BJS results from an autosomal dominant mutation in the *NOD2* (nucleotide-binding oligomerization domain-containing protein two) protein [51]. This gene is also known as *CARD15* (Caspase Recruitment Domain 15) and encodes a cytosolic protein involved in the recognition of muramyl dipeptide in bacterial cell walls, triggering a pro-inflammatory signaling cascade [51]. Seventeen pathogenic *NOD2* variants have been identified and asymptomatic carriers can present with incomplete disease penetrance [51].

7.4.4 Treatment

Given the rarity of the condition, there are no specific treatment guidelines for BJS [51]. Treatment is focused on managing symptoms and suppressing systemic inflammation. Uveitis requires aggressive treatment with topical and systemic corticosteroids with the concurrent start of immunosuppressive agents, with methotrexate as the first-line agent with other DMARDs as alternative therapies when methotrexate is otherwise contraindicated or in refractory disease [51]. As in JIA-associated uveitis, biologic agents including TNF- alpha inhibitors are recommended, except for etanercept, which has not been shown to be clinically effective and its use is not recommended [51].

7.4.5 Complications

Due to the chronic duration and posterior involvement in this disease, BJS is associated with a high rate of vision loss and ocular morbidity. Even with aggressive treatment, an estimated 33% of patients experienced a decline in visual acuity with the development of ocular complications after 3 years of follow-up [51, 52].

7.5 Behçet Disease

7.5.1 Epidemiology

Behçet Disease (BD) is an uncommon multisystem inflammatory disorder of unknown etiology that is rare in Europe and North America, with the greatest prevalence among populations in the Middle East and Asia [54]. BD may present sporadically with no known family history of disease or in the context of known HLA-B51 risk alleles [54]. In addition to uveitis, oral aphthous ulcers are an early common

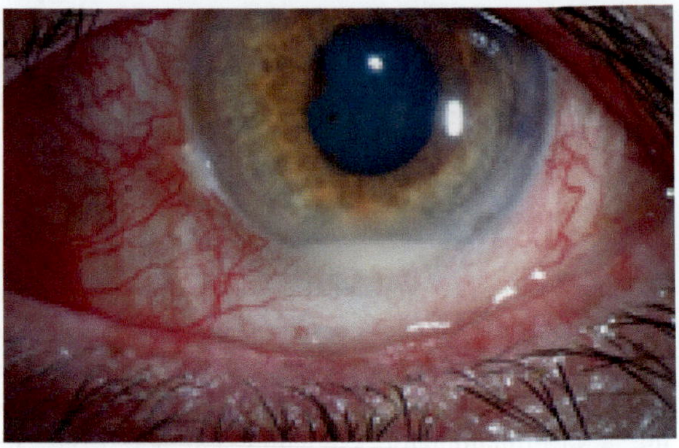

Fig. 7.4 An external photo of a left eye in a patient with Behcet disease with acute hypopyon formation

feature that occurs in the majority of patients along with genital ulcers occur (>80% of patients), and skin abnormalities (70–90%) [55]. An asymmetric polyarthritis mostly affecting the large joints has been estimated to occur in about half of patients. Arthritis and papulopustular lesions often occur simultaneously [54].

The mean childhood onset is estimated to occur from age 13–19 years but may occur into the third decade of life [55, 56]. A large retrospective study of 36 children with childhood onset BD demonstrated bilateral uveitis in 83% of cases with the majority presenting with panuveitis and occlusive retinal vasculitis or retinitis (Fig. 7.4) [56]. A large retrospective study of patients with central nervous system involvement (neuro-BD) found that less than 4% of patients developed symptoms before age 16 years [57]. The majority of childhood onset patients were male with a 5.5:1 ratio and developed BD symptoms and neurologic symptoms at an average of 13 years of age. Of the 26 patients with childhood onset disease, the majority (88.5%) had dural venous sinus thrombosis and only three (11.5%) had involvement of parenchyma within the central nervous system.

7.5.2 Treatment

Compared with the lower rates of posterior pole involvement in JIA and TINU-associated uveitis, immunosuppressive agents are recommended for the treatment of BD given posterior pole involvement and the proclivity for systemic inflammation [25]. In most cases, BD is treated with systemic corticosteroids and one or more immunomodulatory agents [25]. Infliximab and adalimumab are recommended as first-line agents for patients with incompletely controlled uveitis in BD or those who do not tolerate DMARDs [25].

7.5.3 Complications

Complications in BD are similar to the other autoimmune-related uveitis with cataract being quite common (47% of eyes), CME (45%), and optic atrophy (39%) [56].

The visual prognosis is poor, with 23% of pediatric-onset patients experiencing loss above a LogMAR vision of 0.1 in affected eyes [56].

7.6 Intermediate Uveitis

7.6.1 Epidemiology

Intermediate uveitis is an inflammatory disease that affects the peripheral retina and vitreous [5, 58]. Pars planitis is a subset of chronic, idiopathic intermediate uveitis that is characterized by inflammatory aggregates in the pars plana or vitreous in the absence of systemic and inflammatory diseases such as Lyme disease, syphilis, sarcoidosis, and MS [5, 58]. Pars planitis is predominantly seen in the early pediatric and adolescent population, where it is the most common form of intermediate uveitis, accounting for 5–26.7% of uveitis cases in this group [59]. The etiology of pars planitis remains unknown, but a genetic predisposition of HLA-DR2, -DR15, -B51, and -DRB1*0802 has been suggested [59–61]. Of note, multiple sclerosis is also associated with HLA-DR2 and -DR15, and patients may present with MS-associated intermediate uveitis, which needs to be differentiated from pars planitis. Patients with pars planitis are estimated to have a 2–3% annual risk of subsequently developing MS [62]. Most patients have bilateral involvement, but inflammation can be asymmetric. Presenting symptoms include blurred vision, floaters, pain, photophobia, and redness [58]. The disease can also be asymptomatic and incidentally diagnosed on routine examination [59].

7.6.2 Screening

Pars planitis is a clinical diagnosis. Inflammatory and infectious etiologies must be ruled out through serologic workup and imaging [59]. As of this year, the Standardization of Uveitis Nomenclature (SUN) Working Group proposed a set of classification criteria for pars planitis including vitreous cells or haze, vitreous inflammation greater than that in the anterior chamber when both are present, no evidence of retinitis or choroiditis, no retinal vascular occlusion in posterior pole and mid-periphery, and evidence of pars planitis—vitreous snowballs or pars plana snowbanks. Exclusions for pars planitis consisted of any of the following: MS per McDonald criteria, a positive treponemal test, sarcoidosis diagnosed via chest imaging or tissue biopsy, and positive Lyme serology [62]. This classification criteria was found to be clinically reliable with a low misclassification rate [62].

7.6.3 Treatment

Currently, there is no consensus regarding treatment in pars planitis with mild disease [59]. Some have suggested that in the absence of ocular complications and visual acuity of at least 20/40, treatment is not required and the patient can be routinely monitored [59, 63]. More recently, it has been argued that early and aggressive treatment of inflammation is critical, irrespective of visual acuity [59, 64]. Initial treatment strategies for non-infectious intermediate uveitis include use of the intravitreal dexamethasone implant or intravitreal injection of triamcinolone [59, 65–68]. The largest series employing these local management strategies was by Tomkin-Netzer et al. in 2016, which consisted of 16 pediatric patients (22 eyes) with intermediate or posterior uveitis [68]. Intravitreal dexamethasone resulted in significant BCVA improvement (0.55–0.38 logMAR), central retinal thickness reduction by 219 μm, and vitreous haze resolution in an additional 47% subjects by 1–2 months post-implantation [68]. Relapse of inflammation occurred about 9 months after implantation, but it was controlled with reimplantation [68]. Cataract progression was observed in 4 eyes, while elevated IOP was observed in 6 eyes [68]. Of note, the PeriOcular versus INTravitreal corticosteroids for uveitic macular edema (POINT) Trial showed that intravitreal dexamethasone implant and intravitreal triamcinolone are superior to periocular triamcinolone for treating uveitic macular edema at 8 weeks post-treatment [69]. However, caution should be exercised with the use of local therapy alone as the Systemic Immunosuppressive Therapy for Eye Diseases (SITE) Study showed that peri- and intraocular corticosteroid injections increase the risk of elevated IOP between 7- and 20-fold [70]. The use of topical corticosteroids is reserved for concurrent anterior segment inflammation with the exception of difluprednate. It has been shown that difluprednate penetrates into the vitreous and reduces cystoid macular edema in pediatric patients with non-infectious uveitis, but clinicians need to be wary of IOP elevation as seen with other local corticosteroids [59, 71–73].

When long-term treatment is required, immunomodulatory therapy should be implemented. As in the treatment of JIA and TINU, patients requiring systemic disease treatment or who are intolerant of local corticosteroid therapy, due to a lack of response or the development of side effects, require the start of corticosteroid sparing immunosuppressive agents [59]. DMARDs remain the first-line agents followed by TNF-α inhibitors for use in refractory cases [59].

7.6.4 Complications

The most common cause of vision loss in patients with pars planitis is CME [59]. Other complications requiring the need for escalation of treatment include the development of increased vitreous cell and haze, vitreous hemorrhage, exudative retinal detachments, and peripheral retinal neovascularization [59]. If a non-clearing vitreous hemorrhage or tractional membranes develop, then pars plana vitrectomy is indicated [59]. Laser photocoagulation and intravitreal injections of anti-vascular endothelial growth factor agents can be used as adjunctive therapy for peripheral neovascularization or vitreous hemorrhage [59, 74–78]. Cryotherapy is no longer favored due to disruption of the blood-ocular barrier and induction of vitreous contraction, which may predispose to retinal detachment [59].

7.7 Pediatric Infectious Uveitis: Ocular Tuberculosis and Toxocariasis

7.7.1 Ocular Tuberculosis

7.7.1.1 Epidemiology

Mycobacterium tuberculosis is the pathogen responsible for tuberculosis, which is a rare cause of uveitis. The prevalence of ocular tuberculosis (Tubercular Uveitis, TBU) varies widely across the globe, implicated in an estimated 0.6% of uveitis cases in a Boston-based study and 10% of uveitis patients in northern India [79].

7.7.2 Clinical Overview

Ocular tuberculosis can affect any part of the eye including the orbit and anterior segment but is most commonly associated with posterior or panuveitis [80]. TBU can present with chronic granulomatous uveitis with mutton-fat keratic precipitates, nodules on the iris, posterior synechiae, choroidal tubercles, or pseudo-serpiginous choroiditis [79].

A retrospective study of 29 pediatric patients with TBU from the Collaborative Ocular Tuberculosis Study-1 (COTS-1) cohort showed a mean age at disease onset of 12 years (range 4–18), 70% male, and 86% Asian ethnicity. TBU was most commonly associated with posterior uveitis (50%) with extension into the choroid in 65% of cases [81]. Edema of the optic nerve head and macula were more commonly found in children with TBU than adults within COTS-1 [81].

7.7.3 Screening

No standardized diagnostic approach exists to guide the workup or diagnosis of TBU [79]. The COTS Workshop created a consensus definition for the diagnosis of ocular tuberculosis, which requires a positive Mantoux test, interferon-gamma release assay, and/or chest computerized tomography consistent with prior tuberculosis infection [82]. Confirmatory histopathology or polymerase chain reaction testing of ocular fluids is not required [82].

7.7.4 Treatment

Because of the severity of intraocular inflammation associated with pediatric TBU, uveitis must be diagnosed and treated expediently with anti-tuberculosis therapy and corticosteroids to control infection, reduce intraocular inflammation, and prevent vision loss through the development of ocular complications [81]. All pediatric patients with TBU in the COTS-1 study received oral corticosteroids and most received anti-tuberculosis antibiotic treatment [81]. Less than 5% of pediatric patients failed treatment, although this has been estimated to be as high as 16% in adult populations on four-drug combination anti-tubercular therapy and corticosteroids or 46% on corticosteroids alone [74, 78].

Patients with uveitis living in or originating from endemic areas must have latent or active tuberculosis infection ruled out prior to initiation of immunosuppressive therapy. While a positive Mantoux test or interferon-gamma release assay may suggest systemic TB infection, they are not necessarily indicative of TBU. It is important to note that in patients with non-specific uveitis findings in the setting of positive TB test, obtaining TB culture or PCR from ocular fluids is unlikely to confirm TBU diagnosis. The classic presentations for TBU are limited to pseudo-serpiginous choroiditis and choroidal granuloma, and in cases with these clinical findings, systemic laboratory tests are more useful in confirming TB as the etiology.

7.7.5 Complications

Similar to noninfectious uveitis, infections within the eye can lead to serious sight-threatening complications including the development of cataracts and glaucoma [83].

7.7.6 Ocular Toxocariasis

7.7.6.1 Epidemiology

Ocular toxocariasis is an uncommon cause of uveitis, accounting for only 1% of cases in several studies [84, 85]. Ocular toxocariasis is a zoonotic disease caused by *Toxocara* spp. It is transmitted through the consumption of developing parasitic embryos from dog or cat feces [86]. Less commonly, it may also occur through the consumption of undercooked meat of an infected host. Patients most often only have either ocular or visceral toxocariasis, affecting the lungs or liver, rather than both [86]. Reported risk factors include young age, lower economic status, male sex, and cat or dog ownership [84, 86–88]. Seroprevalence in the United States is estimated around 14%, with a disproportionate impact on African Americans and children in the Southern regions [88, 89]. A retrospective 20-year study of pediatric patients diagnosed with ocular toxocariasis in Costa Rica found that most patients were diagnosed around age 6–7 years where mean estimates in the United States have ranged from 8–16 years [86, 89]. Prevention techniques include proper hand hygiene, pet deworming, and proper feces disposal [86].

7.7.7 Clinical Overview

Clinically, the most common presentation is unilateral vision loss or blurred vision [90]. However, strabismus, leukocoria, photophobia, eye pain, floaters, and redness may also occur [86, 90]. Unfortunately, patients often do not present until the disease has caused irreparable damage in the eye. Clinical examination may reveal one of several forms: peripheral or macular granuloma or vitreous inflammation or diffuse infiltrative lesions similar in appearance to retinoblastoma [84, 86, 90, 91]. Peripheral granulomas appear as an elevated white nodule with associated retinal traction. In some cases, fibrous tractional bands may extend to the optic nerve [85]. Unlike granulomas with other retinal diseases, those in ocular toxocariasis can be migratory, which is a pathognomonic finding [85].

7.7.8 Screening

For ocular toxocariasis, diagnosis is made based on a history of exposure, clinical evaluation, and serologic testing for serum antibodies. In cases with an obscured fundus, ultrasonography is recommended to detect the reflective granuloma [85]. A serum antibody titer greater than 1/32 against the *T. canis* excretory-secretory antigen on enzyme-linked immunosorbent assay is 78% sensitive [85]. However, antibody testing may not necessarily differentiate between an acute or prior infection [85]. Additionally, laboratory tests may reveal elevated levels of eosinophils or IgE if systemic infection is present [86].

In patients presenting with leukocoria, it is critical to differentiate retinoblastoma from other etiologies, including ocular toxocariasis. Ultrasonography is indicated in these cases as it can detect intratumoral calcifications, which are common in retinoblastoma [92, 93]. Ultrasound findings with toxocariasis include retinal or subretinal mass, vitreous bands, retinal folds, and tractional retinal detachment. Another useful modality to assess retinal complications includes optical coherence tomography [94].

7.7.9 Treatment

Common treatments for ocular toxocariasis include systemic corticosteroids and surgical treatment in late disease (pars plana vitrectomy with or without a scleral buckle or cataract surgery) [86]. Treatment of ocular toxocariasis with anti-helminthic agents remains controversial as no clinical trials for ocular toxocariasis have been performed. The death of the nematodes may contribute to further intraocular inflammation; however, anti-helminthic therapy is used for the treatment of visceral disease [86, 90]. If these agents are used, they should be in combination with corticosteroids [85].

7.7.10 Complications

For untreated ocular toxocariasis, complications may include permanent vision loss, which is often secondary to persistent vitritis, CME, and tractional retinal detachments [84, 85, 90]. The poorest visual outcomes occur with macular involvement of the granuloma [95].

7.8 Cataract in Pediatric Uveitis Patients

Cataract is a common complication in pediatric uveitis. One study found the prevalence to be 44% and estimated that 69% of children would develop cataracts over the following 11 years. Children with panuveitis, chronic anterior uveitis, and intermediate uveitis are most commonly affected [96].

Identification of cataracts in children is of the utmost importance given the association with amblyopia and ultimately decreased academic performance [96]. Increased frequency of uveitis flares, cystoid macular edema, posterior synechiae at presentation, and local corticosteroid injections were all shown to be independent risk factors for cataracts secondary to pediatric uveitis of any etiology [96].

As discussed previously, achieving quiescence of the uveitis is critical to prevent surgery-requiring ocular complications, including cataracts [96, 97]. One retrospective review found that early initiation of methotrexate within 6 months after the onset of uveitis and addition of biologic agents within 18 months reduced the number of complications requiring surgical interventions over 3.5 years of follow-up [97].

Currently, there is not a standard surgical approach for cataract extraction in pediatric patients with uveitis [98]. One study investigated the efficacy of primary posterior chamber hydrophobic intraocular lens placement in 12 children with chronic uveitis treated with aggressive immunosuppressive agents [99]. This study of 14 eyes demonstrated improvement in mean BCVA (distance) before surgery from 1.11 (0.40–2.30, Standard Deviation 0.57) to 0.48 (0–3, Standard Deviation 0.77, $p = 0.007$) after 35 months of follow-up, indicating postsurgical visual recovery after cataract surgery with lens implantation was possible [99].

However, lens placement during cataract removal in pediatric patients with uveitis remains controversial with or without pre-treatment with corticosteroids [100]. According to a 2020 survey from 47 pediatric ophthalmologists and 62 uveitic specialists, 79% of the experts did not believe that uveitis was a contraindication for primary intraocular lens (IOL) placement [101]. Further, uveitis specialists were significantly more likely than pediatric ophthalmologists to utilize intravitreal corticosteroid injections (65% vs. 30%) and intravenous corticosteroid infusions (60% vs. 35%) for perioperative inflammatory control [101]. Interestingly, there were similar responses between the subspecialists for sub-tenon periocular injections and oral corticosteroids [101]. Regardless of clinician perspective, it is clear that chronic inflammation irreversibly damages ocular structures and early initiation of corticosteroids and immunosuppressive agents are necessary to achieve control of inflammation, prevent complications, and allow for ocular surgeries for vision correction when required [100].

7.9 Risk of Glaucoma

Ocular hypertension and glaucoma are other serious complications of uveitis in both adults and children [70, 102]. Among children with non-infectious uveitis, IOP elevation is not uncommon and has been associated with pressure elevations in the contralateral eye and topical corticosteroid use [70]. The SITE Study examined the potential risk of IOP elevation in pediatric non-infectious uveitis and described predictive risk factors [70]. At baseline, 15.8% and 2.9% of eyes had elevated IOP of ≥21 mmHg and ≥30 mmHg, respectively [70]. Factors significantly associated with IOP elevation at presentation included age of 6–12 years, prior cataract surgery, pars plana vitrectomy, chronic uveitis ≥6 months, contralateral IOP elevation, presenting visual acuity worse than 20/40, and topical corticosteroid use in a dose-response relationship [70]. The risk associated with a presenting IOP of 30 mmHg was nearly 12-fold higher in eyes with ≥5 years of chronic uveitis [70]. Eyes treated with local corticosteroids were noted to have a strong risk of IOP elevation, with the use of >1 drop of prednisolone acetate 1% daily and intravitreous or periocular injections [70]. Eyes receiving 2–3 drops daily of prednisolone acetate 1% or equivalent topical corticosteroids demonstrated a two to threefold increased incidence of IOP elevation and ≥ 4 drops daily conferred an approximately ninefold increase [70]. Finally, this study showed that intraocular corticosteroid injections were the greatest risk factor for IOP elevation, with this route of administration conferring up to a 19.7-fold risk of IOP elevation [70].

In contrast, systemic treatments with immunosuppressive therapy or corticosteroids were not associated strongly with the risk of presenting with an elevated IOP, even after adjusting for topical corticosteroid use [70]. For daily doses of ≤7.5 mg, the risk was similar to or less than that of patients not receiving oral corticosteroids [70]. The estimated incidence of any observed IOP elevation to ≥21 mmHg to ≥30 mmHg, and increase in IOP by ≥10 mmHg was 33.4%, 14.8%, and 24.4%, respectively, within 2 years [70]. The cumulative incidence of eyes with IOP elevation continued to rise with duration of disease [70].

Similar IOP trends have been shown in adult populations [102]. A retrospective study of 5270 uveitic eyes from 3308 adult patients demonstrated a prevalence of baseline IOP elevations of ≥21 mmHg and ≥30 mmHg of 14.4% and 5.1%, respectively. Similar to pediatric studies, pressure elevations in the setting of corticosteroid use were observed in a dose-response relationship in adult eyes [70, 102]. However, risk of pressure elevations with topical steroid was greatest with >8 drops of prednisolone acetate 1% (or equivalent) in adult eyes, suggesting that intraocular pressures in pediatric uveitic eyes may be more responsive to corticosteroids [102]. Furthermore, OHT has been shown to be an important risk factor for the development of glaucoma [103]. Among uveitic eyes with IOP increase of ≥10 mmHg, 24% developed glaucomatous optic neuropathy over a 2 year period in the Multicenter Uveitis Steroid Treatment Trial [103]. Thus, the use of corticosteroids to control inflammation must be assessed against the risk of IOP elevation, especially in pediatric populations.

7.10 Summary

Pediatric uveitis can present with minimal symptoms, requiring screening in patients with systemic diseases at high risk for ocular involvement. The long-term visual prognosis relies on early control of ocular inflammation with escalation of therapies to include oral corticosteroids and immunosuppressive agents in cases refractory to local therapy or with involvement of the posterior pole. Close follow-up and aggressive treatment are required given the high risk for the development of complications and the chronicity of pediatric uveitis.

Key Points

1. With the exception of infectious etiologies, the mainstay of treatment of pediatric uveitis is the use of immunosuppressive agents to limit oral, topical, and regional corticosteroid administration.
2. The rates of glaucoma and cataract increase linearly with the dose topical corticosteroids used.
3. Early initiation of immunosuppressive agents is associated with less ocular surgeries and the development of ocular complications limiting visual acuity and the development of amblyopia.

Acknowledgement This research did not receive any specific grant from no funding agencies in the public, commercial, or not-for-profit sectors.

References

1. Kim L, Li A, Angeles-Han S, Yeh S, Shantha J. Update on the management of uveitis in children: an overview for the clinician. Expert Rev Ophthalmol. 2019;14(4–5):211–8. https://doi.org/10.1080/17469899.2019.1663731.
2. Thorne JE, Suhler E, Skup M, et al. Prevalence of noninfectious uveitis in the United States: a claims-based analysis. JAMA Ophthalmol. 2016;134(11):1237–45. https://doi.org/10.1001/jamaophthalmol.2016.3229.
3. Smith JA, Mackensen F, Sen HN, et al. Epidemiology and course of disease in childhood uveitis. Ophthalmology. 2009;116(8):1544–51, 1551.e1. https://doi.org/10.1016/j.ophtha.2009.05.002.
4. Engelhard SB, Bajwa A, Reddy AK. Causes of uveitis in children without juvenile idiopathic arthritis. Clin Ophthalmol. 2015;9:1121–8. https://doi.org/10.2147/OPTH.S83950.
5. Jabs DA, Nussenblatt RB, Rosenbaum JT, Group SoUNSW. Standardization of uveitis nomenclature for reporting clinical data. Results of the first international workshop. Am J Ophthalmol. 2005;140(3):509–16. https://doi.org/10.1016/j.ajo.2005.03.057.
6. Kalinina Ayuso V, van de Winkel EL, Rothova A, de Boer JH. Relapse rate of uveitis post-methotrexate treatment in juvenile idiopathic arthritis. Am J Ophthalmol. 2011;151(2):217–22. https://doi.org/10.1016/j.ajo.2010.08.021.
7. Jabs DA. Treatment of ocular inflammation. Ocul Immunol Inflamm. 2004;12(3):163–8. https://doi.org/10.1080/09273940490883671.
8. Jabs DA, Rosenbaum JT, Foster CS, et al. Guidelines for the use of immunosuppressive drugs in patients with ocular inflammatory disorders: recommendations of an expert panel. Am J Ophthalmol. 2000;130(4):492–513. https://doi.org/10.1016/s0002-9394(00)00659-0.
9. Jabs DA. Immunosuppression for the Uveitides. Ophthalmology. 2018;125(2):193–202. https://doi.org/10.1016/j.ophtha.2017.08.007.
10. Aljebab F, Choonara I, Conroy S. Systematic review of the toxicity of long-course Oral corticosteroids in children. PLoS One. 2017;12(1):e0170259. https://doi.org/10.1371/journal.pone.0170259.

11. Choi J, Hawley DP, Ashworth J, Edelsten C, Bossuyt ASAM. An update on the modern management of paediatric uveitis. Br J Ophthalmol. 2019;103(12):1685–9. https://doi.org/10.1136/bjophthalmol-2019-314212.
12. Barut K, Adrovic A, Şahin S, Kasapçopur Ö. Juvenile idiopathic arthritis. Balkan Med J. 2017;34(2):90–101. https://doi.org/10.4274/balkanmedj.2017.0111.
13. Durrani OM, Meads CA, Murray PI. Uveitis: a potentially blinding disease. Ophthalmologica. 2004;218(4):223–36. https://doi.org/10.1159/000078612.
14. Kanski JJ. Juvenile arthritis and uveitis. Surv Ophthalmol. 1990;34(4):253–67. https://doi.org/10.1016/0039-6257(90)90026-r.
15. Heiligenhaus A, Niewerth M, Ganser G, Heinz C, Minden K. Group GUiCS. Prevalence and complications of uveitis in juvenile idiopathic arthritis in a population-based nation-wide study in Germany: suggested modification of the current screening guidelines. Rheumatology (Oxford). 2007;46(6):1015–9. https://doi.org/10.1093/rheumatology/kem053.
16. Angeles-Han ST, Ringold S, Beukelman T, et al. 2019 American College of Rheumatology/Arthritis Foundation guideline for the screening, monitoring, and treatment of juvenile idiopathic arthritis-associated uveitis. Arthritis Rheumatol. 2019;71(6):864–77. https://doi.org/10.1002/art.40885.
17. Ramanan AV, Dick AD, Jones AP, et al. Adalimumab plus methotrexate for uveitis in juvenile idiopathic arthritis. N Engl J Med. 2017;376(17):1637–46. https://doi.org/10.1056/NEJMoa1614160.
18. Thorne JE, Woreta F, Kedhar SR, Dunn JP, Jabs DA. Juvenile idiopathic arthritis-associated uveitis: incidence of ocular complications and visual acuity loss. Am J Ophthalmol. 2007;143(5):840–6. https://doi.org/10.1016/j.ajo.2007.01.033.
19. LaMattina KC, Koreishi AF. What is new in paediatric uveitis? Curr Opin Ophthalmol. 2018;29(5):412–8. https://doi.org/10.1097/ICU.0000000000000501.
20. Clarke SL, Sen ES, Ramanan AV. Juvenile idiopathic arthritis-associated uveitis. Pediatr Rheumatol Online J. 2016;14(1):27. https://doi.org/10.1186/s12969-016-0088-2.
21. Thorne JE, Woreta FA, Dunn JP, Jabs DA. Risk of cataract development among children with juvenile idiopathic arthritis-related uveitis treated with topical corticosteroids. Ophthalmology. 2010;117(7):1436–41. https://doi.org/10.1016/j.ophtha.2009.12.003.
22. Simonini G, Paudyal P, Jones GT, Cimaz R, Macfarlane GJ. Current evidence of methotrexate efficacy in childhood chronic uveitis: a systematic review and meta-analysis approach. Rheumatology (Oxford). 2013;52(5):825–31. https://doi.org/10.1093/rheumatology/kes186.
23. Goldberg NR, Lyu T, Moshier E, Godbold J, Jabs DA. Success with single-agent immunosuppression for multifocal choroidopathies. Am J Ophthalmol. 2014;158(6):1310–7. https://doi.org/10.1016/j.ajo.2014.08.039.
24. Ortiz-Alvarez O, Morishita K, Avery G, et al. Guidelines for blood test monitoring of methotrexate toxicity in juvenile idiopathic arthritis. J Rheumatol. 2004;31(12):2501–6.
25. Levy-Clarke G, Jabs DA, Read RW, Rosenbaum JT, Vitale A, Van Gelder RN. Expert panel recommendations for the use of anti-tumor necrosis factor biologic agents in patients with ocular inflammatory disorders. Ophthalmology. 2014;121(3):785–96.e3. https://doi.org/10.1016/j.ophtha.2013.09.048.
26. Hughes DA, Culeddu G, Plumpton CO, et al. Cost-effectiveness analysis of adalimumab for the treatment of uveitis associated with juvenile idiopathic arthritis. Ophthalmology. 2019;126(3):415–24. https://doi.org/10.1016/j.ophtha.2018.09.043.
27. Horton S, Jones AP, Guly CM, et al. Adalimumab in juvenile idiopathic arthritis-associated uveitis: 5-year follow-up of the bristol participants of the SYCAMORE trial. Am J Ophthalmol. 2019;207:170–4. https://doi.org/10.1016/j.ajo.2019.06.007.
28. Acharya NR, Ebert CD, Kelly NK, et al. Discontinuing adalimumab in patients with controlled juvenile idiopathic arthritis-associated uveitis (ADJUST-adalimumab in juvenile idiopathic arthritis-associated uveitis stopping trial): study protocol for a randomised controlled trial. Trials. 2020;21(1):887. https://doi.org/10.1186/s13063-020-04796-z.
29. Ramanan AV, Dick AD, Guly C, et al. Tocilizumab in patients with anti-TNF refractory juvenile idiopathic arthritis-associated uveitis (APTITUDE): a multicentre, single-arm, phase 2 trial. Lancet Rheumatol. 2020;2(3):e135–41. https://doi.org/10.1016/S2665-9913(20)30008-4.

30. Miserocchi E, Modorati G, Berchicci L, Pontikaki I, Meroni P, Gerloni V. Long-term treatment with rituximab in severe juvenile idiopathic arthritis-associated uveitis. Br J Ophthalmol. 2016;100(6):782–6. https://doi.org/10.1136/bjophthalmol-2015-306790.
31. Miserocchi E, Giuffrè C, Cornalba M, Pontikaki I, Cimaz R. JAK inhibitors in refractory juvenile idiopathic arthritis-associated uveitis. Clin Rheumatol. 2020;39(3):847–51. https://doi.org/10.1007/s10067-019-04875-w.
32. Ferrara G, Mastrangelo G, Barone P, et al. Methotrexate in juvenile idiopathic arthritis: advice and recommendations from the MARAJIA expert consensus meeting. Pediatr Rheumatol Online J. 2018;16(1):46. https://doi.org/10.1186/s12969-018-0255-8.
33. Recommended Child and Adolescent Immunization Schedule for ages 18 years or younger, United States, 2021. https://www.cdc.gov/vaccines/schedules/downloads/child/0-18yrs-child-combined-schedule.pdf. Accessed 9 June 2021.
34. Gutierrez JC, Hwang K. The toxicity of methotrexate in male fertility and paternal teratogenicity. Expert Opin Drug Metab Toxicol. 2017;13(1):51–8. https://doi.org/10.1080/17425255.2017.1230198.
35. Emer JJ, Frankel A, Zeichner JA. A practical approach to monitoring patients on biological agents for the treatment of psoriasis. J Clin Aesthet Dermatol. 2010;3(8):20–6.
36. Doeleman MJH, van Maarseveen EM, Swart JF. Immunogenicity of biologic agents in juvenile idiopathic arthritis: a systematic review and meta-analysis. Rheumatology (Oxford). 2019;58(10):1839–49. https://doi.org/10.1093/rheumatology/kez030.
37. Horneff G, Seyger MMB, Arikan D, et al. Safety of adalimumab in pediatric patients with polyarticular juvenile idiopathic arthritis, enthesitis-related arthritis, psoriasis, and Crohn's disease. J Pediatr. 2018;201:166–175.e3. https://doi.org/10.1016/j.jpeds.2018.05.042.
38. Mohan N, Edwards ET, Cupps TR, et al. Demyelination occurring during anti-tumor necrosis factor alpha therapy for inflammatory arthritides. Arthritis Rheum. 2001;44(12):2862–9. https://doi.org/10.1002/1529-0131(200112)44:12<2862::aid-art474>3.0.co;2-w.
39. Rypdal V, Glerup M, Songstad NT, et al. Uveitis in juvenile idiopathic arthritis: 18-year outcome in the population-based nordic cohort study. Ophthalmology. 2021;128(4):598–608. https://doi.org/10.1016/j.ophtha.2020.08.024.
40. Ducos de Lahitte G, Terrada C, Tran TH, et al. Maculopathy in uveitis of juvenile idiopathic arthritis: an optical coherence tomography study. Br J Ophthalmol. 2008;92(1):64–9. https://doi.org/10.1136/bjo.2007.120675.
41. Liang F, Terrada C. Ducos de Lahitte G, et al. foveal serous retinal detachment in juvenile idiopathic arthritis-associated uveitis. Ocul Immunol Inflamm. 2016;24(4):386–91. https://doi.org/10.3109/09273948.2015.1012297.
42. Moradi A, Stroh IG, Reddy AK, et al. Risk of Hypotony in juvenile idiopathic arthritis-associated uveitis. Am J Ophthalmol. 2016;169:113–24. https://doi.org/10.1016/j.ajo.2016.06.026.
43. Stroh IG, Moradi A, Burkholder BM, Hornbeak DM, Leung TG, Thorne JE. Occurrence of and risk factors for ocular hypertension and secondary glaucoma in juvenile idiopathic arthritis-associated uveitis. Ocul Immunol Inflamm. 2017;25(4):503–12. https://doi.org/10.3109/09273948.2016.1142573.
44. Amaro D, Carreño E, Steeples LR, Oliveira-Ramos F, Marques-Neves C, Leal I. Tubulointerstitial nephritis and uveitis (TINU) syndrome: a review. Br J Ophthalmol. 2020;104(6):742–7. https://doi.org/10.1136/bjophthalmol-2019-314926.
45. Regusci A, Lava SAG, Milani GP, Bianchetti MG, Simonetti GD, Vanoni F. Tubulointerstitial nephritis and uveitis syndrome: a systematic review. Nephrol Dial Transplant. 2022;37(5):876–86. https://doi.org/10.1093/ndt/gfab030.
46. Okafor LO, Hewins P, Murray PI, Denniston AK. Tubulointerstitial nephritis and uveitis (TINU) syndrome: a systematic review of its epidemiology, demographics and risk factors. Orphanet J Rare Dis. 2017;12(1):128. https://doi.org/10.1186/s13023-017-0677-2.
47. Pakzad-Vaezi K, Pepple KL. Tubulointerstitial nephritis and uveitis. Curr Opin Ophthalmol. 2017;28(6):629–35. https://doi.org/10.1097/ICU.0000000000000421.
48. Saarela V, Nuutinen M, Ala-Houhala M, Arikoski P, Rönnholm K, Jahnukainen T. Tubulointerstitial nephritis and uveitis syndrome in children: a prospective multicenter study. Ophthalmology. 2013;120(7):1476–81. https://doi.org/10.1016/j.ophtha.2012.12.039.

49. Mackensen F, Billing H. Tubulointerstitial nephritis and uveitis syndrome. Curr Opin Ophthalmol. 2009;20(6):525–31. https://doi.org/10.1097/ICU.0b013e3283318f9a.
50. Hettinga YM, Scheerlinck LM, Lilien MR, Rothova A, de Boer JH. The value of measuring urinary β2-microglobulin and serum creatinine for detecting tubulointerstitial nephritis and uveitis syndrome in young patients with uveitis. JAMA Ophthalmol. 2015;133(2):140–5. https://doi.org/10.1001/jamaophthalmol.2014.4301.
51. Suresh S, Tsui E. Ocular manifestations of Blau syndrome. Curr Opin Ophthalmol. 2020;31(6):532–7. https://doi.org/10.1097/ICU.0000000000000705.
52. Sarens IL, Casteels I, Anton J, et al. Blau syndrome-associated uveitis: preliminary results from an international prospective interventional case series. Am J Ophthalmol. 2018;187:158–66. https://doi.org/10.1016/j.ajo.2017.08.017.
53. Poline J, Fogel O, Pajot C, et al. Early-onset granulomatous arthritis, uveitis and skin rash: characterization of skin involvement in Blau syndrome. J Eur Acad Dermatol Venereol. 2020;34(2):340–8. https://doi.org/10.1111/jdv.15963.
54. Yurdakul S, Hamuryudan V, Yazici H. Behçet syndrome. Curr Opin Rheumatol. 2004;16(1):38–42. https://doi.org/10.1097/00002281-200401000-00008.
55. Karincaoglu Y, Borlu M, Toker SC, et al. Demographic and clinical properties of juvenile-onset Behçet's disease: a controlled multicenter study. J Am Acad Dermatol. 2008;58(4):579–84. https://doi.org/10.1016/j.jaad.2007.10.452.
56. Tugal-Tutkun I, Urgancioglu M. Childhood-onset uveitis in Behçet disease:a descriptive study of 36 cases. Am J Ophthalmol. 2003;136(6):1114–9. https://doi.org/10.1016/s0002-9394(03)00791-8.
57. Uluduz D, Kürtüncü M, Yapıcı Z, et al. Clinical characteristics of pediatric-onset neuro-Behçet disease. Neurology. 2011;77(21):1900–5. https://doi.org/10.1212/WNL.0b013e318238edeb.
58. Hersh AO, Cope S, Bohnsack JF, Shakoor A, Vitale AT. Use of immunosuppressive medications for treatment of pediatric intermediate uveitis. Ocul Immunol Inflamm. 2018;26(4):642–50. https://doi.org/10.1080/09273948.2016.1255340.
59. Ozdal PC, Berker N, Tugal-Tutkun I. Pars planitis: epidemiology, clinical characteristics, management and visual prognosis. J Ophthalmic Vis Res. 2015;10(4):469–80. https://doi.org/10.4103/2008-322X.176897.
60. Paroli MP, Spinucci G, Monte R, Pesci FR, Abicca I, Pivetti PP. Intermediate uveitis in a pediatric Italian population. Ocul Immunol Inflamm. 2011;19(5):321–6. https://doi.org/10.3109/09273948.2011.603878.
61. Romero R, Peralta J, Sendagorta E, Abelairas J. Pars planitis in children: epidemiologic, clinical, and therapeutic characteristics. J Pediatr Ophthalmol Strabismus. 2007;44(5):288–93. https://doi.org/10.3928/01913913-20070901-03.
62. The Standardization Of Uveitis Nomenclature Sun Working Group, Jabs DA, Denniston AK, et al. Classification criteria for pars planitis. Am J Ophthalmol. 2021; https://doi.org/10.1016/j.ajo.2021.03.045.
63. Posterior Segment Intraocular Inflammation: guidelines, Forrester JV, Okada AA, BenEzra D, Ohno S, editors. Posterior segment intraocular inflammation: guidelines. Chapter: Pars planitis. KuglerPublications; 1998. p. 93–7.
64. Kump LI, Vitale AT, Foster CS. Diagnosis and treatment of uveitis. In: Foster CS, Vitale AT, editors. Chapter: pediatric uveitis. 2nd ed. Jaypee Brothers Medical Publishers; 2013. p. 1223–5.
65. Lowder C, Belfort R, Lightman S, et al. Dexamethasone intravitreal implant for noninfectious intermediate or posterior uveitis. Arch Ophthalmol. 2011;129(5):545–53. https://doi.org/10.1001/archophthalmol.2010.339.
66. Taylor SR, Tomkins-Netzer O, Joshi L, Morarji J, McLoone E, Lightman S. Dexamethasone implant in pediatric uveitis. Ophthalmology. 2012;119(11):2412–2412.e2. https://doi.org/10.1016/j.ophtha.2012.07.025.
67. Winterhalter S, Behrens UD, Salchow D, Joussen AM, Pleyer U. Dexamethasone implants in paediatric patients with noninfectious intermediate or posterior uveitis: first prospective exploratory case series. BMC Ophthalmol. 2017;17(1):252. https://doi.org/10.1186/s12886-017-0648-3.

68. Tomkins-Netzer O, Talat L, Seguin-Greenstein S, Bar A, Lightman S. Outcome of treating pediatric uveitis with dexamethasone implants. Am J Ophthalmol. 2016;161:110–5.e1–2. https://doi.org/10.1016/j.ajo.2015.09.036.
69. Thorne JE, Sugar EA, Holbrook JT, et al. Periocular triamcinolone vs. intravitreal triamcinolone vs. intravitreal dexamethasone implant for the treatment of uveitic macular edema: the PeriOcular vs. INTravitreal corticosteroids for uveitic macular edema (POINT) Trial. Ophthalmology. 2019;126(2):283–95. https://doi.org/10.1016/j.ophtha.2018.08.021.
70. Kothari S, Foster CS, Pistilli M, et al. The risk of intraocular pressure elevation in pediatric noninfectious uveitis. Ophthalmology. 2015;122(10):1987–2001. https://doi.org/10.1016/j.ophtha.2015.06.041.
71. Sheppard JD, Toyos MM, Kempen JH, Kaur P, Foster CS. Difluprednate 0.05% versus prednisolone acetate 1% for endogenous anterior uveitis: a phase III, multicenter, randomized study. Invest Ophthalmol Vis Sci. 2014;55(5):2993–3002. https://doi.org/10.1167/iovs.13-12660.
72. Schallhorn JM, Niemeyer KM, Browne EN, Chhetri P, Acharya NR. Difluprednate for the treatment of uveitic cystoid macular edema. Am J Ophthalmol. 2018;191:14–22. https://doi.org/10.1016/j.ajo.2018.03.027.
73. Slabaugh MA, Herlihy E, Ongchin S, van Gelder RN. Efficacy and potential complications of difluprednate use for pediatric uveitis. Am J Ophthalmol. 2012;153(5):932–8. https://doi.org/10.1016/j.ajo.2011.10.008.
74. Faisal SM, Tahir MA, Cheema AM, Anjum MI. Pars plana vitrectomy in vitreous hemorrhage with or without Intravitreal Bevacizumab a comparative overview. Pak J Med Sci. 2018;34(1):221–5. https://doi.org/10.12669/pjms.341.12683.
75. Mansour AM, Mackensen F, Arevalo JF, et al. Intravitreal bevacizumab in inflammatory ocular neovascularization. Am J Ophthalmol. 2008;146(3):410–6. https://doi.org/10.1016/j.ajo.2008.05.024.
76. Mansour AM, Arevalo JF, Ziemssen F, et al. Long-term visual outcomes of intravitreal bevacizumab in inflammatory ocular neovascularization. Am J Ophthalmol. 2009;148(2):310–316.e2. https://doi.org/10.1016/j.ajo.2009.03.023.
77. Mansour AM, Arevalo JF, Fardeau C, et al. Three-year visual and anatomic results of administrating intravitreal bevacizumab in inflammatory ocular neovascularization. Can J Ophthalmol. 2012;47(3):269–74. https://doi.org/10.1016/j.jcjo.2012.03.042.
78. Kurup S, Lew J, Byrnes G, Yeh S, Nussenblatt R, Levy-Clarke G. Therapeutic efficacy of intravitreal bevacizumab on posterior uveitis complicated by neovascularization. Acta Ophthalmol. 2009;87(3):349–52. https://doi.org/10.1111/j.1755-3768.2008.01208.x.
79. Agrawal R, Gunasekeran DV, Grant R, et al. Clinical features and outcomes of patients with tubercular uveitis treated with antitubercular therapy in the collaborative ocular tuberculosis study (COTS)-1. JAMA Ophthalmol. 2017;135(12):1318–27. https://doi.org/10.1001/jamaophthalmol.2017.4485.
80. Yeh S, Sen HN, Colyer M, Zapor M, Wroblewski K. Update on ocular tuberculosis. Curr Opin Ophthalmol. 2012;23(6):551–6. https://doi.org/10.1097/ICU.0b013e328358ba01.
81. Testi I, Agrawal R, Mahajan S, et al. The collaborative ocular tuberculosis study (COTS)-1: a multinational descriptive review of tubercular uveitis in Paediatric population. Ocul Immunol Inflamm. 2020:1–7. https://doi.org/10.1080/09273948.2020.1781197.
82. Agrawal R, Agarwal A, Jabs DA, et al. Standardization of nomenclature for ocular tuberculosis - results of collaborative ocular tuberculosis study (COTS) workshop. Ocul Immunol Inflamm. 2019:1–11. https://doi.org/10.1080/09273948.2019.1653933.
83. Chatterjee S, Agrawal D, Parchand SM, Sahu A. Visual outcome and prognostic factors in cataract surgery in ocular tuberculosis. Indian J Ophthalmol. 2020;68(9):1894–900. https://doi.org/10.4103/ijo.IJO_428_20.
84. Stewart JM, Cubillan LD, Cunningham ET. Prevalence, clinical features, and causes of vision loss among patients with ocular toxocariasis. Retina. 2005;25(8):1005–13. https://doi.org/10.1097/00006982-200512000-00009.

85. Ahn SJ, Ryoo NK, Woo SJ. Ocular toxocariasis: clinical features, diagnosis, treatment, and prevention. Asia Pac Allergy. 2014;4(3):134–41. https://doi.org/10.5415/apallergy.2014.4.3.134.
86. Woodhall DM, Fiore AE. Toxocariasis: a review for pediatricians. J Pediatric Infect Dis Soc. 2014;3(2):154–9. https://doi.org/10.1093/jpids/pit066.
87. Marmor M, Glickman L, Shofer F, et al. Toxocara canis infection of children: epidemiologic and neuropsychologic findings. Am J Public Health. 1987;77(5):554–9. https://doi.org/10.2105/ajph.77.5.554.
88. Lee RM, Moore LB, Bottazzi ME, Hotez PJ. Toxocariasis in North America: a systematic review. PLoS Negl Trop Dis. 2014;8(8):e3116. https://doi.org/10.1371/journal.pntd.0003116.
89. Won KY, Kruszon-Moran D, Schantz PM, Jones JL. National seroprevalence and risk factors for zoonotic Toxocara spp. infection. Am J Trop Med Hyg. 2008;79(4):552–7.
90. Martinez J, Ivankovich-Escoto G, Wu L. Pediatric ocular toxocariasis in costa rica: 1998-2018 experience. Ocul Immunol Inflamm. 2021;297:1246–51. https://doi.org/10.1080/09273948.2020.1792513.
91. Ponce-Macotela M, Martínez-Gordillo MN. Toxocara: seroprevalence in Mexico. Adv Parasitol. 2020;109:341–55. https://doi.org/10.1016/bs.apar.2020.01.012.
92. Afshari MA, Hart L, Afshari NA, Mukai S. Ophthalmic ultrasonography in children. Int Ophthalmol Clin. 2001;41(4):153–64. https://doi.org/10.1097/00004397-200110000-00014.
93. Gupta A, Tripathy K. Ocular Toxocariasis. Stat Pearls. Accessed May 8, 2021.
94. Arevalo JF, Espinoza JV, Arevalo FA. Ocular toxocariasis. J Pediatr Ophthalmol Strabismus. 2013;50(2):76–86. https://doi.org/10.3928/01913913-20120821-01.
95. Zhang T, Guo D, Xu G, Jiang R. Ocular Toxocariasis: long-term follow-up and prognosis of patients following vitrectomy. Ocul Immunol Inflamm. 2020;28(3):517–23. https://doi.org/10.1080/09273948.2019.1597897.
96. Blum-Hareuveni T, Seguin-Greenstein S, Kramer M, et al. Risk factors for the development of cataract in children with uveitis. Am J Ophthalmol. 2017;177:139–43. https://doi.org/10.1016/j.ajo.2017.02.023.
97. Cheung CSY, Mireskandari K, Ali A, Silverman E, Tehrani N. Earlier use of systemic immunosuppression is associated with fewer ophthalmic surgeries in paediatric non-infectious uveitis. Br J Ophthalmol. 2020;104(7):938–42. https://doi.org/10.1136/bjophthalmol-2019-314875.
98. Moshirfar M, Somani AN, Motlagh MN, Ronquillo YC. Management of cataract in the setting of uveitis: a review of the current literature. Curr Opin Ophthalmol. 2020;31(1):3–9. https://doi.org/10.1097/ICU.0000000000000626.
99. Guindolet D, Dureau P, Terrada C, et al. Cataract surgery with primary lens implantation in children with chronic uveitis. Ocul Immunol Inflamm. 2018;26(2):298–304. https://doi.org/10.1080/09273948.2016.1213855.
100. Agrawal R, Murthy S, Ganesh SK, Phaik CS, Sangwan V, Biswas J. Cataract surgery in uveitis. Int J Inflam. 2012;2012:548453. https://doi.org/10.1155/2012/548453.
101. Carpentier SJ, Jung JL, Patnaik JL, Pecen PE, Palestine AG. A cross-sectional online survey identifies subspecialty differences in the Management of Pediatric Cataracts Associated with uveitis. Ophthalmol Ther. 2020;9(2):293–303. https://doi.org/10.1007/s40123-020-00245-x.
102. Daniel E, Pistilli M, Kothari S, et al. Risk of ocular hypertension in adults with non-infectious uveitis. Ophthalmology. 2017;124(8):1196–208. https://doi.org/10.1016/j.ophtha.2017.03.041.
103. Friedman DS, Holbrook JT, Ansari H, et al. Risk of elevated intraocular pressure and glaucoma in patients with uveitis: results of the multicenter uveitis steroid treatment trial. Ophthalmology. 2013;120(8):1571–9. https://doi.org/10.1016/j.ophtha.2013.01.025.

Update of Retinoblastoma Management 8

Carley K. Tarallo, Todd Abruzzo, and Aparna Ramasubramanian

8.1 Introduction

Retinoblastoma is the most common pediatric ocular malignancy, with a majority of cases being diagnosed before age of 5 years [1–3]. In recent studies, the incidence is approximately 12 children in one million children under 4 years old and 0.49 cases per million in children between the ages of 4–9 years old [4]. This cancer is exceptionally notable for its rapid growth rate, with tumors doubling approximately every 15 days [5, 6]. While there are approximately 7000–9000 new cases documented worldwide each year, the mortality rates vary greatly between developed and developing countries [3, 7]. Nearly 100% of patients diagnosed with retinoblastoma in developed countries will survive; however, in developing countries, the death rates are as high as 39–70% [2, 3, 7]. If retinoblastoma is recognized and treatment is initiated at an early age, the prognosis is generally very good. On the other hand, severe morbidity and mortality are common when definitive treatment is delayed [2, 6, 8].

Retinoblastoma arises within immature retinal tissue when loss of function mutations affect both copies of the RB1 tumor suppressor gene in a neuroectodermal photoreceptor progenitor cell of the cone cell lineage. In 40% of retinoblastoma patients, one of the two contributory mutations originates in a germline

Aparna Ramasubramanian, M.D. has had full access to all the data in the study and takes responsibility for the integrity of the data.

C. K. Tarallo
University of Arizona College of Medicine, Tucson, AZ, USA
e-mail: c.kcoopirood@email.arizon.edu

T. Abruzzo · A. Ramasubramanian (✉)
Phoenix Children's Hospital, Phoenix, AZ, USA
e-mail: tabruzzo@phoenixchildrens.com; aramasubramanian@phoenixchildrens.com

A. Ramasubramanian (ed.), *Pediatric Ophthalmology*, Current Practices in Ophthalmology, https://doi.org/10.1007/978-981-19-4963-0_8

cell, and the second mutation is somatic. Since most germline mutations occur in utero, only 10% of retinoblastoma is familial. In other words, not all patients with germline RB1 mutations have familial retinoblastoma, though all patients with familial retinoblastoma have a germline mutation. Notably, if a child has a germline RB1 mutation, there is a 95% chance that they will develop retinoblastoma as a result of an acquired somatic mutation in a second allele of the RB1 gene. All patients with germline RB1 mutations have an increased risk of developing secondary cancers in their lifetime. Of these cancers, the most common secondary cancers include melanoma, osteosarcoma, and soft tissue sarcomas [8, 9]. This chapter focuses on the genetic components, clinical features, diagnostic tools, treatment, long-term outcomes, and future directions concerning patients with retinoblastoma.

8.2 Genetics of Retinoblastoma

Retinoblastoma is a cancer that has been studied rigorously by its genetic components. It was the cancer that proposed the idea of the infamous "two hit hypothesis" formulated by Alfred Knudson in 1971 [10]. This hypothesis suggested that there must be two inactivating mutations that cause unregulated cell proliferation in retinal cells leading to retinoblastoma. The hypothesis was later confirmed in 1987 when RB1, a tumor suppressor gene key in the development of retinoblastoma, was cloned [11, 12]. The RB1 gene is located on chromosome 13q14 which encodes for a protein called pRB. pRB is a protein responsible for regulation of the cell cycle from the G1 to S phase, the phase responsible for DNA replication and cell growth [12–14]. This protein regulates cell activity via binding and inhibiting the function of E2F and DP transcription factors that are required for cell division. With mutations in pRB, there is limited inhibition of these transcription factors (E2F and DP) leading to unregulated cell proliferation and eventually tumor formation [15].

The pathophysiology of retinoblastoma requires inactivation of both alleles of the RB1 gene. This exemplifies the model of a "two hit hypothesis" for tumorigenesis in this childhood cancer. Several different mechanisms of inactivation of RB1 have been recorded ranging from single point mutations to large base deletions or substitutions, DNA rearrangements, mutations in RNA splicing, chromothripsis, or methylation of the RB1 promoter with a majority of these mechanisms resulting in a diminished effect, if any effect at all, of RB1 and subsequently the pRB protein [16–18].

Two forms of retinoblastoma exist: nonhereditary or hereditary. Nonhereditary disease accounts for approximately 60% of all retinoblastoma cases and results from two separate somatic mutations that occur within retinal cells during retinal development of a child. Patients with nonhereditary retinoblastoma typically present at older ages, with a median age of 22 months, no family history of retinoblastoma, and unilateral eye involvement. Because these patients do not harbor the RB1 mutation in any other cells other than retinal progenitor cells, they are not at increased risk of developing second malignancies or to pass down mutated RB1 genes to their offspring [8].

Hereditary pattern of disease is responsible for the other 40% of all retinoblastoma cases. Heritable retinoblastoma can be further classified into familial or sporadic retinoblastoma. In familial disease, there is inheritance of a mutated RB1 gene from either of the patient's biological parents. The familial, heritable form of retinoblastoma makes up approximately 10% of all retinoblastoma cases. Sporadic, heritable retinoblastoma occurs in about 30% of all retinoblastoma patients. With this, parents will have normal RB1 genes, but patients will harbor the RB1 mutation in all of their cells. This is believed to be caused by a new mutation in a parent's gamete prior to conception [7, 19, 20]. Up to 90% of patients with bilateral retinoblastoma are thought to have the hereditary form of the disease [1]. Patients with hereditary retinoblastoma usually present at an earlier age, with a median age of diagnosis at 11 months old [8]. Due to the fact that every cell in these patients' bodies will have the RB1 mutation, they are also at risk for other cancers later in life [9]. Regardless of sporadic or familial heritable retinoblastoma, patients have a 50% chance of passing down the RB1 mutation down to their offspring in an autosomal dominant fashion.

At diagnosis of retinoblastoma, it is very important to screen for and differentiate between hereditary and nonhereditary disease given the consequences that can arise with hereditary disease. Because of this, typically tumor tissue and blood lymphocyte samples will be tested for mutations in RB1. These mutations may be alterations in the RB1 exons itself, the introns surrounding the RB1 gene or in the promoter region for the RB1 gene. This has a sensitivity of approximately 75% for finding inactivating RB1 mutations [8, 21]. When a negative test results, quantitative PCR may be used to look for entire or partial gene deletions as well as gene duplications with a sensitivity of about 95% [22]. Generally, if there are no RB1 mutations in lymphocyte DNA, the patient's retinoblastoma is determined to be nonheritable without the chance of passing down mutations to offspring. In cases of patients with heritable retinoblastoma, the RB1 mutation is passed down in an autosomal dominant fashion; however, there in some cases, carriers of the RB1 mutation will show reduced expression or incomplete penetrance resulting in either unilateral eye involvement or later onset of disease [23–26].

With new technology arising, prenatal genetic testing has been made possible to test retinoblastoma susceptibility in utero. This is generally done in patients with a positive family history of retinoblastoma via DNA analysis of fetal cells from either chorion sampling or amniocentesis. For parents with known RB1 mutations, preimplantation techniques have also been designed where specific DNA mutations are screened for in the sperm and ova and then implanted via in vitro fertilization. While this makes the likelihood small that the child will have retinoblastoma in a parent with a germline mutation, these techniques can be very expensive and take expertise that is not available at all institutions [27–29].

In conclusion, genetic testing is very important in the clinical course of retinoblastoma as it can indicate the risk of developing future neoplasms as well as determine treatment courses.

8.3 Clinical Features and Staging of Disease

The most common presentation of retinoblastoma is leukocoria followed by strabismus. Rarely it can present as a red inflamed eye, microphthalmos, or orbital cellulitis [2]. In a review by Fang et al., the median age of presentation of retinoblastoma in patients at a tertiary hospital in China was 17.2 months with the most common symptoms being leukocoria in 57% of patients and strabismus in 16.1% of patients [30].

Tumors themselves are typically round and opaque with translucent thickening of the sensory retina. As the tumor grows, they develop vascular supply and often lose adhesion to the retina. This will disseminate into surrounding ocular tissues leading to seeding which can occur in the subretinal or vitreous space. As disease advances, patients may also develop extraocular disease, proptosis, or metastatic disease [18, 31].

Retinoblastoma conveys three main growth patterns including exophytic, endophytic, and diffuse infiltrating. With exophytic growth, there is a growth of the tumor from the retina into the subretinal space resulting in retinal detachment [32]. Endophytic growth consists of tumor growth into the vitreous cavity. Lastly, diffuse infiltrating, which only occurs in about 2% of all retinoblastoma cases consists of a flat pattern of tumor growth usually in the posterior retina. With these, calcifications are rarely visible and are often misdiagnosed as uveitis [33, 34].

The tumor is staged using the International Classification of Retinoblastoma. Each eye is staged separately.

- **Group A**: tumors smaller than 3 mm away from the optic nerve of macula (Fig. 8.1a).
- **Group B**: Tumors larger than 3 mm, macular or juxtapapillary retinal tumors, tumors with subretinal fluid (Fig. 8.1b).
- **Group C**: Tumors with focal subretinal or vitreous seeding within 3 mm of edge of the tumor (Fig. 8.1c).
- **Group D:** Tumors with diffuse subretinal or vitreous seeding >3 mm from edge of the tumor (Fig. 8.1d).
- **Group E:** Large tumor touching the lens, tumor involving the ciliary body or aqueous, neovascular glaucoma, phthisis or cellulitis (Fig. 8.1e, f) [35–37].

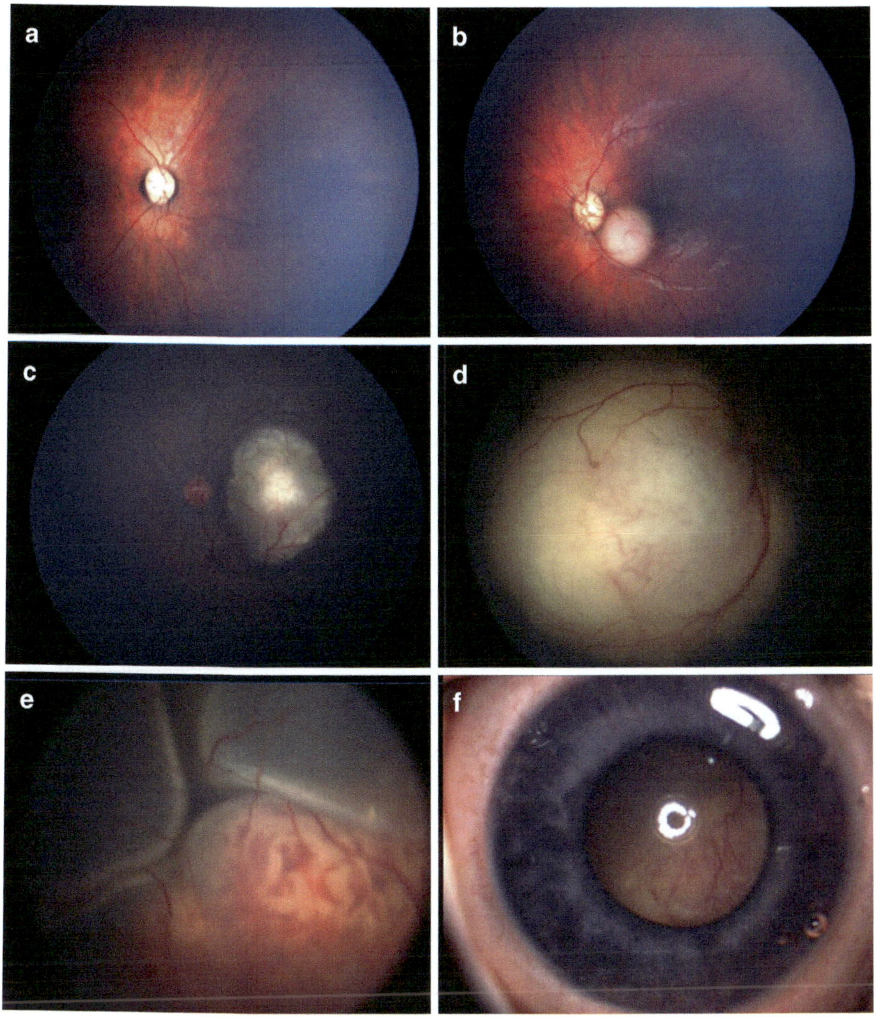

Fig. 8.1 Staging of retinoblastoma. International Classification of retinoblastoma characterizes eyes as small Group A tumor (**a**) and Group B tumor (**b**). Tumors with localized seeds are classified as Group C (**c**) and tumors with diffuse seeds are classified as Group D (**d**). Large tumors with total retinal detachment (**e**) and neovascularization of the iris (**f**) are classified as Group E

8.4 Pathology

Retinoblastoma is a small blue cell tumor. The cells characteristically are arranged in a ring around the central lumen and this arrangement of cells is called Flexner Wintersteiner rosette. Homer Wright rosettes are cells arranged around a fibrillary center. Cells that undergo photoreceptor differentiation are called Fleurettes.

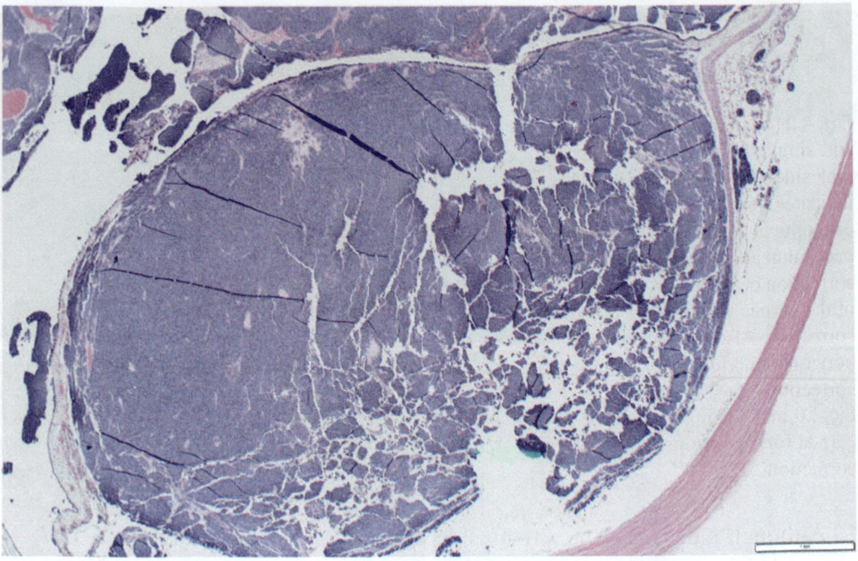

Fig. 8.2 Pathology of retinoblastoma. Pathology of retinoblastoma shows clumps of small blue cells and calcification appears purple

Retinoblastoma tumor can invade the optic nerve, choroid, anterior chamber, iris, ciliary bodies, or sclera [37–39]. These high-risk features are very important to diagnose early on as they carry a risk of systemic metastasis in 24% of patients [40] (Fig. 8.2).

8.5 Diagnosis

Retinoblastoma is diagnosed clinically with the aid of ancillary testing. Lesions that appear similar or mimic retinoblastoma are known as "pseudo-retinoblastomas." [41] According to a study by Huang et al., retinoblastoma is misdiagnosed in about 6–30% of cases resulting in an unnecessary enucleation [42]. Patients who are suspected of having retinoblastoma may undergo several other diagnostic imaging techniques such as ultrasonography, fluorescein angiography, computed tomography, MRI, ultrasound biomicroscopy, and optical coherence tomography.

In order to take pictures for further evaluation, RetCam™ was designed as a wide-angle fundus camera to capture and save fundoscopic images [43]. Fluorescein angiography works with RetCam™ to show the vascular pattern of retinoblastoma. With this, fluorescein dye is injected peripherally and then recorded on the instrument showing the arterial and venous phases of the vessels associated with the tumor [43, 44].

Ultrasonography is a noninvasive and very useful modality to diagnose retinoblastoma. In 90% of retinoblastoma tumors, there is calcification, and the ultrasound detection of calcium is key to the diagnosis (Fig. 8.3a). Ultrasound is also useful for tumor monitoring and detection of recurrence [45, 46].

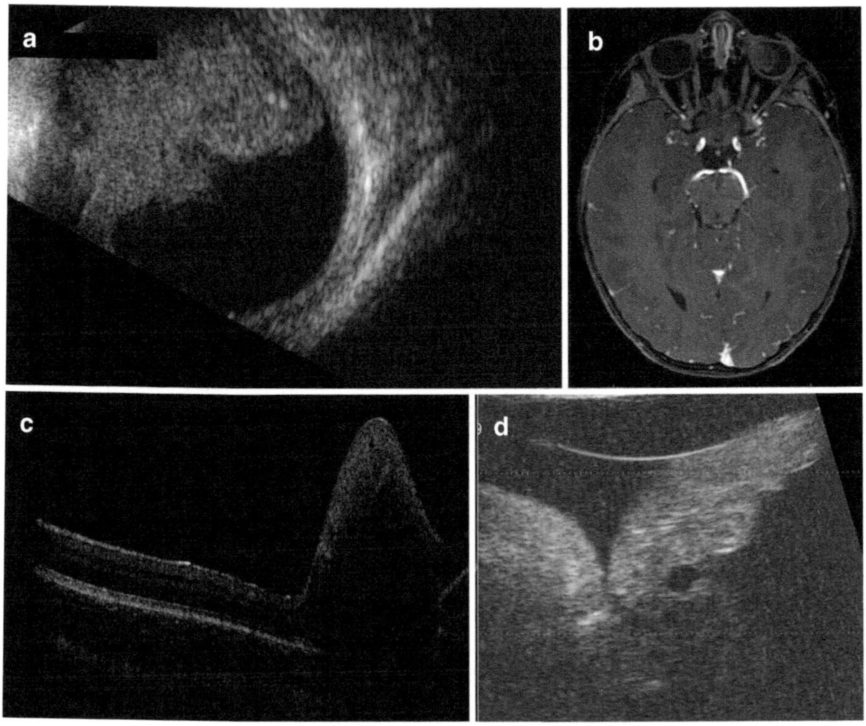

Fig. 8.3 Imaging of retinoblastoma. Ultrasonography shows an elevated retinal tumor with hyperreflective echo suggestive of calcification (**a**). Magnetic resonance imaging of retinoblastoma shows a hyperintense mass on T1 imaging (**b**). Optical coherence tomography shows an elevated intraretinal tumor (**c**). Ultrasound biomicroscopy is useful to rule out ciliary body infiltration in retinoblastoma (**d**)

MRI is a very common modality used to diagnose and routinely image patients with new or treated retinoblastoma. Tumors will show as hyperintense in comparison to the vitreous humor on T1 weighted imaging (Fig. 8.3b) and hypointense on T2 weighted images. On T2 imaging and after contrast, tumors will still appear hypointense and surrounding retinal fluid will not enhance [53]. MRI has the advantage of also estimating optic nerve involvement or choroidal infiltration [54]. Patients with retinoblastoma, especially hereditary form, are screened with cerebral MRI every 6 months until the age of 3 years to detect tumors in the pineal or Sella turcica region (pineoblastoma) which can arise with retinoblastoma [55, 56].

Optical Coherence tomography (OCT) is a diagnostic technique that utilizes light echoes to produce high-resolution, cross-sectional images of the eye. This is exceptionally valuable in diagnosing retinoblastoma as it can detail the structure and depth of the tumor (Fig. 8.3c) [48, 49]. OCT is routinely used to monitor treatment outcomes and look for small tumors or seeding [50]. Lastly, OCT is superior in identifying changes in foveal anatomy posttreatment which can often impact visual function [51, 52].

Ultrasound biomicroscopy is a high-resolution ultrasound that is useful to image the anterior ocular structures (Fig. 8.3d). For retinoblastoma patients, it is useful to detect ciliary body invasion. It is also useful prior to intravitreal chemotherapy to ensure the location of the injection is free of tumor [11, 47].

8.6 Treatment

Treatment for retinoblastoma has made remarkable improvements in the past 25 years. The goals of treating retinoblastoma are to salvage the life of the child, to prevent metastatic disease, and to preserve vision the best possible [37]. Prior to advances in therapy, enucleation and external beam radiotherapy were the treatment of choice to eradicate retinoblastoma. These treatments come with costs though both physically and psychologically. This section will focus on different categories of treatment including local, systemic, intra-arterial/intravitreal, radiation, and surgical therapies of retinoblastoma.

8.6.1 Local

Local therapy of retinoblastoma are treatment options that are typically done under ophthalmoscopic guidance to treat tumors as seen through indirect ophthalmoscopy. The two main local therapies done by ophthalmologists are cryotherapy and laser therapy.

Cryotherapy is a treatment that acts to freeze the tumor itself facilitating tumor death and better chemotherapy penetration. This is usually done to treat tumors that are less than 3 mm in thickness anterior to the equator. In one session, tumors are treated under indirect ophthalmoscope three times using the "freeze and thaw" technique. Tumors may be treated in several sessions with cryotherapy and the objective is to create a flat scar with no more viable tumor tissue [57–59]. Chemo-cryo therapy can also be used which describes a treatment process in which cryotherapy is done on the same day as systemic or intra-arterial chemotherapy to increase drug concentration at the tumor site [59].

Laser transpupillary thermotherapy (TTT) is another commonly used therapy and can be used as the primary treatment of retinoblastoma tumors when the tumor is less than 3 mm or it can be used in combination with other therapies for larger or more complex tumors [60, 61]. With this therapy, a small laser is focalized on the tumor site and the temperature output from the laser is raised over the course of the treatment. The temperature increase is designed to kill the tumor cells that the laser focalizes on. This treatment may last anywhere from 10 to 20 min and may take several different sessions to achieve tumor eradication [59]. It is important to note that the clinical response may appear earlier in patients with more pigmented retinal epithelium and therefore settings of the laser should be adjusted depending on the patients' pigmentations [62]. Chemothermotherapy is another advantageous treatment option that combines the use of chemotherapy and TTT. With this treatment, chemotherapy, usually carboplatin or recently a combination of etoposide and carboplatin is given 1–2 h before TTT. The point of this is to allow better penetration of the chemotherapy into the tumor cells. The course of chemothermotherapy treatment is anywhere from 1 to 6 cycles each separated by 28 days [63].

8.7 Systemic Chemotherapy

Systemic intravenous chemotherapy (IVC) is often used as primary or adjunct therapy in the treatment of retinoblastoma. The indications to use systemic chemotherapy include extraocular retinoblastoma, prophylaxis for extraocular or metastatic spread, in cases of hereditary/bilateral disease, to decrease the risk of trilateral retinoblastoma, and in combination with local therapy to shrink the tumor [59]. To be effective, the chemotherapeutic agent must be able to cross the blood-brain barrier and/or the blood-retinal barrier. Drug choices for systemic chemotherapy in retinoblastoma take expertise as many factors such as age, tumor type, resistances, and complications must be taken into consideration. IVC usually involves a 2–4 drug regimen for anywhere from 6 to 9 months [59]. The drug classes that are most effective against retinoblastoma include alkylating agents, topoisomerase inhibitors, and anthracyclines. This includes vincristine, etoposide, and carboplatin. Systemic chemotherapy is often combined with local transpupillary thermotherapy and cryotherapy for tumor regression (Fig. 8.4). The

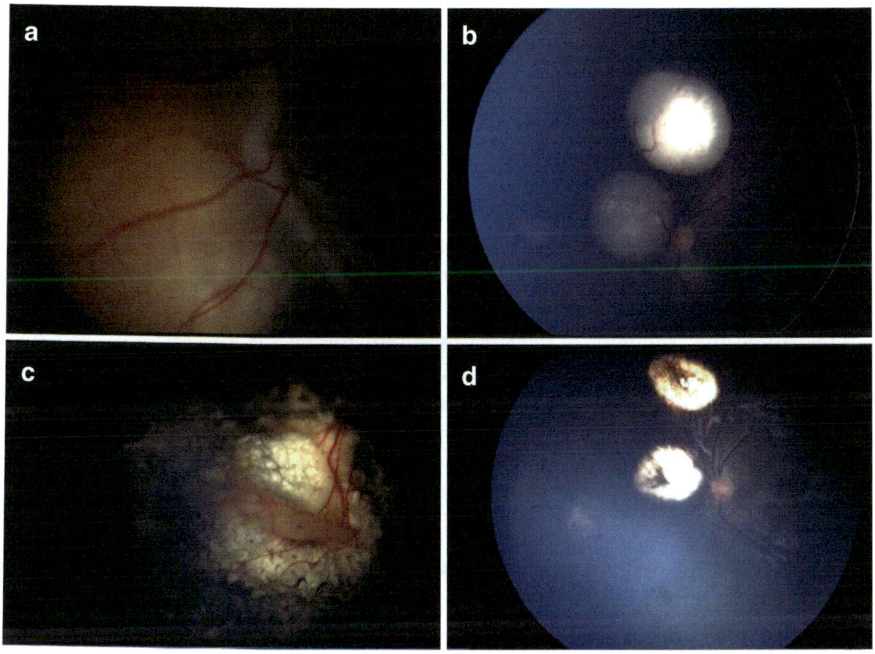

Fig. 8.4 Systemic chemotherapy for retinoblastoma. Bilateral retinoblastoma presented with Group E (**a**) in the right eye and Group B (**b**) in the left eye. Following 6 cycles of systemic chemotherapy and local therapy, both eyes showed a nice response (**c**, **d**)

outcome of retinoblastoma defined as the absence of enucleation and external beam radiation in a large study was Group A (96%), Group B (91%), Group C (91%), Group D (71%), and Group E (32%) [37].

8.8 Intra-Arterial Chemotherapy

Intra-arterial chemotherapy (IAC) has revolutionized the treatment of retinoblastoma and is the primary treatment for unilateral retinoblastoma and for recurrence of retinoblastoma after systemic chemotherapy [70]. The remarkable success of IAC in achieving high rates of clinical remission without significant local or systemic toxicity is owed to the very high concentration of drug produced in tumor tissue when drug is infused directly into the circulation of the eye. Since the chemotherapeutic is not diluted into the systemic circulation, there is a very high first-pass drug concentration. The small blood volume of the eye, and removal of dilution effects associated with systemic administration, allows for a 300-fold increase in chemotherapeutic concentration despite a 90% total dose reduction. IAC is performed by a neuroendovascular surgeon under general anesthesia [71]. In current clinical practice, IAC is usually administered directly into the ophthalmic artery (in 95–97% of cases). In some patients with atypical anatomical variations (3–5%), IAC may be administered into an external carotid artery branch that anastomoses with the ophthalmic artery, most commonly the middle meningeal artery. To administer chemotherapy into the infusion vessel (ophthalmic artery or middle meningeal artery), a microcatheter (≤3 French) is placed into the infusion vessel over a microguidewire (0.008″ to 0.014″). In most cases, the surgeon initially advances a larger guiding catheter (i.e., 4 French outer diameter with 0.038″ lumen) from the femoral artery to the ipsilateral common carotid artery under fluoroscopic guidance [70, 72, 73]. Angiography is performed to delineate the ophthalmic artery circulation and select the infusion vessel. The guiding catheter is then stationed in the internal carotid artery or external carotid artery to support the coaxial microcatheter. After the microcatheter is introduced into the guiding catheter, it is placed into the infusion vessel using fluoroscopic guidance further aided by a mask image of the target infusion vessel superimposed on the live fluoroscopic image.

Once the microcatheter is placed in the infusion vessel, the anatomy and flow dynamics of the ophthalmic circulation are assessed by microcatheter angiography. Particular attention is given to the identification of retrograde or competitive countercurrent flow that may compromise the chemotherapy dose reaching the target tumor tissue. A variety of methods have been described to optimize ocular hemodynamics, including balloon occlusion of the external carotid artery to suppress countercurrent competitive flow [74–76].

Melphalan is an alkylating agent with a short half-life that is commonly used in IAC because retinoblastoma cell lines are very sensitive to it in small doses [77]. In an in vivo rabbit model by Daniels et al., melphalan was proven to have excellent vitreous and retinal drug penetration when administered via IAC [78]. When melphalan is administered systemically for the treatment of retinoblastoma, prohibitively severe adverse effects are common. While melphalan is the first-line medication for IAC, combination multi-agent chemotherapy may also be used for IAC if there is a poor response to melphalan IAC or a previous exposure to systemic chemotherapy. Melphalan is typically combined with topotecan and carboplatin for combination multi-agent IAC therapy [70]. Recent studies also show that administration of verapamil before administering melphalan increases the sensitivity of tumors to melphalan, rendering treatment more successful [79]. The limitations of IAC include the need for repeated treatments (also true for other retinoblastoma treatments) and potential lack of access to advanced neuroendovascular surgical care [80, 81]. Notably, IAC carries a small risk of stroke, retinal ischemia, retinal hemorrhage, femoral artery occlusion, and ophthalmic artery occlusion. Procedure-related ophthalmic artery occlusion may preclude additional IAC treatments. In theory, exposure to ionizing radiation during IAC may increase the risk of secondary malignancy in children with germline RB1 mutations. Overall, IAC is advantageous in treating retinoblastoma as it incurs less systemic side effects, higher rates of clinical remission, and ultimately lower risk of resistance to chemotherapy [70]. In an analysis of 70 eyes treated with IAC, the treatment was primary in 36 eyes and secondary in 34 eyes [81]. After treatment with IAC and a mean follow-up of 19 months, globe salvage was achieved in 72% of primary-treated cases and in 62% of secondary-treated cases. By the international classification of retinoblastoma, the globe salvage rate was group B (100%), group C (100%), group D (94%), and group E (36%). In the study, the combined incidence of ophthalmic, retinal, and choroidal vascular ischemia was 1%. There was no patient with stroke, seizure, neurologic impairment, limb ischemia, secondary leukemia, metastasis, or death.

8.9 Intravitreal Chemotherapy

Intravitreal chemotherapy (IVitC) is a treatment option for retinoblastoma which involves administering chemotherapy directly through the vitreous in order to achieve maximum drug concentration [82, 83]. It is used for recurrent and persistent vitreous seeds There is a risk of tumor dissemination and hence after needle withdrawal, cryotherapy is performed. Typically, melphalan or topotecan are administered intravitreally every 1–4 weeks. Munier et al. reported the first few patients with intravitreal chemotherapy with this modified technique and had a global retention rate of 87% [84]. The most common side effect of intravitreal chemotherapy is the development of RPE changes in the quadrant of injection.

8.10 Radiation

Radiation is a modality that has been used to treat retinoblastoma throughout the years. In 1931, retinoblastoma was termed a radiosensitive tumor [64]. External Beam Radiotherapy (EBRT) has been used in the past to treat retinoblastoma, but due to its lack of specificity, retinal toxicity, induction of cosmetic deformities, and ability to induce other neoplasms in individuals with hereditary disease, it is sparingly used. Sarcomas have been identified as the most common secondary malignancy to occur following EBRT [65]. There are also several reports of decreased visual acuity ranging from 5/200 to 20/50 with the use of EBRT. The most common encountered intraocular problems associated with EBRT include cataract formation, retinopathy, and optic neuropathy [66, 67]. Because of the sensitivity of radiation therapy, plaque radiation therapy was introduced as a viable option to treat retinoblastoma.

Plaque radiation therapy also known as brachytherapy is designed to give direct radiation to tumor tissue. Iodine-125 or Ruthenium-106 are the most commonly used radioactive materials for this treatment [68]. The plaques are commonly custom-made for retinoblastoma tumors consisting of several radioactive seeds that are concave to reflect the curvature of the surface of the eye. The ideal tumor candidate for this therapy is typically less than 16 mm in diameter and less than 9 mm in thickness (Fig. 8.5c, d). It is also preferred that there be no vitreous or subretinal seeding [69]. The globe salvage rate following plaque brachytherapy has been reported to be 95% [85]. The most common complications with plaque brachytherapy include radiation retinopathy and cataract.

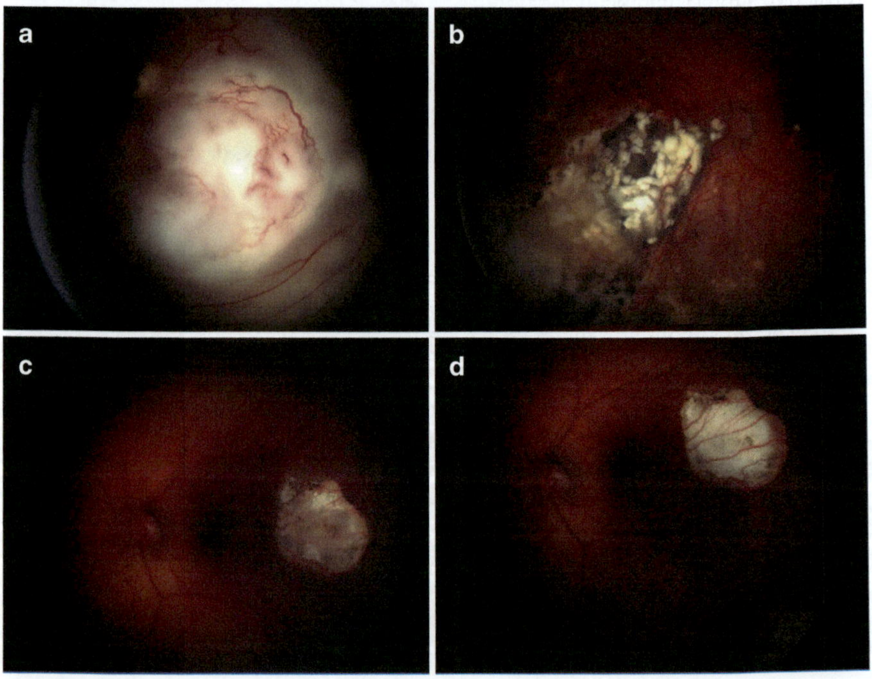

Fig. 8.5 Treatment of retinoblastoma. Large Group D retinoblastoma (**a**) treated with intra-arterial chemotherapy showing a good tumor regression (**b**). Recurrent retinoblastoma (**c**) treated with plaque brachytherapy showing a flat tumor (**d**)

8.11 Enucleation

Enucleation is the treatment of choice for advanced unilateral Group E retinoblastoma with high-risk features. Enucleation is also the treatment of choice when other therapies have failed [84, 85]. During enucleation the extraocular muscles are attached to an implant to provide symmetric ocular motility. For best cosmetic outcomes, the implant should replace 70–80% of the volume originally maintained by the enucleated eye. A prosthetic eye will then be placed on top of this implant [7, 86].

8.12 Extraocular Retinoblastoma

Orbital retinoblastoma encompasses the spectrum of primary clinical manifestation (primary), orbital recurrence following enucleation (secondary), inadvertent perforation or intraocular surgery in an eye with unsuspected retinoblastoma (accidental), intraoperative discovery of extraocular or optic nerve extension (overt), and full-thickness scleral, extrascleral, and optic nerve transection involvement on histopathology (microscopic) [87]. Extraocular retinoblastoma is generally more common in developing countries in part by decreased medical services but also the lack of comprehensive management for retinoblastoma in advanced disease [88]. Orbital invasion has a 10–27 times higher risk of systemic metastasis [89]. The treatment of orbital retinoblastoma involves a combination of high-dose chemotherapy, exenteration, and radiation therapy.

8.13 Metastatic Retinoblastoma

While uncommon in developed countries, metastatic retinoblastoma is a complication of untreated and/or advanced retinoblastoma. This occurs in less than 5% of retinoblastoma cases [90]. Unfortunately, a large majority of metastatic cases take place in developing countries due to inadequate access to medical care [2]. Metastatic disease is the leading cause of death in children with retinoblastoma. The most common sites of metastasis are CNS, bone, and bone marrow [91]. Tumor spread may occur directly via the extension of the optic nerve, or by the invasion of the choroid or orbit into nearby lymph nodes followed by hematogenous spread. Metastatic retinoblastoma is diagnosed typically with MRI and cerebrospinal fluid analysis. If there is extension into bone, bone marrow biopsies and immune-cytology are recommended [91, 92]. Treatment of metastatic retinoblastoma is usually palliative and involves chemotherapy and radiotherapy [93]. According to a study by Hu et al. the median survival time post-diagnosis of metastatic retinoblastoma is 6 months [91].

8.14 Long-Term Visual Outcomes

Recall that the goals of treatment of retinoblastoma are to eradicate tumors for survival, preserve the eye both externally and internally, and to maximize visual outcomes. Best treatment outcomes tend to stem from earlier disease presentation. In a study by Suzuki et al., the long-term visual outcomes after IAC therapy detected no severe eye damage or systemic events and for those eyes without macular involvement, visual acuity remained over 20/60 [94]. In another study, 50% of group D tumors that were salvaged via IAC, had less than 20/200 vision, 60% had strabismus, and 22% had nystagmus. This study also noted that TTT was the biggest risk factor for worsened visual outcomes [95]. While not all eyes affected by retinoblastoma can be salvaged (especially group D and E tumors), the presence of factors that may already cause diminished visual acuity should be fully understood while deciding treatment plans. If a patient already has lost visual acuity due to macular involvement, retinal detachment, or extensive seeding, salvage therapy may not be necessary as the visual outcomes will not improve. This is to be taken into consideration when determining treatment plans and counseling caretakers [96].

Patients with retinoblastoma will be monitored closely with frequent eye exams until the age of 7 [37]. Notably, most recurrences of retinoblastoma reappear within 3 years after treatment with a small likelihood of recurrence thereafter [97]. For patients with hereditary disease, close surveillance and monitoring are necessary to identify and treat secondary malignancies if they are to appear later in life [9].

Key Points

1. Retinoblastoma is the most common intraocular malignancy of childhood and is transmitted as an autosomal dominant condition.
2. Early detection is key for long-term survival and for the preservation of vision.
3. The treatment options include local therapy, systemic chemotherapy, intra-arterial chemotherapy, intravitreal chemotherapy, plaque brachytherapy, external radiation, and enucleation.
4. Patients with retinoblastoma are at a risk of second cancer and hence external radiation use must be minimized and these patients should be monitored for second malignancy.

Acknowledgment This research did not receive any specific grant from funding agencies in the public, commercial, or not-for-profit sectors.

References

1. MacCarthy A, Draper GJ, Steliarova-Foucher E, et al. Retinoblastoma incidence and survival in European children (1978–1997). Report from the Automated Childhood Cancer Information System project. Eur J Cancer. 2006;42(13):2092–102. https://doi.org/10.1016/j.ejca.2006.06.003.

2. Global Retinoblastoma Study G, Fabian ID, Abdallah E, et al. Global retinoblastoma presentation and analysis by national income level. JAMA Oncol. 2020;6(5):685–95. https://doi.org/10.1001/jamaoncol.2019.6716.
3. Kivela T. The epidemiological challenge of the most frequent eye cancer: retinoblastoma, an issue of birth and death. Br J Ophthalmol. 2009;93(9):1129–31. https://doi.org/10.1136/bjo.2008.150292.
4. Fernandes AG, Pollock BD, Rabito FA. Retinoblastoma in the United States: a 40-year incidence and survival analysis. J Pediatr Ophthalmol Strabismus. 2018;55(3):182–8. https://doi.org/10.3928/01913913-20171116-03.
5. Abramson DH, Schefler AC, Beaverson KL, et al. Rapid growth of retinoblastoma in a premature twin. Arch Ophthalmol. 2002;120(9):1232–3. https://doi.org/10.1001/archopht.120.9.1232.
6. Shah PK, Narendran V, Kalpana N. In vivo growth of retinoblastoma in a newborn infant. Indian J Ophthalmol. 2010;58(5):421–3. https://doi.org/10.4103/0301-4738.67066.
7. Dimaras H, Corson TW, Cobrinik D, et al. Retinoblastoma. Nat Rev Dis Primers. 2015;1:15021. https://doi.org/10.1038/nrdp.2015.21.
8. Lohmann DR, Gallie BL. Retinoblastoma: revisiting the model prototype of inherited cancer. Am J Med Genet C Semin Med Genet. 2004;129C(1):23–8. https://doi.org/10.1002/ajmg.c.30024.
9. Schonfeld SJ, Kleinerman RA, Abramson DH, et al. Long-term risk of subsequent cancer incidence among hereditary and nonhereditary retinoblastoma survivors. Br J Cancer. 2021;124(7):1312–9. https://doi.org/10.1038/s41416-020-01248-y.
10. Knudson AG Jr. Mutation and cancer: statistical study of retinoblastoma. Proc Natl Acad Sci U S A. 1971;68(4):820–3. https://doi.org/10.1073/pnas.68.4.820.
11. Dimaras H, Corson TW. Retinoblastoma, the visible CNS tumor: a review. J Neurosci Res. 2019;97(1):29–44. https://doi.org/10.1002/jnr.24213.
12. Friend SH, Bernards R, Rogelj S, et al. A human DNA segment with properties of the gene that predisposes to retinoblastoma and osteosarcoma. Nature. 1986;323(6089):643–6. https://doi.org/10.1038/323643a0.
13. Dryja TP, Friend S, Weinberg RA. Genetic sequences that predispose to retinoblastoma and osteosarcoma. Symp Fundam Cancer Res. 1986;39:115–9.
14. Toguchida J, McGee TL, Paterson JC, et al. Complete genomic sequence of the human retinoblastoma susceptibility gene. Genomics. 1993;17(3):535–43. https://doi.org/10.1006/geno.1993.1368.
15. Engeland K. Cell cycle arrest through indirect transcriptional repression by p53: I have a DREAM. Cell Death Differ. 2018;25(1):114–32. https://doi.org/10.1038/cdd.2017.172.
16. Dyson NJ. RB1: a prototype tumor suppressor and an enigma. Genes Dev. 2016;30(13):1492–502. https://doi.org/10.1101/gad.282145.116.
17. McEvoy J, Nagahawatte P, Finkelstein D, et al. RB1 gene inactivation by chromothripsis in human retinoblastoma. Oncotarget. 2014;5(2):438–50. https://doi.org/10.18632/oncotarget.1686.
18. Kaewkhaw R, Rojanaporn D. Retinoblastoma: etiology, modeling, and treatment. Cancers (Basel). 2020;12(8) https://doi.org/10.3390/cancers12082304.
19. Dryja TP, Morrow JF, Rapaport JM. Quantification of the paternal allele bias for new germline mutations in the retinoblastoma gene. Hum Genet. 1997;100(3–4):446–9. https://doi.org/10.1007/s004390050531.
20. Knudson AG. Antioncogenes and human cancer. Proc Natl Acad Sci U S A. 1993; 90(23):10914–21. https://doi.org/10.1073/pnas.90.23.10914.
21. Nichols KE, Houseknecht MD, Godmilow L, et al. Sensitive multistep clinical molecular screening of 180 unrelated individuals with retinoblastoma detects 36 novel mutations in the RB1 gene. Hum Mutat. 2005;25(6):566–74. https://doi.org/10.1002/humu.20184.
22. Richter S, Vandezande K, Chen N, et al. Sensitive and efficient detection of RB1 gene mutations enhances care for families with retinoblastoma. Am J Hum Genet. 2003;72(2):253–69. https://doi.org/10.1086/345651.

23. Ahmad NN, Melo MB, Singh AD, et al. A possible hot spot in exon 21 of the retinoblastoma gene predisposing to a low penetrant retinoblastoma phenotype? Ophthalmic Genet. 1999;20(4):225–31. https://doi.org/10.1076/opge.20.4.225.2269.
24. Cowell JK, Bia B, Akoulitchev A. A novel mutation in the promotor region in a family with a mild form of retinoblastoma indicates the location of a new regulatory domain for the RB1 gene. Oncogene. 1996;12(2):431–6.
25. Cowell JK, Cragg H. Constitutional nonsense germline mutations in the RB1 gene detected in patients with early onset unilateral retinoblastoma. Eur J Cancer. 1996;32A(10):1749–52. https://doi.org/10.1016/0959-8049(96)00201-8.
26. Yilmaz S, Horsthemke B, Lohmann DR. Twelve novel RB1 gene mutations in patients with hereditary retinoblastoma. Mutations in brief no. 206. Online. Hum Mutat. 1998;12(6):434. https://doi.org/10.1002/(SICI)1098-1004(1998)12:6<434::AID-HUMU16>3.0.CO;2-7.
27. Skalet AH, Gombos DS, Gallie BL, et al. Screening children at risk for retinoblastoma: consensus report from the American Association of Ophthalmic Oncologists and Pathologists. Ophthalmology. 2018;125(3):453–8. https://doi.org/10.1016/j.ophtha.2017.09.001.
28. Soliman SE, Dimaras H, Khetan V, et al. Prenatal versus postnatal screening for familial retinoblastoma. Ophthalmology. 2016;123(12):2610–7. https://doi.org/10.1016/j.ophtha.2016.08.027.
29. Schofield D, Zeppel MJB, Staffieri S, et al. Preimplantation genetic diagnosis for retinoblastoma survivors: a cost-effectiveness study. Reprod Biomed Soc Online. 2020;10:37–45. https://doi.org/10.1016/j.rbms.2020.03.001.
30. Fang X, Wang H, Ma X, et al. Clinical features of children with retinoblastoma and Neuroblastoma. J Ophthalmol. 2020;2020:9315784. https://doi.org/10.1155/2020/9315784.
31. Soliman SE, Eldomiaty W, Goweida MB, et al. Clinical presentation of retinoblastoma in Alexandria: a step toward earlier diagnosis. Saudi J Ophthalmol. 2017;31(2):80–5. https://doi.org/10.1016/j.sjopt.2017.03.003.
32. Shields JA, Shields CL. Intraocular tumors: an atlas and textbook. 3rd edition ed. 2015. Lippincott Williams & Wilkins (LWW).
33. Dikkaya F, Sarıcı AM, Erbek F, et al. Evaluation of high-risk features of primary enucleation of patients with retinoblastoma in a tertiary center of a developing country in the era of intra-arterial chemotherapy. Int Ophthalmol. 2018;38(1):151–6. https://doi.org/10.1007/s10792-016-0436-8.
34. Nawaiseh I, Al-Hussaini M, Alhamwi A, et al. The impact of growth patterns of retinoblastoma (endophytic, exophytic, and mixed patterns). Turk Patoloji Derg. 2015;31(1):45–50. https://doi.org/10.5146/tjpath.2014.01278.
35. Linn MA. Intraocular retinoblastoma: the case for a new group classification. Ophthalmol Clin North Am. 2005;18(1):41–53, viii. https://doi.org/10.1016/j.ohc.2004.11.003.
36. Shields CL, Shields JA. Basic understanding of current classification and management of retinoblastoma. Curr Opin Ophthalmol. 2006;17(3):228–34. https://doi.org/10.1097/01.icu.0000193079.55240.18.
37. Ancona-Lezama D, Dalvin LA, Shields CL. Modern treatment of retinoblastoma: a 2020 review. Indian J Ophthalmol. 2020;68(11):2356–65. https://doi.org/10.4103/ijo.IJO_721_20.
38. Chantada GL, Doz F, Orjuela M, et al. World disparities in risk definition and management of retinoblastoma: a report from the international retinoblastoma staging working group. Pediatr Blood Cancer. 2008;50(3):692–4. https://doi.org/10.1002/pbc.21427.
39. Kaliki S, Srinivasan V, Gupta A, et al. Clinical features predictive of high-risk retinoblastoma in 403 Asian Indian patients: a case-control study. Ophthalmology. 2015;122(6):1165–72. https://doi.org/10.1016/j.ophtha.2015.01.018.
40. Kaliki S, Shields CL, Shah SU, et al. Postenucleation adjuvant chemotherapy with vincristine, etoposide, and carboplatin for the treatment of high-risk retinoblastoma. Arch Ophthalmol. 2011;129(11):1422–7. https://doi.org/10.1001/archophthalmol.2011.289.
41. Ghassemi F, Bazvand F, Makateb A. Lesions simulating retinoblastoma at a tertiary care center. J Ophthalmic Vis Res. 2015;10(3):316–9. https://doi.org/10.4103/2008-322x.170351.

42. Huang S, Rutar T, Bloomer M, et al. Analysis of clinical misdiagnoses in children treated with enucleation. Arch Ophthalmol. 2010;128(8):1009–13. https://doi.org/10.1001/archophthalmol.2010.153.
43. Callaway NF, Mruthyunjaya P. Widefield imaging of retinal and choroidal tumors. Int J Retina Vitreous. 2019;5(Suppl 1):49. https://doi.org/10.1186/s40942-019-0196-5.
44. Kim JW, Ngai LK, Sadda S, et al. Retcam fluorescein angiography findings in eyes with advanced retinoblastoma. Br J Ophthalmol. 2014;98(12):1666–71. https://doi.org/10.1136/bjophthalmol-2014-305180.
45. National Retinoblastoma Strategy Canadian Guidelines for Care. Stratégie thérapeutique du rétinoblastome guide clinique canadien. Can J Ophthalmol. 2009;44(Suppl 2):S1–88. https://doi.org/10.3129/i09-194.
46. Kendall CJ, Prager TC, Cheng H, et al. Diagnostic ophthalmic ultrasound for radiologists. Neuroimaging Clin N Am. 2015;25(3):327–65. https://doi.org/10.1016/j.nic.2015.05.001.
47. Vasquez LM, Giuliari GP, Halliday W, et al. Ultrasound biomicroscopy in the management of retinoblastoma. Eye (Lond). 2011;25(2):141–7. https://doi.org/10.1038/eye.2010.193.
48. Fujimoto J, Swanson E. The development, commercialization, and impact of optical coherence tomography. Invest Ophthalmol Vis Sci. 2016;57(9):OCT1–OCT13. https://doi.org/10.1167/iovs.16-19963.
49. Soliman SE, VandenHoven C, MacKeen LD, et al. Optical coherence tomography-guided decisions in retinoblastoma management. Ophthalmology. 2017;124(6):859–72. https://doi.org/10.1016/j.ophtha.2017.01.052.
50. Rootman DB, Gonzalez E, Mallipatna A, et al. Hand-held high-resolution spectral domain optical coherence tomography in retinoblastoma: clinical and morphologic considerations. Br J Ophthalmol. 2013;97(1):59–65. https://doi.org/10.1136/bjophthalmol-2012-302133.
51. Cao C, Markovitz M, Ferenczy S, et al. Hand-held spectral-domain optical coherence tomography of small macular retinoblastoma in infants before and after chemotherapy. J Pediatr Ophthalmol Strabismus. 2014;51(4):230–4. https://doi.org/10.3928/01913913-20140603-01.
52. Samara WA, Pointdujour-Lim R, Say EA, et al. Foveal microanatomy documented by SD-OCT following treatment of advanced retinoblastoma. J AAPOS. 2015;19(4):368–72. https://doi.org/10.1016/j.jaapos.2015.02.019.
53. Razek AA, Elkhamary S. MRI of retinoblastoma. Br J Radiol. 2011;84(1005):775–84. https://doi.org/10.1259/bjr/32022497.
54. Cho SJ, Kim JH, Baik SH, et al. Diagnostic performance of MRI of post-laminar optic nerve invasion detection in retinoblastoma: a systematic review and meta-analysis. Neuroradiology. 2021;63(4):499–509. https://doi.org/10.1007/s00234-020-02538-1.
55. Chen S, Ji X, Liu M, et al. The value of MRI in evaluating the efficacy and complications with the treatment of intra-arterial chemotherapy for retinoblastoma. Oncotarget. 2017;8(24):38413–25. https://doi.org/10.18632/oncotarget.16423.
56. Kamihara J, Bourdeaut F, Foulkes WD, et al. Retinoblastoma and neuroblastoma predisposition and surveillance. Clin Cancer Res. 2017;23(13):e98–e106. https://doi.org/10.1158/1078-0432.Ccr-17-0652.
57. Murphree AL, Villablanca JG, Deegan WF 3rd, et al. Chemotherapy plus local treatment in the management of intraocular retinoblastoma. Arch Ophthalmol. 1996;114(11):1348–56. https://doi.org/10.1001/archopht.1996.01100140548005.
58. Gallie BL, Budning A, DeBoer G, et al. Chemotherapy with focal therapy can cure intraocular retinoblastoma without radiotherapy. Arch Ophthalmol. 1996;114(11):1321–8. https://doi.org/10.1001/archopht.1996.01100140521001.
59. Shields CL, Lally SE, Leahey AM, et al. Targeted retinoblastoma management: when to use intravenous, intra-arterial, periocular, and intravitreal chemotherapy. Curr Opin Ophthalmol. 2014;25(5):374–85. https://doi.org/10.1097/icu.0000000000000091.
60. Cohen VM, Kingston J, Hungerford JL. The success of primary chemotherapy for group D heritable retinoblastoma. Br J Ophthalmol. 2009;93(7):887–90. https://doi.org/10.1136/bjo.2008.142679.

61. Soliman S, Feng ZX, Gallie B. Primary laser therapy as monotherapy for discrete retinoblastoma. Br J Ophthalmol. 2021; https://doi.org/10.1136/bjophthalmol-2020-317885.
62. Ibarra MS, Hsu J, Mirza N, et al. Retinal temperature increase during transpupillary thermotherapy: effects of pigmentation, subretinal blood, and choroidal blood flow. Invest Ophthalmol Vis Sci. 2004;45(10):3678–82. https://doi.org/10.1167/iovs.04-0436.
63. Lumbroso-Le Rouic L, Aerts I, Hajage D, et al. Conservative treatment of retinoblastoma: a prospective phase II randomized trial of neoadjuvant chemotherapy followed by local treatments and chemothermotherapy. Eye (Lond). 2016;30(1):46–52. https://doi.org/10.1038/eye.2015.179.
64. Moore RF, Stallard HB, Milner JG. Retinal gliomata treated by radon seeds. Br J Ophthalmol. 1931;15(12):673–96. https://doi.org/10.1136/bjo.15.12.673.
65. Ketteler P, Hülsenbeck I, Frank M, et al. The impact of RB1 genotype on incidence of second tumours in heritable retinoblastoma. Eur J Cancer. 2020;133:47–55. https://doi.org/10.1016/j.ejca.2020.04.005.
66. Chan MP, Hungerford JL, Kingston JE, et al. Salvage external beam radiotherapy after failed primary chemotherapy for bilateral retinoblastoma: rate of eye and vision preservation. Br J Ophthalmol. 2009;93(7):891–4. https://doi.org/10.1136/bjo.2007.129981.
67. Kim JY, Park Y. Treatment of retinoblastoma: the role of external beam radiotherapy. Yonsei Med J. 2015;56(6):1478–91. https://doi.org/10.3349/ymj.2015.56.6.1478.
68. Echegaray JJ, Al-Zahrani YA, Singh A. Episcleral brachytherapy for retinoblastoma. Br J Ophthalmol. 2020;104(2):208–13. https://doi.org/10.1136/bjophthalmol-2019-313985.
69. Shields CL, Shields JA, De Potter P, et al. Plaque radiotherapy for retinoblastoma. Int Ophthalmol Clin. 1993;33(3):107–18. https://doi.org/10.1097/00004397-199303330-00016.
70. Manjandavida FP, Stathopoulos C, Zhang J, et al. Intra-arterial chemotherapy in retinoblastoma - a paradigm change. Indian J Ophthalmol. 2019;67(6):740–54. https://doi.org/10.4103/ijo.IJO_866_19.
71. Wyse E, Handa JT, Friedman AD, et al. A review of the literature for intra-arterial chemotherapy used to treat retinoblastoma. Pediatr Radiol. 2016;46(9):1223–33. https://doi.org/10.1007/s00247-016-3554-6.
72. Dilenge D, Ascherl GF Jr. Variations of the ophthalmic and middle meningeal arteries: relation to the embryonic stapedial artery. AJNR Am J Neuroradiol. 1980;1(1):45–54.
73. Shields CL, Ramasubramanian A, Rosenwasser R, et al. Superselective catheterization of the ophthalmic artery for intraarterial chemotherapy for retinoblastoma. Retina. 2009;29(8):1207–9. https://doi.org/10.1097/IAE.0b013e3181b4ce39.
74. Abruzzo T, Patino M, Leach J, et al. Cerebral vasoconstriction triggered by sympathomimetic drugs during intra-arterial chemotherapy. Pediatr Neurol. 2013;48(2):139–42. https://doi.org/10.1016/j.pediatrneurol.2012.10.005.
75. Abruzzo TA, Geller JI, Kimbrough DA, et al. Adjunctive techniques for optimization of ocular hemodynamics in children undergoing ophthalmic artery infusion chemotherapy. J Neurointerv Surg. 2015;7(10):770–6. https://doi.org/10.1136/neurintsurg-2014-011295.
76. Yamane T, Kaneko A, Mohri M. The technique of ophthalmic arterial infusion therapy for patients with intraocular retinoblastoma. Int J Clin Oncol. 2004;9(2):69–73. https://doi.org/10.1007/s10147-004-0392-6.
77. Inomata M, Kaneko A. In vitro chemosensitivity assays of retinoblastoma cells. Int J Clin Oncol. 2004;9(1):31–5. https://doi.org/10.1007/s10147-003-0370-4.
78. Daniels AB, Froehler MT, Pierce JM, et al. Pharmacokinetics, tissue localization, toxicity, and treatment efficacy in the first small animal (rabbit) model of intra-arterial chemotherapy for retinoblastoma. Invest Ophthalmol Vis Sci. 2018;59(1):446–54. https://doi.org/10.1167/iovs.17-22302.
79. Abruzzo T, Abraham K, Karani KB, et al. Correlation of technical and adjunctive factors with quantitative tumor reduction in children undergoing selective ophthalmic artery infusion chemotherapy for retinoblastoma. AJNR Am J Neuroradiol. 2021;42(2):354–61. https://doi.org/10.3174/ajnr.A6905.

80. Rishi P, Sharma T, Sharma M, et al. Intra-arterial chemotherapy for retinoblastoma: two-year results from tertiary eye-care center in India. Indian J Ophthalmol. 2017;65(4):311–5. https://doi.org/10.4103/ijo.IJO_843_16.
81. Shields CL, Manjandavida FP, Lally SE, et al. Intra-arterial chemotherapy for retinoblastoma in 70 eyes: outcomes based on the international classification of retinoblastoma. Ophthalmology. 2014;121(7):1453–60. https://doi.org/10.1016/j.ophtha.2014.01.026.
82. Manjandavida FP, Shields CL. The role of intravitreal chemotherapy for retinoblastoma. Indian J Ophthalmol. 2015;63(2):141–5. https://doi.org/10.4103/0301-4738.154390.
83. Shields CL, Alset AE, Say EA, et al. Retinoblastoma control with primary intra-arterial chemotherapy: outcomes before and during the intravitreal chemotherapy era. J Pediatr Ophthalmol Strabismus. 2016;53(5):275–84. https://doi.org/10.3928/01913913-20160719-04.
84. Munier FL, Gaillard MC, Balmer A, Soliman S, Podilsky G, Moulin AP, Beck-Popovic M. Intravitreal chemotherapy for vitreous disease in retinoblastoma revisited: from prohibition to conditional indications. Br J Ophthalmol. 2012 Aug;96(8):1078–83.
85. Shields CL, Mashayekhi A, Sun H, Uysal Y, Friere J, Komarnicky L, Shields JA. Iodine 125 plaque radiotherapy as salvage treatment for retinoblastoma recurrence after chemoreduction in 84 tumors. Ophthalmology. 2006;113(11):2087–92.
86. Shah V, Yadav L, Singh M, et al. Custom ocular prosthesis in rehabilitation of a child operated for retinoblastoma. Natl J Maxillofac Surg. 2015;6(2):232–6. https://doi.org/10.4103/0975-5950.183871.
87. Honavar SG, Manjandavida FP, Reddy VAP. Orbital retinoblastoma: an update. Indian J Ophthalmol. 2017;65(6):435–42. https://doi.org/10.4103/ijo.IJO_352_15.
88. The Committee for the National Registry of Retinoblastoma. Survival rate and risk factors for patients with retinoblastoma in Japan. Jpn J Ophthalmol. 1992;36(2):121–31.
89. Friedman DN, Sklar CA, Oeffinger KC, et al. Long-term medical outcomes in survivors of extra-ocular retinoblastoma: the Memorial Sloan-Kettering Cancer Center (MSKCC) experience. Pediatr Blood Cancer. 2013;60(4):694–9. https://doi.org/10.1002/pbc.24280.
90. Berry JL, Kogachi K, Aziz HA, et al. Risk of metastasis and orbital recurrence in advanced retinoblastoma eyes treated with systemic chemoreduction versus primary enucleation. Pediatr Blood Cancer. 2017;64(4) https://doi.org/10.1002/pbc.26270.
91. Hu H, Zhang W, Wang Y, et al. Characterization, treatment and prognosis of retinoblastoma with central nervous system metastasis. BMC Ophthalmol. 2018;18(1):107. https://doi.org/10.1186/s12886-018-0772-8.
92. Chantada GL, Sampor C, Bosaleh A, et al. Comparison of staging systems for extraocular retinoblastoma: analysis of 533 patients. JAMA Ophthalmol. 2013;131(9):1127–34. https://doi.org/10.1001/jamaophthalmol.2013.260.
93. Dunkel IJ, Khakoo Y, Kernan NA, et al. Intensive multimodality therapy for patients with stage 4a metastatic retinoblastoma. Pediatr Blood Cancer. 2010;55(1):55–9. https://doi.org/10.1002/pbc.22504.
94. Suzuki S, Yamane T, Mohri M, et al. Selective ophthalmic arterial injection therapy for intraocular retinoblastoma: the long-term prognosis. Ophthalmology. 2011;118(10):2081–7. https://doi.org/10.1016/j.ophtha.2011.03.013.
95. Fabian ID, Naeem Z, Stacey AW, et al. Long-term visual acuity, strabismus, and nystagmus outcomes following multimodality treatment in group D retinoblastoma eyes. Am J Ophthalmol. 2017;179:137–44. https://doi.org/10.1016/j.ajo.2017.05.003.
96. Berry JL, Jubran R, Wong K, et al. Factors predictive of long-term visual outcomes of group D eyes treated with chemoreduction and low-dose IMRT salvage: the Children's Hospital Los Angeles experience. Br J Ophthalmol. 2014;98(8):1061–5. https://doi.org/10.1136/bjophthalmol-2013-304411.
97. Shah SU, Shields CL, Lally SE, et al. Hydroxyapatite orbital implant in children following enucleation: analysis of 531 sockets. Ophthalmic Plast Reconstr Surg. 2015;31(2):108–14. https://doi.org/10.1097/iop.0000000000000207.

Pseudotumor Cerebri Syndrome in Children: Current Diagnosis and Treatment

9

Ryan Gise, Eric D. Gaier, and Gena Heidary

9.1 Introduction

Suspicion of papilledema or swelling of the optic nerves from elevated intracranial pressure (ICP) is a common reason for referral to pediatric neuro-ophthalmology. The pediatric neuro-ophthalmologist is tasked with confirming the presence or absence of papilledema and if present, determining the next steps in evaluation and management. Increased ICP, in the absence of a mass, has been labeled pseudotumor cerebri syndrome [1–4]. This designation encompasses idiopathic intracranial hypertension (IIH; used interchangeably with primary pseudotumor cerebri syndrome in this chapter) as well as elevated ICP secondary to etiologies including exposure to certain medications, in association with underlying systemic disease, and cerebral venous system abnormalities. This chapter outlines the epidemiology, pathophysiology, and etiologies of pseudotumor cerebri syndrome (PTCS). Further, this chapter reviews the most recent diagnostic criteria, disease monitoring methods, treatment approaches, and visual outcomes for PTCS. Having a systematic strategy in place to evaluate patients with papilledema and presumed pseudotumor cerebri is crucial for the timely identification of an underlying etiology, if present, and for the prevention of visual loss with effective treatment.

R. Gise · G. Heidary (✉)
Department of Ophthalmology, Boston Children's Hospital, Boston, MA, USA

Harvard Medical School, Boston, MA, USA
e-mail: Ryan.Gise@Childrens.harvard.edu; Gena.Heidary@Childrens.harvard.edu

E. D. Gaier
Department of Ophthalmology, Boston Children's Hospital, Boston, MA, USA

Harvard Medical School, Boston, MA, USA

Picower Institute for Learning and Memory, Massachusetts Institute of Technology, Boston, MA, USA
e-mail: Eric.Gaier@Childrens.harvard.edu

A. Ramasubramanian (ed.), *Pediatric Ophthalmology*, Current Practices in Ophthalmology, https://doi.org/10.1007/978-981-19-4963-0_9

9.2 Epidemiology

The incidence of IIH in the pediatric population (<18 years of age) has been estimated at 0.63–0.90 per 100,000 children [5–7]. This is similar to estimates for IIH in the general adult population estimated at 0.9 per 100,000 [8]. Within the traditional IIH demographic of obese women aged 20–44 years, the incidence rises to 19.3 per 100,000 [8]. By contrast, the demographics of pediatric IIH vary depending on age and pubertal status. There is a predilection for obese females in the pubertal population, but prepubertal children demonstrate equal proportions of male and female patients [4]. Notably, these estimates do not include cases of secondary pseudotumor cerebri syndrome, only those of an idiopathic etiology.

The interplay between pubertal status and obesity in the incidence of IIH has been highlighted in several studies. Tepe et al. performed a prospective study where the authors performed ophthalmologic exams on 1058 obese children, uncovering 14 cases of IIH (prevalence of 1.3%). Considering pubertal status as defined by Tanner stage, the prevalence among postpubertal subjects was 1.5% vs. 0.9% in prepubertal subjects [9]. Sheldon et al. performed a multicenter retrospective review of 233 pediatric IIH cases. While they found associations between age and body mass index (BMI) in both boys and girls, the likelihood of obesity among patients increased when among those diagnosed at age 12 on average [10]. They highlighted three specific subgroups of pediatric patients: a preadolescent group that was younger and had no association with weight, an early adolescent group that tended to be overweight or obese, and a late adolescent group that tended to be more obese similar to the adult phenotype [10]. These anthropomorphic features of pediatric IIH are corroborated by other studies demonstrating that obesity is a risk factor for IIH in and after puberty [11, 12]. Brara et al. found that among children between the ages of 11 and 19, the risk of developing IIH was much higher in overweight and obese children [13]. While these studies agree that the important risk factor of obesity depends on age, and/or pubertal status, only a prospective study with detailed pubertal staging will allow us to reliably define the anthropomorphic features of pediatric IIH.

The important role of pubertal status in governing the prevalence and features of IIH intuitively suggests a potential hormonal role in IIH pathogenesis. Notably, endocrine disorders such as Addison's disease, hypoparathyroidism, adrenal insufficiency, and hypo/hyperthyroidism as well as exogenous growth hormone use have been associated with secondary pseudotumor cerebri syndrome [1, 3, 14, 15]. Tepe et al. found that 14 obese patients with IIH had evidence of metabolic syndrome, including transaminitis, evidence of insulin resistance, elevated cortisol, and fasting insulin levels [9]. Cerebrospinal fluid production may be influenced by metabolic and hormonal signaling [16, 17], suggesting a potential direct role for hormonal dysregulation in intracranial hypertension. However, no single hormonal factor has been identified as causative in pediatric or adult IIH. Future research in this area is warranted which could potentially enable the identification of at-risk individuals by serologic testing.

9.3 Symptoms

Symptoms of pseudotumor cerebri syndrome reflect those secondary to elevated ICP including headache (often positional), transient visual obscurations, pulsatile tinnitus, and binocular diplopia. While the spectrum of symptomology is similar between children and adults, pediatrics poses added diagnostic challenges in teasing out these symptoms. Depending on patient age, the children may not be able to specifically or accurately express symptoms as well as their adult counterparts. As such, the predictive values of typical symptoms are lower in children than in adults.

Pediatric patients may present without the classic symptoms of elevated ICP. Aylward et al. performed a retrospective review of 152 patients with pseudotumor cerebri syndrome and found that 14.5% did not endorse headaches [18]. This group was younger (mean age 9.7 without headache vs. 13.4 years with headache) and less likely to be overweight or obese. Importantly, cerebral spinal fluid opening pressures on lumbar puncture were not different between these groups [18]. Among patients with secondary pseudotumor syndrome in this study, 35/37 patients (95%) reported headaches. The authors did not specifically comment on the age of patients with secondary pseudotumor cerebri and if that may have influenced symptomology. Glatstein et al. retrospectively evaluated patients younger than 17 who presented to a tertiary care hospital emergency department over an 8-year period and were subsequently diagnosed with IIH. Of the 63 patients that were identified, 47(75%) presented with headaches. Headache was less common in children <11 years of age compared to those in the 11–17-year-old group [11]. Thus, headache is less commonly reported among pediatric patients with pseudotumor cerebri syndrome, particularly among younger children.

Pediatric patients may present entirely without symptoms. In their study, Ayward et al. noted that 8/22 (36%) patients were referred because of incidental discovery of papilledema during a routine eye exam [18]. Bassan et al. evaluated 45 pediatric patients with IIH and found that 14 (31%) were asymptomatic. As in the aforementioned studies, asymptomatic patients were younger and less likely to be obese. They also noted a male predominance (10/14, 71%) in the asymptomatic group [19]. A retrospective review of 86 patients with PTCS at Boston Children's Hospital found that 21% were asymptomatic. Asymptomatic patients were more likely to be younger and have lower body mass indices compared to symptomatic patients [20]. Thus, the literature is consistent in showing that a significant population of IIH patients are asymptomatic (may be discovered incidentally) and that these patients tend to be younger.

Secondary pseudotumor cerebri patients can also present with or without symptoms. To our knowledge, no study has examined potential differences in symptomology between primary and secondary pseudotumor cerebri syndrome specifically in children. Orme et al. evaluated adult patients with pseudotumor cerebri syndrome secondary to tetracycline use and compared the clinical features to traditional IIH patients. They found that patients with tetracycline-induced pseudotumor cerebri were less likely to be obese (43.8% vs. 79.2%) and were more likely to present with double vision [21]. There was no statistically significant difference in the rate of headaches reported at presentation between the two groups. The disease course was shorter in the secondary pseudotumor cerebri patients (mean duration of 18.3 weeks vs. 62.9 weeks) and the risk of recurrence was higher in the IIH group (16.5% vs. 4.0%) [21]. Liu et al. evaluated 65 patients of all ages who presented with cerebral venous sinus thrombosis and found 87.7% of patients presented with headache and 23.1% with pulsatile tinnitus [22]. As mentioned previously, Aylward et al. included 37 pediatric patients with secondary pseudotumor cerebri syndrome and 35/37 (95%) had headache on presentation. Secondary pseudotumor seems more likely to present with headache in children but this is an area that needs further explanation as it has not been evaluated based on age or pubertal status in children [18]. Clinicians should have a high index of suspicion for secondary causes in prepubertal patients who present with symptoms of elevated ICP.

9.4 Diagnosis

9.4.1 Examination

Findings on ophthalmic examination of pediatric patients are identical to those of adults with pseudotumor cerebri syndrome, including papilledema with or without afferent visual dysfunction (decreased vision, visual field defects, and dyschromatopsia) and abduction limitations with esotropia (Figs. 9.1 and 9.2) [1, 3]. Comprehensive neuro-ophthalmic examination and testing are essential in the evaluation of suspected elevated ICP so that more malignant presentations can be identified. For example, patients presenting with fulminant IIH are at risk for serious visual morbidity if not treated quickly and aggressively [23]. Fulminant IIH is defined as an acute development of symptoms of increased ICP with rapidly progressive vision loss within 4 weeks of symptom onset and in the setting meeting clinical criteria for IIH. Thambisetty et al. described 16 cases of fulminant idiopathic intracranial hypertension in patients ranging in age from 14 to 39 who presented with acute symptoms (mean onset 16.1 days) and suffered subsequent irreversible vision loss within 4 weeks of symptom onset. Aggressive interventions included multiple lumbar punctures, and optic nerve sheath fenestration or CSF diversion in 11/16 patients. Despite these measures, all were left with severe, bilateral visual field deficits and 8/16 (50%) remained legally blind [23].

Although papilledema ICP is a hallmark ICP examination finding, its absence does not preclude the diagnosis of pseudotumor cerebri syndrome [1]. A subset of pediatric patients with PTCS may present without papilledema, just as in adults. Aylward et al. noted that 27/152 (17.8%) patients in their retrospective review did not have papilledema. Comparing features of those with and without papilledema, they found no differences in age, body mass indices, or opening pressure on lumbar puncture [24]. Glatstein et al. reported a similar proportion (12/63, 19%) of IIH patients presenting to the emergency department did not have papilledema. Patients with secondary pseudotumor cerebri syndrome can also present without

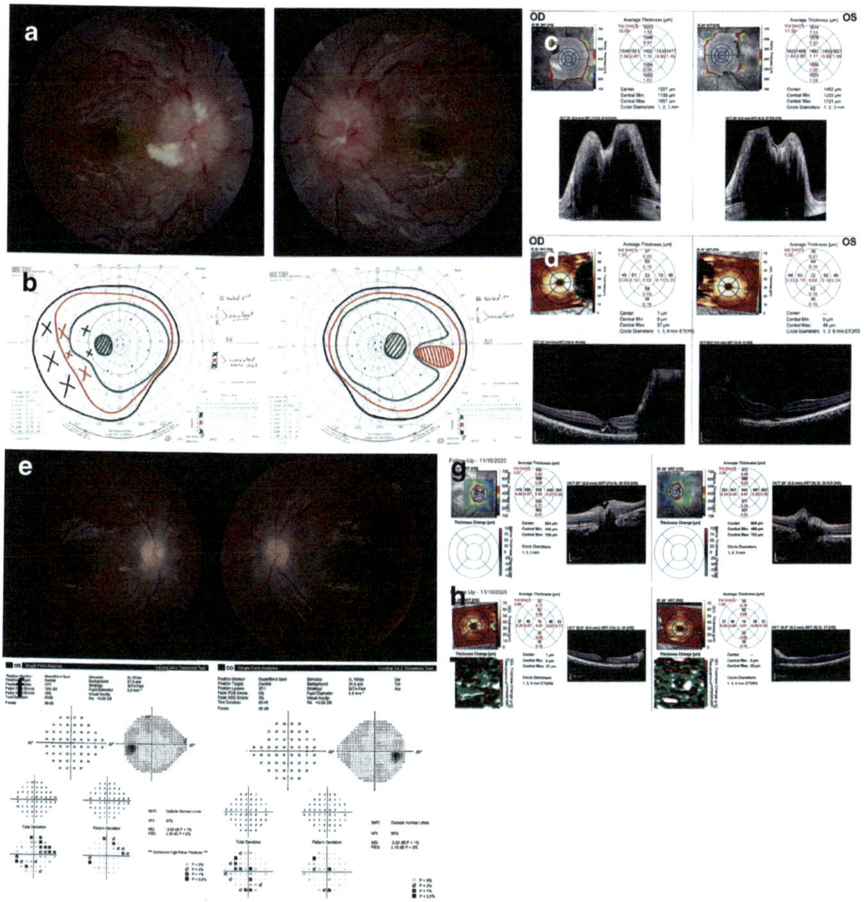

Fig. 9.1 This is a representative case of a 14-year old obese African American female who presented with 3 weeks of progressive headaches and one episode of vomiting. She reported that the headaches would wake her from sleep at times and transient visual obscurations. MRI brain without contrast and MRV were notable for protrusion of the optic nerve head papillae into the globes in both eyes, distention of the optic nerve sheaths, and a partially empty sella. Lumbar puncture with opening pressure revealed bland constituents and an opening pressure of 36 cm H_2O. Visual acuity, pupils, and color vision were normal. She had grade 5 papilledema in both eyes with cotton wool spots. (**a**) She was unable to accurately take an automated perimetry test and kinetic perimetry revealed enlarged blind spots in both eyes. The right eye had a temporal scotoma that was felt to be an extension of the enlarged blind spot (**b**) Her optic nerve head volume was unable to completely capture the degree of swelling. (**c**) Her ganglion cell layer was unable to be properly segmented given the swelling and she had subfoveal fluid in both eyes as well as cystic intraretinal edema in the right eye. (**d**) She was treated aggressively with acetazolamide which was increased to 2 g total per day (24.8 mg/kg/day). She developed a significant and symptomatic metabolic acidosis and was started on sodium bicarbonate supplementation. She was monitored initially twice weekly and then this was slowly spaced out as a concern for vision loss dissipated. On follow-up 2 months later, her optic disc edema had essentially resolved and she was left with significant gliosis in both eyes (**e**). Her visual acuity, color vision, and pupils remained normal. She improved on her ability to take automated visual fields and now there were only scattered nonspecific defects though the left eye reliability was borderline. (**f**) Her optic disc edema had dramatically improved and her optic nerve head volume had returned to essentially normal. (**g**) Her OCT GCL was now low normal indicating some ganglion cell layer loss that was not visually significant (**h**)

papilledema. Liu et al. performed a retrospective multicenter evaluation of adult and pediatric patients with cerebral venous sinus thrombosis and found that only 35/65 (54%) presented with papilledema, though it later manifested in the remainder of patients [22]. Thus, the absence of papilledema should not be considered as an exclusive feature in the diagnosis of pseudotumor cerebri.

The presence of pseudopapilledema can raise concern for and even confound a diagnosis of pseudotumor cerebri syndrome [25]. Pseudopapilledema, caused by optic nerve head drusen and hyperopia, for example, commonly drive referrals to

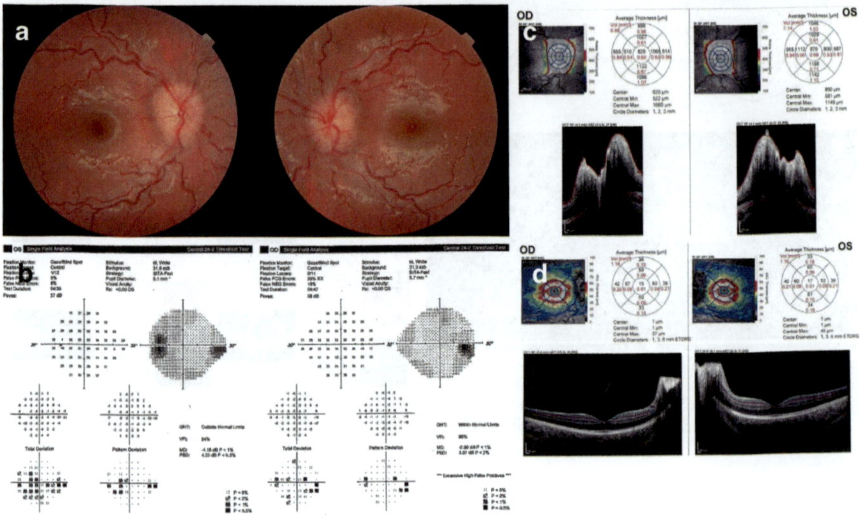

Fig. 9.2 A representative case of a thin, Caucasian 10-year-old girl who presented to the Emergency Department due to worsening headaches. She started to develop headaches, neck pain, and diplopia that progressively worsened over a 3-week period. She had an MRI brain without contrast and MRV that was notable for a partially empty sella, protrusion of the optic nerve heads into the globes, and focal narrowing of the dominant right transverse venous sinus. She had a lumbar puncture performed and her opening pressure was 25 cm H_2O with bland constituents. She was started on acetazolamide in the setting of a borderline opening pressure with other clear signs of increased intracranial pressure. Given the history of headaches, neck pain, and diplopia in the setting of her nontoxic appearance and the fact that she did not fit the typical body habitus for IIH, it was thought that she likely had viral meningitis leading to increased intracranial pressure. On her initial exam, she had normal afferent visual function and bilateral Frisen grade 3 papilledema. (**a**) Her automated perimetry demonstrated an enlarged blind spot bilaterally. (**b**) There is poor reliability of the right eye due to high false positives and this probably served to blunt the presentation of the enlarged blind spot in that eye. The left eye also has a hint of an early nasal step. The optic nerve head volume demonstrates marked elevation in both eyes. (**c**) The ganglion cell layer for both eyes shows no evidence of atrophy in either eye. (**d**) She was started on acetazolamide and had profuse vomiting after each dose. She was transitioned to topiramate and gradually increased to a goal dose of 50 mg twice daily which is approximately 1.5 mg/kg/day). Three months later fundus photography demonstrates resolution of papilledema. (**e**) Her visual fields had normalized with only a hint of an enlarged blind spot in the left eye (**f**). OCT RNFL (**g**) was now performed given the resolution of the edema and her OCT ganglion cell layer (**h**) remained within normal limits though slightly lower than it had been on presentation

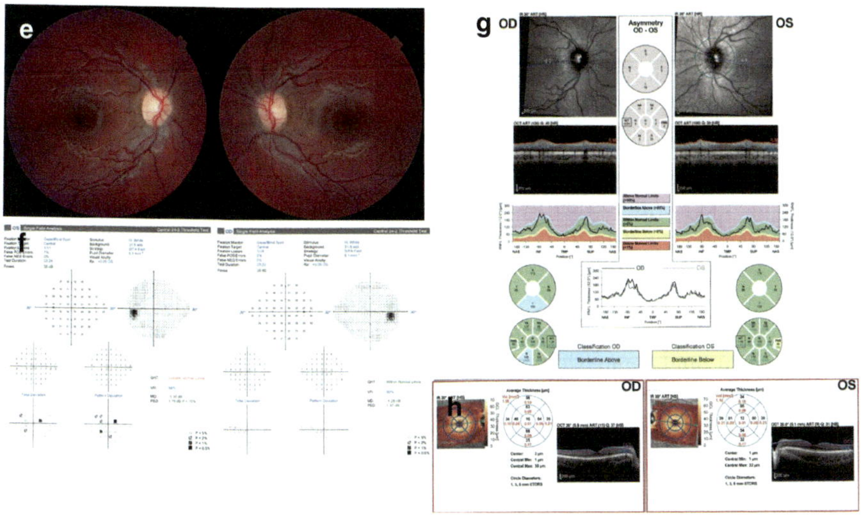

Fig. 9.2 (continued)

pediatric neuro-ophthalmology. Timely distinction between papilledema and pseudopapilledema can be clinically challenging even for the most experienced clinicians.

Optic nerve head drusen are present in 1–2.4% of the population, and their presence is often unknown to the patient [26–28]. Several different methods may be employed to identify optic nerve head drusen, including fundus autofluorescence, extended depth of imaging optical coherence tomography (OCT), B-scan ultrasound, and fluorescein angiography. Though it remains unclear which is the most reliable in children, each has advantages and disadvantages that make their use suitable or impossible in different clinical circumstances [29–31]. Further detail on the approach to diagnosing optic disc drusen is beyond the scope of this chapter. Once a diagnosis of optic disc drusen is made, it is critical for the clinician to remember that this does not preclude the presence of increased ICP. This conundrum places added emphasis on the importance of collecting a complete and thorough history with careful interpretation to accurately identify patients with elevated ICP.

9.4.2 Diagnostic Criteria

The diagnostic criteria for primary and secondary pseudotumor cerebri syndrome have evolved as new diagnostic tools and clear data surrounding their utility become available. Walter Dandy was the first to report a cohort of patients with increased ICP in the absence of brain tumor in 1937 [32]. He described 22 patients with symptomology consistent with increased ICP, normal neurologic examination with the exception of sixth nerve paresis, bland cerebrospinal fluid profiles, and normal ventriculograms [32]. These key features serve as the foundation for the Dandy criteria, later modified by J. Lawton Smith in 1985 [33]. These criteria were further refined in designing the Idiopathic Intracranial Hypertension Treatment Trial (IIHTT) to include specific threshold opening pressure values on lumbar puncture of >25 cm H_2O or between 20 and 25 cm H_2O with other evidence of increased ICP) [34].

Friedman et al. published the most recent diagnostic criteria for pseudotumor cerebri syndrome in 2013 that included specifications for pediatric patients [1] The critical determinant in these criteria is the presence or absence of papilledema. "Definite pseudotumor cerebri" is applied to patients with papilledema, a normal neurologic exam (except for cranial nerve 6 paresis), normal neuroimaging, bland cerebrospinal fluid composition, and an elevated opening pressure. On neuroimaging, evidence of hydrocephalus, mass or structural lesion, or enhancement if contrast was used should be absent. The authors proposed that all patients should undergo neuroimaging with contrast, and MRV should be performed in atypical presentations, such as in male or nonobese patients. For patients who cannot undergo MRI (e.g., those with pacemakers or other MRI-incompatible implanted hardware), a contrast-enhanced CT is acceptable [1].

A diagnosis of pseudotumor cerebri can be made if patients without papilledema when all other diagnostic criteria are met and there is either evidence of sixth nerve paresis or 3/4 signs of increased ICP are evident on MRI. Signs of increased ICP on MRI include flattening of the posterior globes, empty or partially empty sella, distension of the optic nerve sheaths, or evidence of transverse venous sinus stenosis [1]. The inclusion of MRI findings as supportive evidence for pseudotumor cerebri syndrome is based on multiple different adult and pediatric studies. Kohli et al. performed a retrospective review of 119 patients with at least probable pseudotumor cerebri syndrome, no papilledema but increased ICP, and controls. They found that the presence of three or more MRI findings carried 62% sensitivity and 95% specificity [35]. Comparing MRI findings between adults and children with IIH, Hartmann et al. found that while children have similar findings, prepubertal children were less likely to exhibit all four findings [36]. Gilbert et al. performed a retrospective analysis of 38 patients with and 28 patients without IIH to evaluate MRI findings and found that patients with IIH were more likely to exhibit all 4 imaging features. They additionally reported that an optic nerve sheath diameter of $\geq$5.2 mm carried 87% sensitivity and 67% specificity for the diagnosis of IIH [37].

At our institution, we limit the use of gadolinium contrast in children given emerging evidence of long-lasting deposition in the brain and the uncertainty concerning its potential impact [38]. Our neuroimaging protocol for suspected pseudotumor cerebri includes MRI brain and orbits without contrast and MRV head. Contrast can be administered when there is concern for an autoimmune, oncologic, or infectious etiology, and at our institution is done at the radiologist's discretion unless requested [37]. The importance of including MRV in children is underscored by Hollander et al. who performed a retrospective review of 360 patients with IIH or papilledema from another cause and discovered that 10/72 (14%) children imaged by MRV 10 had occult dural venous sinus thromboses. Notably, 6/10 were asymptomatic [39].

The threshold for what is considered an elevated opening pressure on lumbar puncture depends on whether sedation is used and its weight. A cutoff of ≥28 cm H_2O is applied in children who are sedated and/or obese and ≥25 cm H_2O in non-sedated, nonobese children [1]. Applying these criteria to a retrospective cohort spanning 4 years, Gerstl et al. found that only 8/12 patients diagnosed with IIH met the criteria for opening pressure and 4/12 met the criteria for definite IIH [40]. Masri et al. evaluated a cohort of IIH patients aged 7 months to 12 years and found that 5/19 had opening pressures lower than 25 cm H_2O [41]. In a cross-sectional study at Boston Children's Hospital who had a lumbar puncture to evaluate for IIH, we found that only 105/374 (28%) patients met the diagnostic criteria when these opening pressure cutoffs were used [42]. While the guidelines provide a numerical basis for diagnosis, it is important to remember that the utility of any test depends on its accuracy and reliability. Lumbar puncture and measurement of opening pressure can be challenging and may yield spurious results even when seemingly performed correctly by an experienced provider. Clinician expertise, patient positioning, sedation, and number of attempts can all influence the results. Thus, clinical presentation and clinician judgment take precedence in the diagnosis of pseudotumor cerebri.

9.5 Treatment

Treatment of pediatric pseudotumor cerebri syndrome depends on the clinical context. The approach to treatment is multifaceted, with both medical and also surgical interventions available. The initial management is focused on lowering ICP on an appropriate timescale and to a level that will minimize the risk of visual sequelae. Contrary to popular belief, the volume of fluid removed during the diagnostic lumbar puncture as well as the closing pressure measurement do not influence the time to resolution of symptoms or papilledema [43].

Oral acetazolamide is the first-line therapy in non-fulminant case. In the pediatric population, acetazolamide is dosed based on patient weight—typically 10–25 mg/kg divided 2–3 times daily. There is no dedicated study demonstrating the effectiveness of acetazolamide treatment in pediatric PTCS. Practice is guided by data from the Idiopathic Intracranial Hypertension Treatment Trial, which compared oral acetazolamide therapy with weight reduction measures alone in mildly affected adults. Acetazolamide improved visual outcomes and reduced papilledema, though headache was not as responsive to the therapy [44]. Acetazolamide is a carbonic anhydrase inhibitor and is presumed to mediate its effect by reducing CSF production.

While acetazolamide dosing has been dosed up to 100 mg/kg/day, with maximum doses of 2 g per day in children and 4 g per day in adolescents, we have found these ranges to be infeasible because of side effects including lethargy, decreased appetite, paresthesias, gastrointestinal upset, and metabolic acidosis [15]. Although the IIHTT found adverse effects of high acetazolamide doses to be uncommon and did not recommend regular blood testing, in our practice, we have found that pediatric patients tend to be more sensitive to adverse effects of high acetazolamide dosing. We recommend electrolyte testing to evaluate for metabolic acidosis within 2–6 weeks after starting acetazolamide. Depending on symptomology and the degree of acidosis, we replete with oral bicarbonate (usually sodium citrate) with a goal of keeping the bicarbonate level ≥18 mEq/L.

Acetazolamide is widely considered first-line therapy in both adult and pediatric pseudotumor cerebri, but topiramate or furosemide are also used. Topiramate functions as an anticonvulsant by blocking sodium channels, enhancing the activity of GABA (A) and antagonizing certain glutamate receptors, but it also has weak carbonic anhydrase inhibitory activity. Topirimate may be administered a pill or a "sprinkle" for children who are too young to swallow pills. Dosing usually starts between 15 and 25 mg daily and should be up-titrated to 2–4 mg/kg/day divided twice daily to a maximum of 200 mg/day. Topiramate is teratogenic and should be avoided in female patients of childbearing age. Only one open-label study has compared the efficacy of topiramate and acetazolamide and this was an open-label study that found them both efficacious [45]. Topiramate should not be used in combination with acetazolamide due to a theoretical increased risk of kidney stones [46]. Furosemide can also be used as an alternative in patients with intolerance to acetazolamide and topiramate, but its efficacy is also poorly understood [47]. High-dose corticosteroids have been in cases with concern for imminent vision loss, though not for regular or long-term use [48].

Once the ICP is felt to be normalized, as evidenced by resolution of symptoms and papilledema, the question becomes how long to maintain patients on therapy before initiating a medication taper. Unfortunately, the same challenges in diagnosing pediatric patients, such as inability to perform a Snellen visual acuity, to sit for OCT testing or participate reliably with automated perimetry, apply to their follow-up care and limit the data available to guide clinical decision-making. Tovia et al. evaluated 60 pediatric patients with pseudotumor cerebri initially successfully treated (average duration 12 months) with acetazolamide and found that 26% of them suffered a relapse on discontinuation of medication [49]. There remains a great need to define optimal therapeutic practices in pseudotumor cerebri (both primary and secondary).

Clinical considerations that typically guide the initiation of a medical taper are largely focused on whether the driving factor(s) has been adequately addressed and the status of optic nerve health and function. In pubertal/postpubertal IIH, weight loss of 6–10% of body weight is a standard benchmark in adults. In secondary pseudotumor cerebri, discontinuation of a suspected inciting medication or addressing an underlying condition such as anemia or dural venous sinus thrombosis are requisite steps prior to initiating a taper. The clinician may be more conservative in initiating a taper in cases where optic atrophy reaches a significant level or further potential visual morbidity with a relapse would be considered particularly damaging. Orme et al. found that 2/52 (4%) patients diagnosed with pseudotumor cerebri secondary to doxycycline had disease recurrence after cessation of therapy, though the timing and circumstances surrounding these recurrences were not reported. The disease course was significantly shorter (18.3 weeks vs. 62.9 weeks) in the secondary pseudotumor cerebri vs. the IIH subgroup [21]. Liu et al. reported that the time to resolution of papilledema in cerebral venous sinus thrombosis is approximately 6 months [22]. Thus, the duration of anticipated treatment for pseudotumor cerebri depends on the kinetics of resolution of the underlying factor.

Surgical intervention to reduce ICP is considered in patients who either fail medical therapy or present with fulminant signs and cannot risk waiting for medical therapy to take effect. Surgical interventions include optic nerve sheath fenestration, CSF diversion procedures, and venous sinus stenting. Optic nerve sheath fenestration provides a novel pathway for CSF to egress from the subarachnoid space, which extends along the optic nerves, and thus lessens the pressure burden on the optic nerves [50]. This procedure carries the risk of severe vision loss and is typically performed unilaterally in the worse-seeing eye by an experienced oculoplastics-trained surgeon or neurosurgeon.

CSF diversion procedures for elevated ICP (including ventriculoperitoneal and lumboperitoneal shunting) have been used to address refractory or emergent intracranial hypertension for many decades. Implantation of requisite hardware is not without risk; shunts can subsequently become obstructed, migrate attract infection, or otherwise fail [51]. Brune et al. evaluated complications of ventriculoperitoneal shunts initially placed for IIH at their institution and found 6/32 (18.7%) of shunts failed over 10.75 years follow-up [52]. The authors noted 38 Emergency Department presentations across 14 patients because of potential shunt failures subsequently determined to be functional [52]. In pediatric patients, implanted hardware will inherently remain in place for longer periods of time, potentially amplifying the lifetime risk of failure and other complications. Furthermore, signs and symptoms of potential shunt failure may be less apparent in young children, possibly leading to even more hospital visits, testing and anxiety for the patient and family [52]. Therefore, shunt placement in the pediatric population requires special considerations with generally a higher threshold for placement.

One alternative to permanent CSF diversion is placement of a temporary lumbar drain. This provides protection against ongoing pressure-induced vision loss through an immediate lowering of ICP while acetazolamide can be up-titrated. High-dose glucocorticoids are often used as adjuvant therapy during this process as well [53]. Ploof et al. examined 9 patients with fulminant pediatric IIH who received either a temporary lumbar drain [4], a temporary lumbar drain followed by a shunt [2], or only a shunt alone [3, 54]. All 9 were eventually tapered off medication with resolution of papilledema, though 6/9 had mild residual visual field defects. Less favorable outcomes have also been reported with placement of lumbar drains [53]. The potential role of lumbar drains as a temporizing measure in select cases of fulminant IIH is promising, but requires further study to determine the risk-benefit favorability in comparison to permanent CSF diversion surgery [54].

Venous sinus stenting is a recently developed treatment modality for primarily adult patients with pseudotumor cerebri that have failed medical therapy. The potential utility of this novel approach is under active investigation in both adult and pediatric populations. The approach is predicated on the idea that venous sinus stenosis (although generally felt to be secondary to elevated ICP) contributes to elevated ICP by obstructing venous outflow in IIH [55]. Dwyer et al. noted that 76/145 (52%) patients with suspected IIH had evidence of obstruction on the dominant side of their venous systems [56]. Carter et al. described 12 reported pediatric patients undergoing venous sinus stenting for medically refractory IIH and noted that larger decreases in the pressure gradient across the shunted region of stenosis correlated with symptom resolution. Requisite revision of stents has been reported to be 13% at 1 year after insertion, compared to 55% of shunts in that same time frame [57]. Placement of the stent requires cerebral angiography which carries an inherent risk for morbidity and mortality. Anti-platelet therapy for 6 months if required after stent placement, carrying additional risk and/or potentially complicating the feasibility of a shunting procedure if needed [55]. As such, venous stenting is more appropriately considered in patients with more severe diseases.

Schwarz et al. reported 8 patients (4 male and 4 female, aged 4–18) with IIH who were refractory to medical management, intolerant to medications or fulminant at presentation, and underwent venous sinus stenting [58]. All patients had stenosis of the venous sinus system and 7/9 had improvement in symptoms with resolution of papilledema and normalization of CSF pressure. Two patients required a repeat procedure, one of whom responded well and one who went on to require multiple other surgical interventions with poor responses [58]. As with lumbar drains, further dedicated studies are needed to identify the ideal clinical scenarios in which venous stenting may provide patients with optimal benefit in light of the risks inherent to this procedure and its subsequent management.

9.6 Monitoring

Effectiveness of medical or surgical treatment of pseudotumor cerebri must be closely monitored, typically with focus on the optic nerve appearance and visual function. The quality and reliability of these data are inherently lower in pediatric patients, depending on the age and developmental status of the child. Effectiveness of treatment is determined by monitoring for decrease in afferent visual function on visual acuity, color vision, and perimetry testing as well as reduction in papilledema both subjectively on fundus exam as well as quantitatively using ancillary testing. For children who are unable to perform automated perimetry, we attempt kinetic perimetry to define their peripheral vision. OCT has emerged as a very helpful tool in this regard by providing objective measures of optic nerve head anatomy (i.e., the degree of swelling and/or atrophy) as measured through the peripapillary retinal nerve fiber layer (RNFL), optic nerve head volume (ONHV), and macular ganglion cell layer (GCL) or complex (GCC, which summates ganglion cell layer and inner plexiform layer) [25]. Importantly, the increased thickness of the RNFL is not specific to increased ICP and can be seen in other forms of optic disc edema such as optic neuritis which more commonly presents with optic disc edema in children [25, 59].

In the IIHTT, 90% of eyes with papilledema had mean RNFL thickness measurements above the 95th percentile of normal [60]. ICP at 6 months after treatment, mean RNFL thickness decreased more in the acetazolamide group compared to placebo with diet [61]. Similar decreases in both total retinal thickness and optic nerve head volume measurements were also observed [61]. While measurement of RNFL thickness with OCT is often used in neuro-ophthalmologic disease processes, the segmentation algorithm becomes less reliable once the mean RNFL thickness exceeds 200 μm [25]. Thus, whereas RNFL measures mirrored clinically meaningful group differences in the IIHTT, it is not an ideal metric with which to follow patients, particularly if the purpose is to identify treatment response failures. For this reason, we prioritize the use of ONHV as it is less prone to error in the setting of papilledema, though formal evaluation of this remains limited [25, 34, 60–62].

It is important to remember that reductions in retinal nerve fiber layer thickness and optic disc volume may represent the resolution of papilledema, these changes are also seen with the progression toward optic atrophy. Measurement of the macular ganglion cell layer (or ganglion cell complex, which includes the inner plexiform layer) allows for direct assessment of optic atrophy in the setting of a swollen optic nerve. As with the RNFL, atrophy in the form of thinning may not be evident in the acute stage as it typically manifests 6–8 weeks after an axonal insult. Therefore, we recommend performing measurements of the ganglion cell layer or ganglion cell layer complex in addition to formal perimetry (automated or kinetic) at each evaluation. Thinning of the ganglion cell layer is directly representative of optic atrophy and tends to manifest prior to the thinning of the retinal nerve fiber. As with the RNFL however segmentation of the ganglion cell layer/complex may fail in situations where the papilledema is greater than or equal to Frisen grade 3. Failures tend to report artifactual thinning, which was noted in 20% of the study eyes that were enrolled in the IIHTT [25, 60, 63]. Algorithms that may reduce these errors are under investigation [25].

9.7 Outcomes

IIH was initially coined a "benign" condition until the potential for profound vision loss in children became more widely known [64]. This may be at least in part because the same difficulties that arise during examination and diagnosis in children make it more challenging to accrue data on their visual outcomes. One retrospective review at a single tertiary care center of 96 patients demonstrated that there was a higher likelihood of a poor visual outcome in pubertal patients vs. prepubertal or adult patients with IIH [65]. Soiberman et al. evaluated 90 patients <10 years retrospectively and found significant improvement in visual acuity with medical therapy [66]. Using OCT, Gospe et al. evaluated visual and structural outcomes in 31 children with IIH and found that 19% had a permanent visual loss (either visual acuity or visual field) and loss of function correlated with the degree of atrophy [67]. Thus, while the majority of patients with pediatric IIH do well, optic atrophy and permanent vision loss are common.

Data on the visual outcomes of secondary pseudotumor cerebri syndrome in children are limited. Orme et al. found that shunts were placed in 3.8% of both the tetracycline-induced pseudotumor (2/52) and the IIH patients (11/302), while 4/52 (7.7%) of the tetracycline-induced pseudotumor cerebri group underwent optic nerve sheath fenestration compared to 28/302 (9.2%) of the IIH patients [25]. Both groups had a similar rate of afferent pupillary defects (Secondary: 6/52, 12%; IIH: 25/302, 8.3%). The visual outcomes of the tetracycline-induced pseudotumor cerebri group were not described further [21]. In their study of adults and children with cerebral venous sinus thrombosis, Liu et al. noted a mean visual acuity outcome of 20/25, though the range included light perception. Visual field defects were noted in 26/65 (40%) patients at the final visit [22]. Grade ≥ 3 papilledema or progression of papilledema after initiation of treatment were associated with visual field loss at the final follow-up visit [22]. Thus, primary and secondary pseudotumor cerebri syndrome can lead to permanent visual loss in adults and children. Further research characterizing visual outcomes in the pediatric population is greatly needed.

9.8 Conclusion

Primary and secondary pseudotumor cerebri occur in children as well as adults. These diagnoses require a clear and algorithmic approach in their evaluation to identify and address causative factors. It is crucial not to overlook any elements of the work-up, including a detailed patient history, examination, neuroimaging, and lumbar puncture with careful measurement of the opening pressure. Formal diagnostic criteria should be applied in making a diagnosis of primary pseudotumor cerebri syndrome (IIH) et al. [1]. It is important to maintain a high index of suspicion for borderline cases. Prompt recognition and treatment are crucial to prevent permanent vision loss. Interventions include medical therapy, a temporary lumbar drain, or surgical procedures such as csf diversion, optic nerve sheath fenestration, or venous sinus stenting.

Unlike its adult counterpart, pediatric primary pseudotumor cerebri has different risk factors and anthropomorphics depending on age and pubertal status. Prepubertal pseudotumor cerebri is equally common in males and females and there is no association with obesity whereas the anthropomorphics of postpubertal pseudotumor cerebri are more similar to those of adults. Pediatric patients, especially prepuberty, are more likely to present without classic symptoms including headache, visual changes, pulsatile tinnitus, or transient visual obscurations. The difficulty in examination and acquisition of ancillary data make the diagnosis of pseudotumor cerebri more challenging in children. These same limitations hinder the quality and quantity of research in this vulnerable population. Nevertheless, further work in multiple domains of this potentially sight-threatening condition is needed to guide diagnostic and treatment guidelines.

Key Points

1. Pediatric pseudotumor cerebri syndrome can be either primary (idiopathic) or secondary to medications, systemic disease, or venous sinus outflow obstruction.
2. Evaluation of pediatric pseudotumor cerebri syndrome requires a systematic and algorithmic approach including detailed patient history, examination, neuroimaging, and lumbar puncture with measurement of opening pressure.
3. A significant fraction of pediatric patients with pseudotumor cerebri will suffer permanent visual loss and/or optic atrophy, which can be prevented or minimized with timely and appropriate medical and/or surgical intervention.

References

1. Friedman DI, Liu GT, Digre KB. Revised diagnostic criteria for the pseudotumor cerebri syndrome in adults and children. Neurology. 2013;81(13):1159–65.
2. Beres SJ, Digre KB, Friedman DI, Liu GT. Pseudotumor cerebri syndrome is the best term for this condition. Pediatr Neurol. 2018;87:9–10.
3. Mollan SP, Davies B, Silver NC, et al. Idiopathic intracranial hypertension: consensus guidelines on management. J Neurol Neurosurg Psychiatry. 2018;89(10):1088–100.
4. Aylward SC, Waslo CS, Au JN, Tanne E. Manifestations of pediatric intracranial hypertension from the intracranial hypertension registry. Pediatr Neurol. 2016;61:76–82.
5. Gillson N, Jones C, Reem RE, Rogers DL, Zumberge N, Aylward SC. Incidence and demographics of pediatric intracranial hypertension. Pediatr Neurol. 2017;73:42–7.
6. Gordon K. Pediatric pseudotumor cerebri: descriptive epidemiology. Can J Neurol Sci. 1997;24(3):219–21.
7. Matthews YY, Dean F, Lim MJ, et al. Pseudotumor cerebri syndrome in childhood: incidence, clinical profile and risk factors in a national prospective population-based cohort study. Arch Dis Child. 2017;102(8):715–21.
8. Durcan FJ, Corbett JJ, Wall M. The incidence of pseudotumor cerebri. Population studies in Iowa and Louisiana. Arch Neurol. 1988;45(8):875–7.
9. Tepe D, Demirel F, Seker ED, et al. Prevalence of idiopathic intracranial hypertension and associated factors in obese children and adolescents. J Pediatr Endocrinol Metab. 2016;29(8):907–14.
10. Sheldon CA, Paley GL, Xiao R, et al. Pediatric idiopathic intracranial hypertension: age, gender, and anthropometric features at diagnosis in a large, retrospective. Multisite Cohort Ophthalmol. 2016;123(11):2424–31.
11. Glatstein MM, Oren A, Amarilyio G, et al. Clinical characterization of idiopathic intracranial hypertension in children presenting to the emergency department: the experience of a large tertiary care pediatric hospital. Pediatr Emerg Care. 2015;31(1):6–9.
12. Balcer LJ, Liu GT, Forman S, et al. Idiopathic intracranial hypertension: relation of age and obesity in children. Neurology. 1999;52(4):870–2.
13. Brara SM, Koebnick C, Porter AH, Langer-Gould A. Pediatric idiopathic intracranial hypertension and extreme childhood obesity. J Pediatr. 2012;161(4):602–7.
14. Shah V, Hoyos-Martinez A, Horne VE. Association of adrenal insufficiency with pediatric Pseudotumor cerebri syndrome. JAMA Ophthalmol. 2020;138(11):1187–91.

15. Beres SJ. Update in Pediatric Pseudotumor Cerebri Syndrome. Semin Neurol. 2020;40(3):286–93.
16. Sheldon CA, Kwon YJ, Liu GT, McCormack SE. An integrated mechanism of pediatric pseudotumor cerebri syndrome: evidence of bioenergetic and hormonal regulation of cerebrospinal fluid dynamics. Pediatr Res. 2015;77(2):282–9.
17. Kesler A, Fattal-Valevski A. Idiopathic intracranial hypertension in the pediatric population. J Child Neurol. 2002;17(10):745–8.
18. Aylward SC, Aronowitz C, Reem R, Rogers D, Roach ES. Intracranial hypertension without headache in children. J Child Neurol. 2015;30(6):703–6.
19. Bassan H, Berkner L, Stolovitch C, Kesler A. Asymptomatic idiopathic intracranial hypertension in children. Acta Neurol Scand. 2008;118(4):251–5.
20. Whitecross S, Heidary G. Asymptomatic pediatric idiopathic intracranial hypertension. J AAPOS. 2013;17(01):e31.
21. Orme DR, Vegunta S, Miller MA, et al. A comparison between the clinical features of Pseudotumor cerebri secondary to tetracyclines and idiopathic intracranial hypertension. Am J Ophthalmol. 2020;220:177–82.
22. Liu KC, Bhatti MT, Chen JJ, et al. Presentation and progression of papilledema in cerebral venous sinus thrombosis. Am J Ophthalmol. 2020;213:1–8.
23. Thambisetty M, Lavin PJ, Newman NJ, Biousse V. Fulminant idiopathic intracranial hypertension. Neurology. 2007;68(3):229–32.
24. Aylward SC, Aronowitz C, Roach ES. Intracranial hypertension without papilledema in children. J Child Neurol. 2016;31(2):177–83.
25. Sibony PA, Kupersmith MJ, Kardon RH. Optical coherence tomography Neuro-toolbox for the diagnosis and Management of Papilledema, optic disc edema, and Pseudopapilledema. J Neuroophthalmol. 2021;41(1):77–92.
26. Auw-Haedrich C, Staubach F, Witschel H. Optic disk drusen. Surv Ophthalmol. 2002;47(6):515–32.
27. Friedman AH, Gartner S, Modi SS. Drusen of the optic disc. A retrospective study in cadaver eyes. Br J Ophthalmol. 1975;59(8):413–21.
28. Malmqvist L, Li XQ, Eckmann CL, et al. Optic disc Drusen in children: the Copenhagen child cohort 2000 eye study. J Neuroophthalmol. 2018;38(2):140–6.
29. Malmqvist L, Bursztyn L, Costello F, et al. The optic disc Drusen studies consortium recommendations for diagnosis of optic disc Drusen using optical coherence tomography. J Neuroophthalmol. 2018;38(3):299–307.
30. Chang MY, Velez FG, Demer JL, et al. Accuracy of diagnostic imaging modalities for classifying pediatric eyes as papilledema versus Pseudopapilledema. Ophthalmology. 2017;124(12):1839–48.
31. Merchant KY, Su D, Park SC, et al. Enhanced depth imaging optical coherence tomography of optic nerve head drusen. Ophthalmology. 2013;120(7):1409–14.
32. Dandy WE. Intracranial pressure without brain tumor: diagnosis and treatment. Ann Surg. 1937;106(4):492–513.
33. Smith JL. Whence pseudotumor cerebri? J Clin Neuroophthalmol. 1985;5(1):55–6.
34. Wall M, Kupersmith MJ, Kieburtz KD, et al. The idiopathic intracranial hypertension treatment trial: clinical profile at baseline. JAMA Neurol. 2014;71(6):693–701.
35. Kohli AA, Vossough A, Mallery RM, et al. Magnetic resonance imaging findings in pediatric Pseudotumor cerebri syndrome. Pediatr Neurol. 2019;99:31–9.
36. Hartmann AJ, Soares BP, Bruce BB, et al. Imaging features of idiopathic intracranial hypertension in children. J Child Neurol. 2017;32(1):120–6.
37. Gilbert AL, Vaughn J, Whitecross S, Robson CD, Zurakowski D, Heidary G. Magnetic resonance imaging features and clinical findings in pediatric idiopathic intracranial hypertension: a case-control study. Life (Basel). 2021;11(6):487.
38. Gulani V, Calamante F, Shellock FG, Kanal E, Reeder SB, International Society for Magnetic Resonance in M. Gadolinium deposition in the brain: summary of evidence and recommendations. Lancet Neurol. 2017;16(7):564–70.

39. Hollander JPS, Heidary G. Utilization of MRV to evaluate pediatric patients with papilledema. J AAPOS. 2014;18(04):2.
40. Gerstl L, Schoppe N, Albers L, et al. Pediatric idiopathic intracranial hypertension - is the fixed threshold value of elevated LP opening pressure set too high? Eur J Paediatr Neurol. 2017;21(6):833–41.
41. Masri A, Jaafar A, Noman R, Gharaibeh A, Ababneh OH. Intracranial hypertension in children: etiologies, clinical features, and outcome. J Child Neurol. 2015;30(12):1562–8.
42. Delaney AC, Velarde A, Harper MB, et al. Predictors of primary intracranial hypertension in children using a newly suggested opening pressure cutoff of 280 mm H2O. Pediatr Neurol. 2019;91:27–33.
43. Beres SJ, Sheldon CA, Boisvert CJ, et al. Clinical and prognostic significance of cerebrospinal fluid opening and closing pressures in pediatric Pseudotumor cerebri syndrome. Pediatr Neurol. 2018;83:50–5.
44. Committee NIIHSGW, Wall M, McDermott MP, et al. Effect of acetazolamide on visual function in patients with idiopathic intracranial hypertension and mild visual loss: the idiopathic intracranial hypertension treatment trial. JAMA. 2014;311(16):1641–51.
45. Celebisoy N, Gokcay F, Sirin H, Akyurekli O. Treatment of idiopathic intracranial hypertension: topiramate vs acetazolamide, an open-label study. Acta Neurol Scand. 2007;116(5):322–7.
46. Jion YI, Raff A, Grosberg BM, Evans RW. The risk and management of kidney stones from the use of topiramate and zonisamide in migraine and idiopathic intracranial hypertension. Headache. 2015;55(1):161–6.
47. Gaier ED, Heidary G. Pediatric idiopathic intracranial hypertension. Semin Neurol. 2019;39(6):704–10.
48. Liu GT, Glaser JS, Schatz NJ. High-dose methylprednisolone and acetazolamide for visual loss in pseudotumor cerebri. Am J Ophthalmol. 1994;118(1):88–96.
49. Tovia E, Reif S, Oren A, Mitelpunkt A, Fattal-Valevski A. Treatment response in pediatric patients with Pseudotumor cerebri syndrome. J Neuroophthalmol. 2017;37(4):393–7.
50. Thuente DD, Buckley EG. Pediatric optic nerve sheath decompression. Ophthalmology. 2005;112(4):724–7.
51. Hanak BW, Bonow RH, Harris CA, Browd SR. Cerebrospinal fluid shunting complications in children. Pediatr Neurosurg. 2017;52(6):381–400.
52. Brune AJ, Girgla T, Trobe JD. Complications of ventriculoperitoneal shunt for idiopathic intracranial hypertension: a single-institution study of 32 patients. J Neuroophthalmol. 2021;41(2):224–32.
53. Jiramongkolchai K, Buckley EG, Bhatti MT, et al. Temporary lumbar drain as treatment for pediatric fulminant idiopathic intracranial hypertension. J Neuroophthalmol. 2017;37(2):126–32.
54. Ploof J, Aylward SC, Jordan CO, Drapeau AI. Case series of rapid surgical interventions in fulminant intracranial hypertension. J Child Neurol. 2021;36(11):1047–53.
55. Carter LM, Chakraborty AR, McCoy-Stephens TM, Strickland AE, Bohnstedt BN, Gross NL. Venous sinus stenosis treatment in pediatric idiopathic intracranial hypertension: illustrative case and literature review. World Neurosurg. 2021;149:2–7.
56. Dwyer CM, Prelog K, Owler BK. The role of venous sinus outflow obstruction in pediatric idiopathic intracranial hypertension. J Neurosurg Pediatr. 2013;11(2):144–9.
57. Ahmed RM, Zmudzki F, Parker GD, Owler BK, Halmagyi GM. Transverse sinus stenting for pseudotumor cerebri: a cost comparison with CSF shunting. AJNR Am J Neuroradiol. 2014;35(5):952–8.
58. Schwarz J, Al Balushi A, Sundararajan S, et al. Management of idiopathic intracranial hypertension in children utilizing venous sinus stenting. Interv Neuroradiol. 2021;27(2):257–65.
59. Wan MJ, Adebona O, Benson LA, Gorman MP, Heidary G. Visual outcomes in pediatric optic neuritis. Am J Ophthalmol. 2014;158(3):503–7 e2.
60. Group OCTS-SCfNIIHS, Auinger P, Durbin M, et al. Baseline OCT measurements in the idiopathic intracranial hypertension treatment trial, part I: quality control, comparisons, and variability. Invest Ophthalmol Vis Sci. 2014;55(12):8180–8.

61. Optical Coherence Tomography Substudy C, Group NIIHS. Papilledema outcomes from the optical coherence tomography substudy of the idiopathic intracranial hypertension treatment trial. Ophthalmology. 2015;122(9):1939–45 e2.
62. Dreesbach M, Joachimsen L, Kuchlin S, et al. Optic nerve head volumetry by optical coherence tomography in papilledema related to idiopathic intracranial hypertension. Transl Vis Sci Technol. 2020;9(3):24.
63. Group OCTS-SCfNIIHS, Auinger P, Durbin M, et al. Baseline OCT measurements in the idiopathic intracranial hypertension treatment trial, part II: correlations and relationship to clinical features. Invest Ophthalmol Vis Sci. 2014;55(12):8173–9.
64. Lessell S, Rosman NP. Permanent visual impairment in childhood pseudotumor cerebri. Arch Neurol. 1986;43(8):801–4.
65. Stiebel-Kalish H, Kalish Y, Lusky M, Gaton DD, Ehrlich R, Shuper A. Puberty as a risk factor for less favorable visual outcome in idiopathic intracranial hypertension. Am J Ophthalmol. 2006;142(2):279–83.
66. Soiberman U, Stolovitch C, Balcer LJ, Regenbogen M, Constantini S, Kesler A. Idiopathic intracranial hypertension in children: visual outcome and risk of recurrence. Childs Nerv Syst. 2011;27(11):1913–8.
67. Gospe SM 3rd, Bhatti MT, El-Dairi MA. Anatomic and visual function outcomes in paediatric idiopathic intracranial hypertension. Br J Ophthalmol. 2016;100(4):505–9.

Update on Pediatric Glaucoma

10

Rahul Bhola

10.1 Childhood Glaucoma

10.1.1 Introduction

Childhood glaucoma is a relatively rare condition that can have devasting visual consequences if not detected early and managed promptly. Even though it can be secondary to variable etiologies, elevated intraocular pressure (IOP) with resulting optic nerve damage is a common result. There have been significant advancements in the diagnosis and management of childhood glaucoma over the last couple of decades with newer technologies facilitating better IOP measurements and optic nerve health assessment in outpatient settings. The goal of successful glaucoma management in pediatric population is to minimize vision loss by early optimal control of intraocular pressure which is often challenging and is typically achieved surgically. While IOP control is pivotal in glaucoma management, correction of coexistent refractive errors and amblyopia is paramount for a successful visual outcome.

10.1.2 Classification

Childhood glaucoma is a heterogeneous disorder that can be classified as primary, which is caused by an isolated abnormality of the aqueous outflow pathway or secondary, where aqueous outflow is impeded due to a congenital or acquired ocular or

R. Bhola (✉)
Section Chair Ophthalmology, Division Chief Pediatric Ophthalmology, Children's Hospital of Orange County, Orange, CA, USA

A. Ramasubramanian (ed.), *Pediatric Ophthalmology*, Current Practices in Ophthalmology, https://doi.org/10.1007/978-981-19-4963-0_10

systemic abnormality. Childhood glaucoma classification has evolved over the years from simple classifications relating to the age of onset of glaucoma to more complex classifications delineating developmental patterns or anatomical structural maldevelopment of anterior segment. The Childhood Glaucoma Research Network developed a new international classification system for childhood glaucoma which uses a clinical algorithm for classifying a patient with childhood glaucoma (Tables 10.1 and 10.2) [1, 2].

Table 10.1 Classification of childhood glaucoma (childhood glaucoma research network)

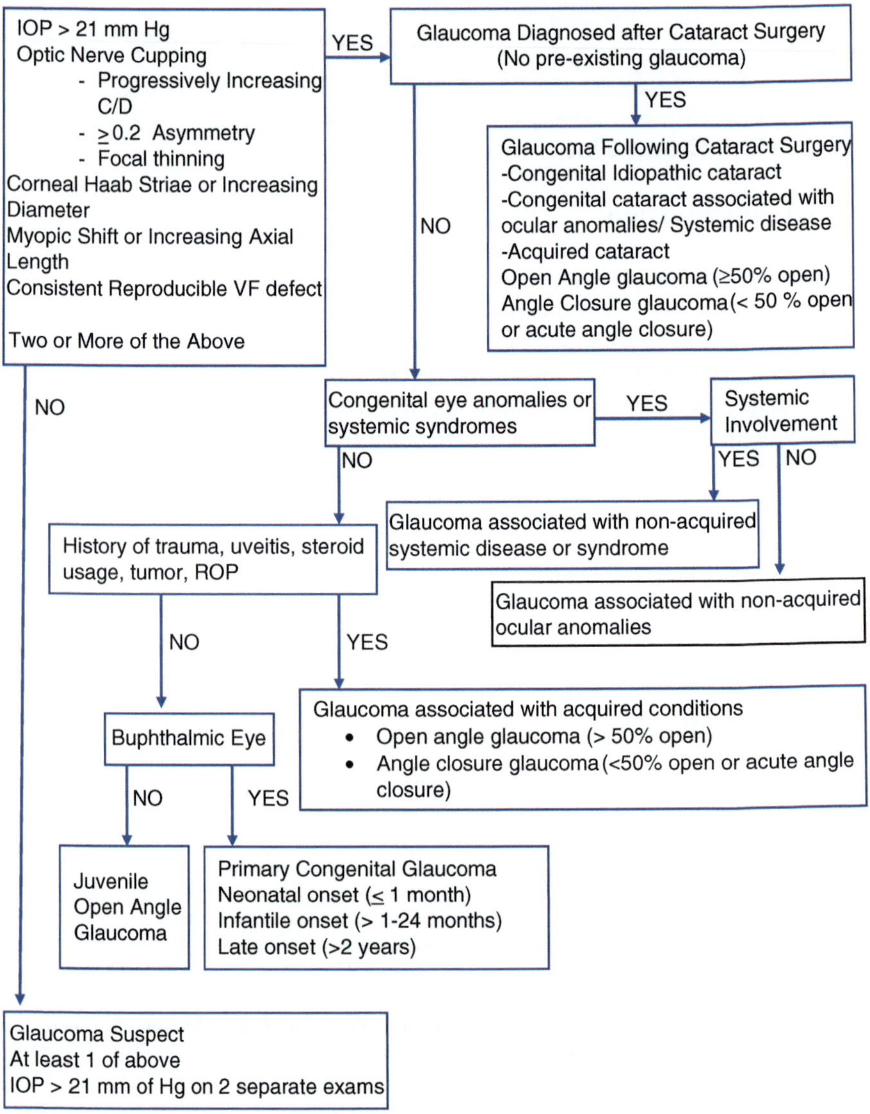

Table 10.2 International classification (CGRN/WGA) of childhood glaucoma

Primary childhood glaucoma
• Primary congenital glaucoma
• Juvenile open-angle glaucoma
Secondary childhood glaucoma
• Glaucoma associated with nonacquired ocular anomalies
• Glaucoma associated with nonacquired systemic anomalies
• Glaucoma associated with acquired condition
• Glaucoma following cataract surgery
Glaucoma associated with nonacquired ocular anomalies
Conditions with predominant ocular anomalies present at birth that may or may not be associated with systemic signs
• Axenfeld Rieger anomaly or syndrome
• Peters anomaly or syndrome
• Ectropion uveae
• Aniridia
• Congenital iris hypoplasia
• Persistent fetal vasculature
• Oculodermal melanocytosis
• Posterior polymorphous dystrophy
• Microphthalmos
• Microcornea
• Ectopia lentis
• Ectopia lentis et pupillae
Glaucoma associated with nonacquired systemic disease or syndrome
Conditions with predominantly known syndromes, systemic anomalies, or systemic disease present at birth that might be associated with ocular signs
• Chromosomal disorders such as trisomy 21
• Connective tissue disorder
• Marfan syndrome
• Weill-Marchesani syndrome
• Stickler syndrome
• Metabolic disorders
• Homocystinuria
• Lowe syndrome
• Mucopolysaccharidoses
• Phacomatoses
• Neurofibromatosis (NF-1, NF-2)
• Sturge weber syndrome
• Klippel-Trenaunay-weber syndrome
• Rubinstein-Taybi
• Congenital rubella
Glaucoma associated with acquired condition
• Uveitis
• Trauma (hyphema, angle recession, ectopia lentis)
• Steroid induced
• Tumors (benign/malignant, ocular/orbital)
• Retinopathy of prematurity
• Prior ocular surgery other than cataract surgery

10.1.3 Genetics

Even though Primary Congenital Glaucoma (PCG) mostly occurs sporadically, patients with a familial pattern usually show a recessive pattern with incomplete or variable penetrance with a possible multifactorial inheritance. Human Genome Organization has established a specific nomenclature for Glaucoma associated genetic loci with GLC3 indicating the loci for primary congenital glaucoma. Four chromosomal loci for PCG have been identified with GLC3A on band 2p21, GLC3B on 1p36, GLC3C on 4q24.3, and GLC3D on 14q24 [3, 4]. GLC3A locus has shown 147 mutations in the gene CYP1B1, coding for the homonymous protein (cytochrome P450, family 1, subfamily B, and polypeptide 1). The mutations showed an autosomal-recessive inheritance pattern and are the most common variations identified among PCG patients, mostly in the consanguineous population. Interestingly patients harboring the same mutations showed a different degree of disease severity, age of onset due to incomplete penetrance, and variable expressivity. Juvenile open-angle glaucoma (JOAG) has been linked to GLC1A myocilin gene (MYOC) [5, 6]. MYOC is a 3-exon gene, located at 1q24.3-1q25.2 and codes for the glycoprotein myocilin. Another PCG-associated gene is FOXC1, a protein expressed in periocular mesenchyme cells [7].

10.2 Clinical Features

Clinical manifestations of childhood glaucoma depend on the age of onset, etiology of glaucoma, and level of intraocular pressure elevation. Neonatal or Infantile glaucoma typically present with the classic triad of epiphora, blepharospasm, and photophobia. Even though most cases of PCG are bilateral, they can be asymmetric or even unilateral in up to 30% of the cases. Enlargement of the eye traditionally referred to as Buphthalmos (Ox Eye) (Fig. 10.1) occurs secondary to chronic elevated intraocular pressure and is mostly present with corneal cloudiness by the time patient is seen by an ophthalmologist. After the age of 3 years, patients may present

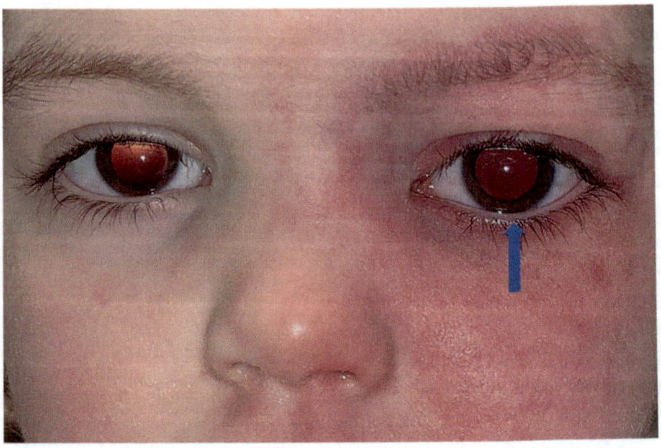

Fig. 10.1 Facial port-wine stain in a child with Sturge-Weber Syndrome associated with ipsilateral buphthalmos and glaucoma (arrow). (Courtsey Parth Shah, MD)

with failed vision screenings and are found to have progressive myopia, strabismus, and/or amblyopia.

10.3 Diagnosis

Even though in majority of cases the diagnosis of childhood glaucoma is made in the outpatient setting, sometimes it is essential to perform a thorough examination under anesthesia for full assessment.

10.3.1 Corneal Examination

Corneal diameter greater than 11.5 mm in the newborn and greater than 12.5 mm by age 1 year is highly suggestive of glaucoma. Increased IOP causes microcystic edema initially involving the epithelium but later extending to the stroma. Breaks in Descemet's membrane (Fig. 10.2, Haab striae) can occur from increased IOP stretching the cornea, these are typically horizontal and linear in the central cornea and curvilinear to the limbus in the periphery. Haab striae are best visualized against the red reflex after pupillary dilation.

10.3.2 Refraction

Myopia and irregular astigmatism (due to corneal irregularity) in a patient with enlarged cornea is highly suggestive of glaucoma.

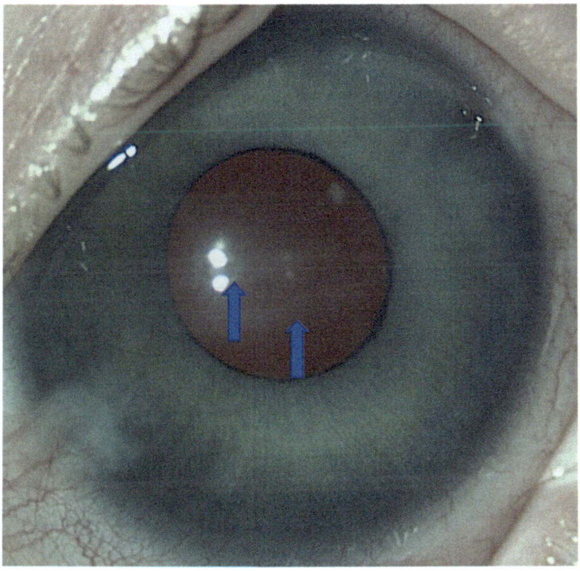

Fig. 10.2 Slit Lamp biomicroscopy showing horizontal breaks in Descemet membrane, arrows (Haab striae). (Courtesy of Parth Shah, MD)

10.3.3 Anterior Segment Examination

PCG typically shows a deep anterior chamber with a hypoplastic peripheral iris stroma. Gonioscopy using Koeppe lens with a hand-hand portable slit lamp provides a great anatomic overview of the angle. In patients with PCG, the iris inserts more anterior than in a normal infant. Also, the details of the ciliary body band, trabecular meshwork, and scleral spur are indistinct.

10.3.4 Intraocular Pressure Measurement

Since long-term health of the optic nerve depends on optimal control and stability of intraocular pressure, it is vital to utilize consistent tools that allow accurate measurement of intraocular pressure. The importance of pachymetry in the assessment of children with glaucoma has also been highlighted in view of the effect of central corneal thickness on intraocular pressure [8, 9]. The advent of iCare tonometry and its greater tolerability in children has resulted in an invigorated interest in gauging its reliability and accuracy. The newer versions (iCare IC200, iCare USA) offer 200° of positional freedom thereby allowing IOP measurements in standing, sitting, elevated or supine positions. In view of its many advantages, it has become an instrument of choice to measure IOP in outpatient clinics.

10.3.5 Optic Nerve Examination

A careful optic nerve exam with comparison of both nerves is essential in assessing the baseline optic nerve involvement as well as following the stability of glaucoma. Glaucomatous cup in childhood glaucoma is commonly round, steep-walled, and central, surrounded by a uniform pink rim (Fig. 10.3). The cup tends to enlarge circumferentially as glaucoma progresses in view of stretching of scleral canal. In

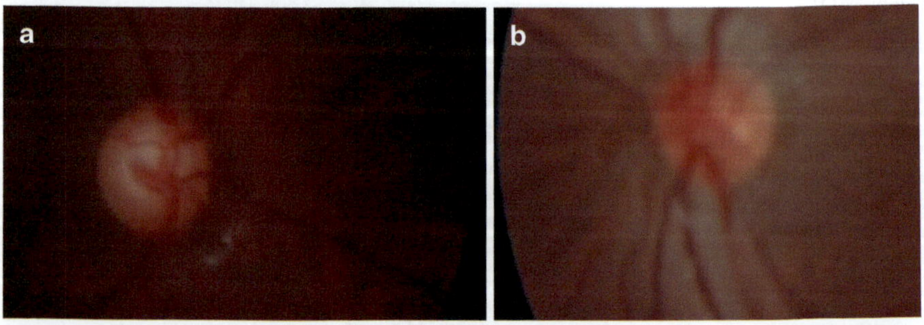

Fig. 10.3 (**a**) Optic nerve in a 4-year old with unilateral aphakic glaucoma shows round, steep-walled central cupping of the Right Eye with healthy Neuroretinal rim. (**b**) The normal left optic nerve is shown for comparison

pediatric populations reversal of cupping with IOP reduction has been repeatedly noticed although OCT has shown irreversible thinning of RNFL despite the reversal of cupping [10].

10.3.6 Optical Coherence Tomography

Optical Coherence Tomography (OCT) has been widely used in the adult glaucoma world for monitoring the stability of Optic nerve head (ONH) over time. It is particularly a great addition to the armamentarium of pediatric glaucoma assessment tools in view of the difficulty of obtaining reliable visual fields in children. Over the last few years measuring the Retinal Nerve Fiber layer thickness for childhood glaucoma has gained traction and in some centers is used routinely to monitor ONH parameters. It has been shown to correlate well with the severity of optic nerve head cupping with reasonable reproducibility. In one study, peripapillary RNFL remained thinned in pediatric glaucoma patients despite reversal of cupping following successful glaucoma surgery highlighting the role of OCT as a more sensitive method of assessing severity of glaucomatous damage in children in comparison to gross optic nerve exam [10]. Recently great effort has been made to obtain normative database of macular thickness, retinal nerve fiber layer (RNFL) thickness, and optic nerve topography in healthy pediatric eyes using OCT measurements [11]. Even though pediatric normative values are yet to be integrated into most OCT machines, many pediatric glaucoma specialists have incorporated this tool for managing glaucoma in pediatric patients.

10.4 Management

Early diagnosis and prompt management are vital in cases of pediatric glaucoma to minimize visual impairment. The first and foremost step in management after confirming the diagnosis and obtaining baseline parameters is IOP control followed by correction of coexisting refractive errors and aggressive amblyopia management. An aggressive approach to glaucoma detection and management with effective utilization of medical, surgical, or a combination of these therapies can result in good long-term visual outcome even in some difficult subtypes of glaucoma [12].

10.4.1 Medical Therapy

Even though childhood glaucoma is primarily managed surgically, medical therapy usually plays a supportive role. IOP lowering drugs are typically used preoperatively to reduce IOP temporarily allowing corneal clarity and better visualization of angle to facilitate surgical intervention. They are sometimes also used to delay surgical intervention in medically fragile patients and sometimes for additional IOP control after surgical intervention. The potential for side effects in the pediatric population should always be addressed prior to starting medical therapy.

Beta-Blockers: Use of timolol in childhood glaucoma has been extensively studied. In view of risk of side effects like bronchospasm and bradycardia from 0.5% timolol, β-1 selective antagonist betaxolol and timolol gel 0.25% have been extensively used to control IOP with a safer risk tolerance profile. Once daily dosing with timolol 0.25% in gel formulation has shown adequate IOP reduction with a better safety profile. Timolol 0.1% has also been safely used in neonates for immediate IOP reduction. Punctal occlusion may greatly reduce systemic absorption and should be employed 3–5 min after instilling drops.

Carbonic anhydrase inhibitors: Topical carbonic anhydrase inhibitors are useful as a second-line drug and may be considered on a short-term basis prior to surgery or when beta-blockers are contraindicated. Topical dorzolamide and brinzolamide are both useful second-line drugs. Local side effects include corneal decompensation and care must be taken when the corneal endothelial function is compromised. Although oral acetazolamide is very efficacious in IOP reduction, its long-term use in the pediatric population is limited due to the potential of serious systemic side effects such as metabolic acidosis and failure to thrive. For older children, fixed combination of dorzolamide with timolol may be employed to simply medical regimen.

Prostaglandin analogs: Even though few researchers have studied the effect of topical latanoprost in pediatric glaucoma, it was found to be less efficacious in children both as a monotherapy and in combination with other medications [13]. Another study showed that majority of eyes did not respond to favorable IOP reduction after latanoprost usage. Majority of responders in this study were more likely diagnosed with juvenile onset open-angle glaucoma and were older than nonresponders [14]. There is a possibility of side effects such as permanent iris pigmentation and longer thicker hyperpigmented eyelashes.

Alpha-2 agonist: Topical alpha-2 agonist like Brimonidine can cause central nervous mediated side effects such as drowsiness and extreme fatigue in younger children that limits its usage in younger pediatric glaucoma patients.

10.4.2 Surgical Therapy

Early surgical intervention in cases of childhood glaucoma can prevent progression thereby achieving visual preservation if optimal IOP control is obtained. Strict follow-up in these patients with IOP and Optic nerve function monitoring is required as gradual IOP elevation can happen even after early surgical success. There are many approaches to glaucoma surgery with the common goal of achieving optimal IOP control. The choice of surgery is determined by the type of glaucoma, any associated ocular or systemic disease, and most importantly the surgeon's level of comfort and experience. Corneal clarity, degree of optic neuropathy, prior ocular surgeries, state of fellow eye, and availability of specialized staff and equipment largely determines the type of surgery performed [15].

10.4.3 Angle Surgery

10.4.3.1 Goniotomy

Traditionally Goniotomy has always been considered the treatment of choice for PCG in patients with satisfactory visualization of angle. In recent years 360° trabeculotomy has been gaining popularity as the primary procedure of choice. Goniotomy restores the access of aqueous to Schlemm's canal by removing the obstructing tissue over trabecular meshwork. Even though goniotomy has a steep learning curve, it offers many advantages and once mastered is a rapid procedure. It allows direct visualization of the angle structures, is less traumatic, and does not violate conjunctiva allowing future surgery if needed. To improve visualization of the angle in the presence of hazy cornea, coaxial endoscopic goniotomy has been described [16].

10.4.3.2 Trabeculotomy

Trabeculotomy is the procedure of choice when the cornea is hazy with inadequate visualizing of the angle. In recent years it has gained popularity and in some centers is being performed as the primary procedure for childhood glaucoma. Trabeculotomy ab externo offers many advantages over goniotomy [17]. It can be performed with poor visibility of the anterior chamber, is anatomically precise in rupturing the inner wall of Schlemm's canal, and there is decreased risk of damage to intraocular tissues as it does not require introduction of sharp instruments across anterior chamber. Conventional trabeculotomy using trabeculotome opens about one-third of drainage angle, the angle can be opened circumferentially using a 6/0 Polypropylene suture passed through the Schlemm's canal. This technique has been associated with many complications including creation of a false passage, misdirected suture, iris tear, and prolonged hypotony. To avoid these complications, an illuminated microcatheter with a nontraumatic tip has gained popularity. Illuminated microcatheter-assisted circumferential trabeculotomy has shown to have better IOP reduction both in early and long-term follow-up as compared to both goniotomy and conventional trabeculotomy [18–21]. Illuminated microcatheter-facilitated trabeculotomy was combined with trabeculectomy for childhood glaucoma (congenital, juvenile, and aphakic glaucoma) with excellent IOP reduction (Fig. 10.4) [22].

10.4.3.3 Trabeculectomy

Trabeculectomy is primarily used in patients with failed angle surgeries or in certain subsets of secondary glaucoma. It is a more technically demanding procedure and is more likely to fail in children due to a more aggressive healing response and thicker Tenon's capsule with its large reserve of fibroblasts [23, 24]. It has a variable success rate influenced by factors such as ethnicity and history of prior surgeries. Intraoperative beta radiation to the surgical site showed improved outcomes with diffuse bleb formation [25]. The use of Mitomycin-C in children has been associated with higher complications including early complications related to hypotony and late complications associated with thin avascular, cystic blebs prone to leakage and infection [26, 27].

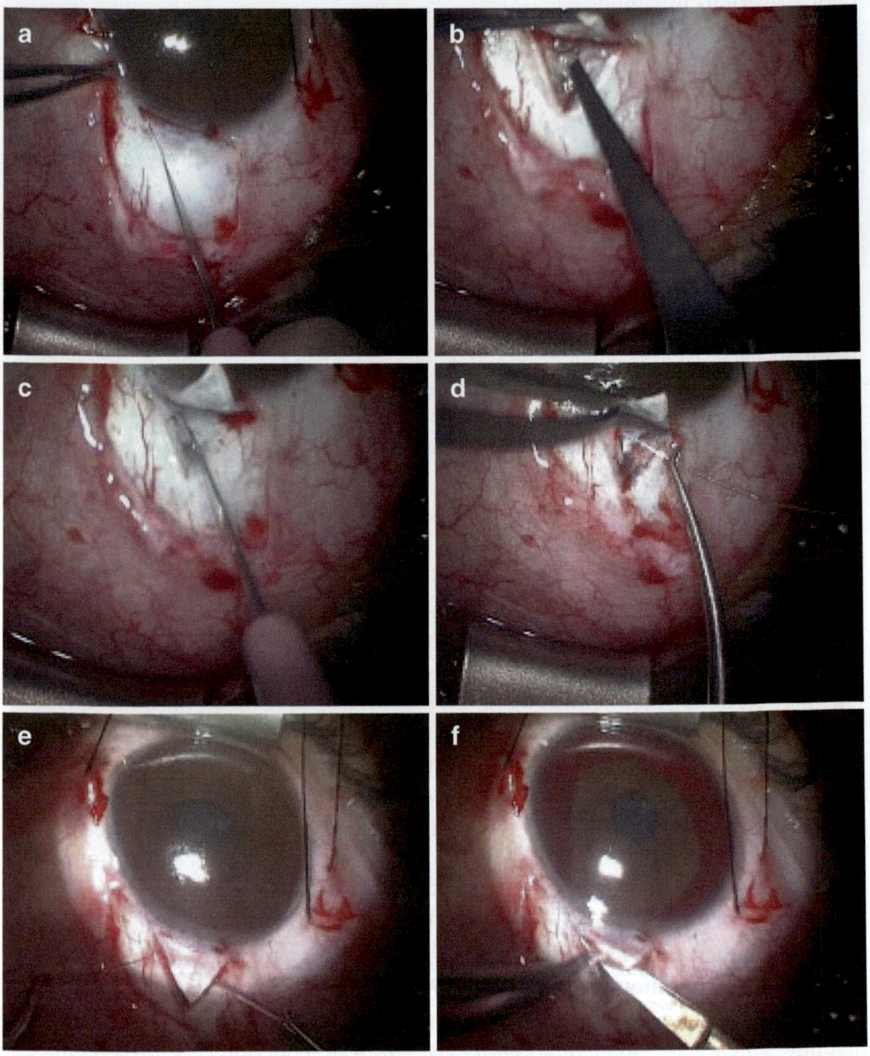

Fig. 10.4 Illuminated microcatheter-facilitated trabeculotomy and trabeculectomy for pediatric Glaucoma. (**a**, **b**) Superficial scleral flaps outlined and advanced. (**c**) Deep scleral flap created. (**d**) I-track catheter inserted into Schlemm's canal. (**e**) I-track catheter pulled like a purse string to open Schlemm's canal into anterior chamber. (**f**) Deep sclerectomy with trabeculectomy, note blood in the anterior chamber signifying rupture of the trabecular meshwork

10.4.4 Glaucoma Drainage Devices

Tube drainage devices are useful when other surgical treatments are associated with poor surgical outcome or when prior conventional surgeries have failed to achieve optimal IOP control. It offers the best chance of long-term IOP control in such patients. The most used devices currently are Ahmed implant (96 mm^2 and 184 mm^2) with unidirectional flow restriction, which theoretically reduces the risk of early hypotony and the Baerveldt implant (250 mm^2 and 350 mm^2) which is an unrestricted implant. Success rate of GDD is very variable with good early control of IOP but reduced optimal IOP control over time with the need for adjunctive medication. In children, there is no superiority of one type of GDD over the other, the Baerveldt implant has shown better long-term IOP control and the Ahmed implant has fewer short-term complications [28, 29]. Plate encapsulation is a major cause of late failure.

10.4.5 Cyclodestruction

Cyclodestruction, with the aim of reducing aqueous production, is typically reserved for blind painful eyes, those with poor visual potential and those where surgery has a poor prognosis or is technically not possible. Cyclocryotherapy has essentially been replaced by less destructive laser cyclophotocoagulation, specially transscleral diode laser (810 mm) which is better tolerated and is associated with fewer complications. Placement in buphthalmic eyes with distorted landmarks causing difficulty in the titration of laser energy is one of the major drawbacks of this procedure. Endoscopic diode laser allows precise treatment of ciliary processes but requires an intraocular approach and is risky in phakic patients.

10.4.6 Visual Rehabilitation

Long-term care of pediatric glaucoma is important with continued attention on refractive correction and amblyopia management. The visual outcome is dependent on the laterality, age of onset, age of treatment, intraocular pressure control, and surgical outcomes. Long-term outcomes of children with glaucoma have shown that 25% of patients achieve a visual acuity of 20/40 and better [30]. The mean refraction was −2.90 ± 3.83 diopters and 66% of the eye required refractive correction [30]. Patients with pediatric glaucoma can achieve a satisfactory visual outcome but continued management of refractive error and amblyopia is important.

Key Points

1. In patients with childhood glaucoma, an aggressive approach to glaucoma detection and management with effective utilization of medical, surgical, or a combination of these therapies can result in good long-term visual outcomes even in some difficult subtypes of glaucoma.
2. Incorporation of newer diagnostic techniques like iCare tonometer for measurement of Intraocular pressure and Optical coherence tomography for morphometric evaluation of optic nerve and retinal nerve fiber layer can significantly facilitate the diagnosis and follow-up of pediatric glaucoma patients.

3. Safer and newer surgical techniques like Illuminated microcatheter-facilitated trabeculotomy are a great addition to the armamentarium of pediatric glaucoma management. Glaucoma Drainage Devices continue to have a role in the management of childhood glaucoma patients that do not achieve adequate IOP control despite maximal medical therapy or after angle or filtration surgical procedures.

References

1. Beck AD, Chang TCP, Freedman SF. Definition, classification, differential diagnosis. In: Weinreb RN, et al., editors. Childhood Glaucoma: Consensus Series 9. Amsterdam: Kugler; 2013.
2. Thau A, Lloyd M, Freedman S, et al. New classification system for pediatric glaucoma: implication for clinical care and a research registry. Curr Opin Ophthalmol. 2018;29:385–94.
3. Khan AO. Genetics of primary glaucoma. Curr Opin Ophthalmol. 2011;22:347–55.
4. Sharafieh AR, Child H, Sarafarazi M. Molecular genetics of primary congenital glaucoma. Gen Dis Eye. 2011;17:295–307.
5. Kaur K, Reddy AB, Mukhopadhyay A, et al. Myocilin gene implicated in primary congenital glaucoma. Clin Genet. 2005;67(4):335–40.
6. Fingert JH, Stone EM, Sheffield VC, et al. Myocilin glaucoma. Surv Ophthalmol. 2002;47(6):547–61.
7. Siggs OM, Souzeau E, Pasutto F, et al. Prevalence of FOXC1 variants in individuals with a suspected diagnosis of primary congenital glaucoma. JAMA Ophthalmology. 2019;137:348–55.
8. Henriques MJ, Vessani RM, Reis FA, et al. Corneal thickness in congenital glaucoma. J Glaucoma. 2004;13:185–8.
9. Muir KW, Jin J, Freedman SF. Central corneal thickness and its relationship to intraocular pressure in children. Ophthalmology. 2004;111:2220–3.
10. Ely AL, El-Dairi MA, Freedman SF. Cupping reversal in pediatric glaucoma-evaluation of the retinal nerve fiber layer and visual field. Am J Ophthalmol. 2014;158(5):905–15.
11. El-Dairi MA, Asrani SG, Enyedi LB. Optical coherence tomography in the eyes of normal children. Arch Ophthalmol. 2009;127(1):50–8.
12. Bhola R, Keech RV, Olson RJ, et al. Long-term outcome of pediatric aphakic glaucoma. J AAPOS. 2006;10:243–8.
13. Enyadi LB, Feedman SF. Latanoprost for the treatment of pediatric glaucoma. Surv Ophthal. 2002;47(suppl 1):S129–32.
14. Enyedi LB, Freedman SF, Buckley EG. The effectiveness of Latanoprost for the treatment of pediatric glaucoma. J AAPOS. 1999;3:33–9.
15. Mandal AK, Chakrabati D. Update on congential glaucoma. India J Ophthalmol. 2011 Jan;59(Suppl1):S148–57.
16. Joos KM, Shen JH. An ocular endoscope enables a goniotomy despite a cloudy cornea. Arch Opthalmol. 2001;119:134–5.
17. Luntz MH. The advantages of trabeculotomy over goniotomy. J Pediatr Ophthamol Strabismus. 1984;21(4):150–3.
18. Sarkisian J Sr. An illuminated microcatheter for 360-degree trabeculotomy in congenital glaucoma: a retrospective case series. J AAPOS. 2010;14(5):412–6.
19. Girkin CA, Rhodes L, McGwin G, et al. Goniotomy versus circumferential trabeculotomy with an illuminated microcatheter in congenital glaucoma. J AAPOS. 2012;16(5):424–7.

20. Girkin CA, Marchase N, Cogen MS. Circumferential trabeculotomy with an illuminated microcatheter in congenital glaucoma. J Glaucoma. 2012;21(3):160–3.
21. Shakrawal J, Bali S, Sidhu T. Randomized trial on illuminated-microcatheter circumferential trabeculotomy versus conventional trabeculotomy in congenital glaucoma. Am J Ophthalmol. 2017;180:158–64.
22. Syed R, Bhola R. Illuminated Microcather-facilitated trabeculotomy and trabeculectomy for pediatric glaucoma. Poster presentation at AAO annual meeting 2015, Las Vegas.
23. Beauchamp GR, Parks MM. Filtering surgery in children: barriers to success. Ophthalmology. 1979;86:170–80.
24. Gressel MG, Heuer DF, Parish RK. Trabeculectomy in young patients. Ophthalmology. 1984;91:1242–6.
25. Miller MH, Rice NS. Trabeclectomy combined with beta irradiation for congential glaucoma. Br J Ophthalmol. 1991;75:584–90.
26. Freedman SF, McCormick K, Cox TA. Mitomycin C-augmented trabeculectomy with postoperative wound modulation in pediatric glaucoma. J AAPOS. 1999;3:117–24.
27. Sidoti PA, Belmonte SJ, Liebmann JM, Ritch R. Trabeculectomy with mitomycin-C in the treatment of pediatric glaucomas. Ophthalmology. 2000;107:422–9.
28. Budenz DL, Barton K, Feuer WJ, et al. Ahmed Baerveldt comparison study group. Treatment outcomes in the Ahmed Baerveldt comparison study after 1 year of follow up. Ophthalmology. 2011;118:443–52.
29. Christakis PG, Tsai JC, Kalenak JW, et al. The Ahmed versus Baerveldt study: three year treatment outcomes. Ophthalmology. 2013;120:2232–40.
30. Esfandiari H, Prager A, Hassanpour K, et al. The long-term visual outcomes of primary congenital glaucoma. J Ophthalmic Vis Res. 2020;15(3):326–30. https://doi.org/10.18502/jovr.v15i3.7451.

28. [illegible]

Update on Congenital Cataract

11

Michael C. Struck

11.1 Introduction

Vision 2020: The Right to Sight has identified the control of congenital cataract and blindness in children as a priority in its global initiative to reduce the burden of avoidable blindness [1]. Congenital cataract (CC) (Fig. 11.1), which refers to the opacity of the lens detected at birth or in early childhood [2] is a leading cause, along with retinopathy of prematurity (ROP), of treatable childhood blindness worldwide [3].

The epidemiological impact is often confused in the literature [4–6] but it is estimated that the prevalence of children worldwide that are bilaterally blind from cataracts is about 190,000, and an additional number suffer from partial or unilateral cataracts that cause differing levels of visual impairment [1, 7]. Of 1.4 million children worldwide who are blind, cataract is responsible for an estimated 14% [8]. A blind child is more likely to live in socioeconomic deprivation, to be more frequently hospitalized during childhood, and to die in childhood than a child not living with blindness.

Since Dr. Gregg Norman published the observation that CC is associated with material Rubella infection in 1941, a great deal of progress has been made in the epidemiology, etiology, diagnosis, and management of CC. This update on congenital cataract and the related burden of visual impairment focuses on emerging knowledge and therapies for children with severe visual disabilities. Much of this progress has been in recent years, and the goal of this chapter is to provide an update.

M. C. Struck (✉)
University of Wisconsin, Madison, WI, USA
e-mail: mcstruck@wisc.edu

A. Ramasubramanian (ed.), *Pediatric Ophthalmology*, Current Practices in Ophthalmology, https://doi.org/10.1007/978-981-19-4963-0_11

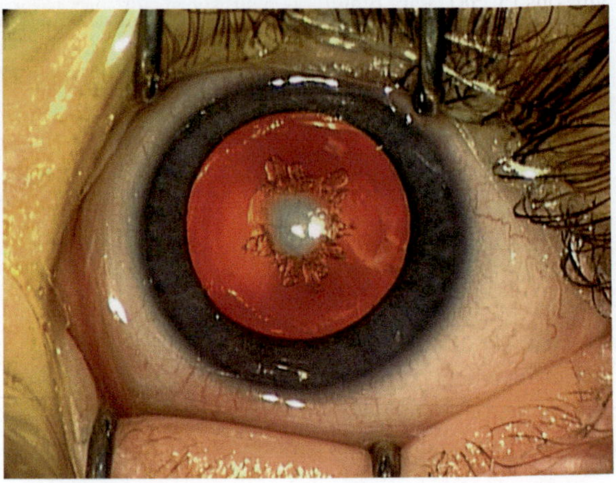

Fig. 11.1 Central congenital cataract with clear peripheral lens

11.2 Epidemiology

In most studies, cerebral visual impairment and optic nerve anomalies remain the most common causes of childhood severe vision impairment and blindness, while retinopathy of prematurity (ROP) and cataract is now the most common avoidable causes [9–11]. The constellation of causes of childhood blindness in lower income settings is shifting from infective and nutritional corneal opacities and congenital anomalies to more resemble the patterns seen in higher income settings.

In a study of 231,000 children (aged under 16 years) examined in a population-based study, 8 per 10,000 had vision worse than 3/60; almost half of the blind children had retinal disorders, the most common being retinopathy of prematurity. Cataract (28%) and globe anomaly (11%) were the next most common blinding disorders [10, 12]. These findings have been reproduced with minor variations in the incidence of etiology in multiple studies [12].

In a meta-analysis of the epidemiology of CC, the prevalence was estimated to be 4.2/10,000 children worldwide, which makes it a rare disease based on WHO (<6.5/10,000) and European (<5/10,000) standards. In contrast with common disorders, rare diseases have a much lower population prevalence, resulting in greater demands for documenting disease data and a greater reliance on accurate and comprehensive epidemiological information [13].

The incidence, or the number of new cases that develop over a specific time period (typically 1 year), is a harder figure to obtain. Estimates suggest an incidence of bilateral CC between 2.2 and 3.2/10,000 births per year worldwide, or about 20–30,000 new cases globally per year [14, 15].

Although relatively rare compared with age-related cataracts, CC tends to alter the quality of sensory information available to the child during sensitive periods of visual system development and causes irreversible visual defects [16, 17]. Children who are born blind and are not effectively treated have a lifetime of irreversible blindness. The resulting loss, expressed in blindness years, has a dramatic impact on the socioeconomics of the child, family, and community.

Genetic, metabolic, traumatic, and infectious factors can all lead to childhood cataracts.

Unfortunately, few large-scale epidemiological studies have provided a complete synthesis of the population, disease etiology, heritability of the evidence, and epidemiological traits. The common understanding for many years has been that roughly one-third of CC cases are inherited, one-third are associated with environmental risk factors and the remaining one-third are idiopathic [18]. However, more recent examination of the data suggests that idiopathic CC accounts for as much as two-thirds (62%) of all CC cases, while hereditary (22%) and nonhereditary (11%) are substantially less [13]. These older studies did not have the benefit of newer genetic testing. At the time of this writing, mutation screening of inherited congenital cataracts has identified nearly 200 locus and more than 100 causative genes, which are well summarized in the "Cat-Map" website (http://cat-map.wustl.edu/) (Messina-Baas and Cuevas-Covarrubias, 2017; Shiels et al., 2010). Newer genetic analysis would predict that, in the isolated bilateral CC category, 75% of cases have a genetic etiology [19]. Evaluation of the idiopathic aspects of this condition leave room for progress in this area of research in terms of both cataractogenesis and clinical considerations.

At this point, it may be beneficial for the reader to segregate bilateral and unilateral CC into separate categories of CC. The heritability, etiology, and visual consequences roughly separate along this distinction. Bilateral CC constituted only a slightly higher pooled proportion (54%) than unilateral CC. However, the proportions were quite different in subsets formed according to hereditary factors. Unilateral CC constitutes 56% of idiopathic CC but just 6% of hereditary CC [14, 20].

Bilateral congenital cataracts are often associated with monogenetic gene defects, systemic diseases, and infectious factors. Unilateral cataracts are more often related to local anomaly, such as persistent fetal vasculature (PFV). PFV is a congenital ocular dysgenesis in which the hyaloid embryonal vasculature is unable to regress completely [21, 22]. PFV was found in 22–46.5% of unilateral congenital cataract patients undergoing surgery [20, 23, 24]. A number of pathogenic gene mutations have been identified in animal models with bilateral PFV, including CRYBA3/A1, TSPAN12, and FZD5, but no genetic basis has been identified for unilateral PFV [25–27].

In regard to comorbidity associated with CC, isolated CC accounted for the highest percentage (62%), followed by CC associated with ocular disorder (23%), and CC associated with systemic disorders (17%) [13].

While the amassed knowledge on the genetics of congenital cataracts and associated systemic diseases has expanded dramatically in the last two decades; [4, 28] there is limited knowledge on the prevalence of systemic disorders in patients with unilateral congenital cataracts.

In the infantile aphakia treatment study (IATS), a very low percentage 8/217 (3.7%) of patients with a significant unilateral cataract had a significant associated systemic disorder. Including two patients with Down's syndrome, one with cerebral atrophy and delayed maturation, and one with Conradi–Hunermann syndrome, one patient with a mitochondrial disorder, another with autism, and one with Stickler syndrome. Finally, one adopted patient was found to have a profound hearing impairment and the cataract was presumed to be the result of congenital rubella [23].

Of the infectious causes of CC, Rubella and Herpes simplex virus (HSV) are the most common etiology [29, 30]. Congenital Rubella Syndrome (CRS), is the most important worldwide preventable cause of CC. In many countries, Rubella (German measles) has been virtually eliminated through childhood vaccination programs. The Rubella infection in adults is generally mild; however, if infected in the first trimester the rate of fetal infection is 90% with severe fetal detrimental effects. It is estimated that more than 100,000 infants worldwide are born each year with CRS [31]. According to a survey of the member countries in the World Health Organization (WHO), the number of countries that have incorporated rubella-containing vaccines into their routine national immunization programs increased from 83 in 1996 to 148 (76%) of countries in 2016. As of December 2016, the WHO Region of the Americas and the European Region have established rubella elimination goals, verified by the Region of the Americas in 2015 [32]. The South-East Asia region has rubella/CRS reduction goal (95%) by 2020; [33] the Western Pacific Region has established a rubella elimination target without a specific date, and the Eastern Mediterranean and African Regions do not currently have elimination targets (https://www.cdc.gov/vaccines/pubs/surv-manual/chpt15-crs.html).

Despite the great efforts made to improve the management of CC and a giant leap in surgical techniques, CC treatment is among the most difficult and cost-intensive interventions in ophthalmology, and the etiology of this condition remains largely unknown [34].

11.3 Genetics

Over the last 10 years, the progress and integration of diverse genetic approaches have accelerated the research of inherited cataracts to try to identify genetic defects that are associated with a specific phenotype. The molecular basis of congenital cataract is generally considered monogenetic, with causative mutations identified in genes encoding many different proteins.

Monogenic CC is of particular importance, as it is associated with high recurrence risk in affected families. It has been estimated that approximately 22–40% of CC are caused by single-gene mutations [13, 35, 36]. Monogenic CC is a genetically heterogeneous disorder, as mutations in over 100 genes have been associated with isolated pediatric cataract (Cat-Map; https://cat-map.wustl.edu/). Notably, mutations in a particular CC gene can result in different lens phenotypes even among subjects from the same family, this clinical heterogeneity precludes a genotype–phenotype correlation which could facilitate molecular diagnosis [37, 38].

The clinical phenotypes of childhood cataract are complex and diverse, categorized under a variety of classifications according to the lesion location and morphology, with a significant disparity in clinical outcome and visual compromise. Morphologic subtypes include anterior lenticonus, anterior polar, anterior pyramidal, anterior subcapsular, posterior polar, posterior lentiglobus, posterior lenticonus, posterior subcapsular, nuclear, cortical, lamellar, zonular, pulverulent, cerulean, sutural, polymorphic, membranous, and total cataracts [39, 40]. The main phenotypes of CC epidemiologically are (1) total (37%), (2) nuclear (27%), and (3) posterior subcapsular (27%) [13].

Morphology of cataract can help to reveal the cataractogenesis mechanisms in different stages of lens development, and, hence, help with diagnosing the cause and treating the disease properly. However, hereditary cataracts have significant clinical heterogeneity, both genetically and phenotypically, and reveal considerable changes among family members [37].

A great many pathogenic genes and mutations of congenital cataract have been successfully characterized by linkage analysis, DNA probe microarray, gene sequencing, and other screening strategies [35, 41]. Genes responsible for distinct isolated cataract can be divided into five main groups based on the encoded proteins: (1) *Crystallins*: including intracellular lens proteins, (2) *Connexins:* membrane gap junction proteins, (3) *Major Intrinsic Protein (MIP) or Aquaporins:* membrane water channel proteins, (4) *Cytoskeletal proteins:* (e.g., BFSP1 (filensin), BFSP2 (phakinin) and vimentin), and (5) *Transcription factors:* (TFs) (e.g., FOXE3, PAX6, PITX3, and MAFA) [6] see Fig. 11.2.

First-generation sequencing is based on the Sanger chain termination method, while Next Generation Sequencing (NGS), also known as High-throughput

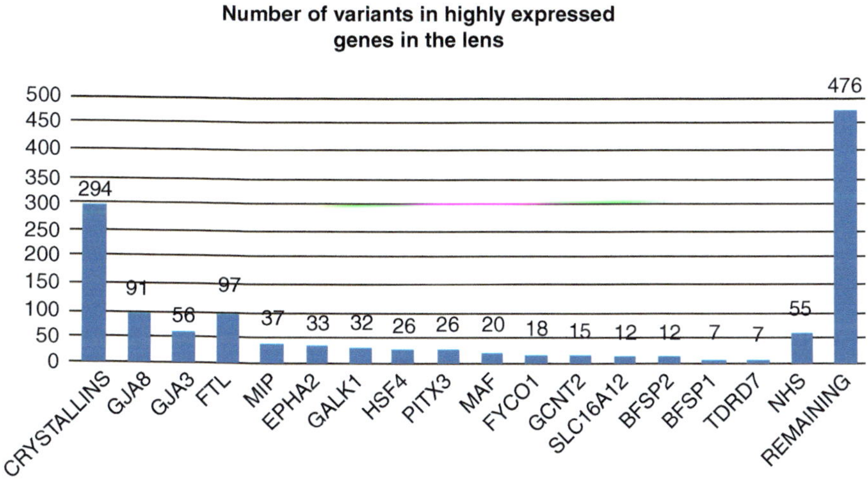

Fig. 11.2 Cataract-causing variants by gene. Total number of 1314 disease-causing variants (novel and recurrent) are shown in various highly expressed genes to date (http://cat-map.wustl.edu/), including crystallins, gap junction proteins, membrane proteins, developmental and cytoskeletal proteins in the lens; the remaining 476 variants are found in various other genes important for the normal function of the crystalline lens

sequencing, has been gradually applied in congenital cataract detection [19], such as genome sequencing, whole exome sequencing [42], sure select target enrichment [19, 43], and targeted exome sequencing [44]. NGS improves the yield in diagnosis of small deletions beyond the resolution of microarray and improves the detection of defects in genomically complex regions. NGS, which has gained acceptance as the testing method of choice, has demonstrated the efficiency of gene panel NGS testing in CC diagnosis with impressive mutation pick-up rates, ranging from 70 to 85% for isolated cataract [4, 28, 45], and 63% for syndromic CC [4, 19]. However, this still leaves approximately 25% of bilateral isolated CC of unknown etiology (Fig. 11.3). Moreover, these studies have highlighted the enormous clinical utility of ascertaining the precise cause of CC. Examples of this include where genetic diagnosis has (1): altered the clinical hypothesis regarding predicted mode of inheritance thereby redefining recurrence risk and informing genetic counseling (2); directed clinical management and patient care via presymptomatic diagnosis of significant multisystemic disease (3); diagnosed an unsuspected metabolic disease that is amenable to treatment where early treatment significantly reduces morbidity [46]. Furthermore, a study of 50 patients by CC panel testing found that over 15% of cases were due to mutations in genes associated with inborn errors of metabolism [19].

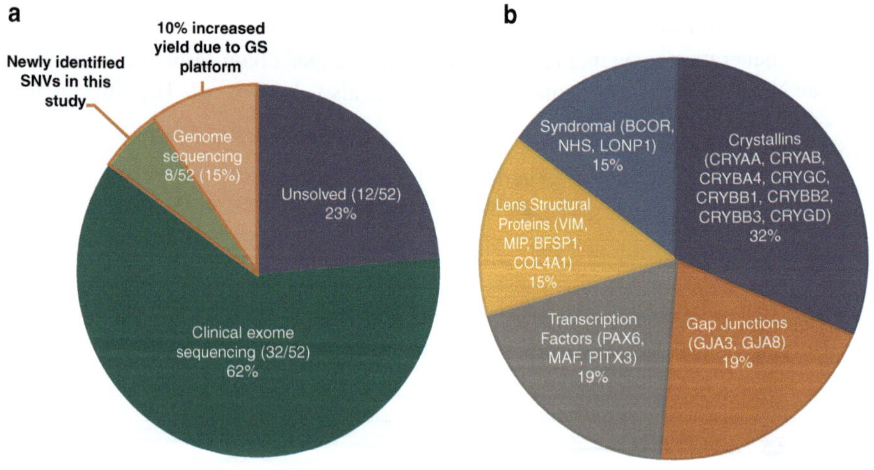

Fig. 11.3 Overall yield and gene breakdown in combined cataract cohort of 52 patients. (**a**) The overall yield in the congenital cataract cohort studied in this and our previous publication. In 52 patients, pathogenic variants were found in an additional 10% of cases using the genome sequencing (GS) platform due to detection of small copy number variants (CNVs) (2), indels in repetitive regions (2), and single-nucleotide variants (SNVs) in GC-rich regions (1). Additional SNVs were identified in this study due to the use of an extended gene list (2) and identification of an SNV in a known disease gene in a previously uninvestigated case (1). In total, 62% were identified previously on clinical ES. (**b**) The chart demonstrates the overall breakdown, by gene category, in the entire cataract cohort. Over half the responsible variants are still in the frequently reported crystallin and gap junction genes. However, an increasing role of rarely reported genes such as the transcription factors and lens structural proteins has been found. Also, syndromal genes are increasingly reported, even in cases referred initially as nonsyndromal cataracts. (From Ma [47])

The Cat-Map and iSyTE (integrated Systems Tool for Eye gene discovery) databases are effective tools for exploring the molecular genetics and mechanism of inherited cataracts. The Cat-Map, a web-based database and chromosome map, summarizes the spectrum of mutations associated with hereditary and age-related cataract and updates the data in real-time [48] (Cat-Map, http://cat-map.wustl.edu/). Further, the eye gene expression database iSyTE uses a microarray data set of the mouse embryonic lens to identify genes associated with lens growth and cataract, and to indicate the potential regulatory pathways of these genes [49, 50].

The crystallin proteins constitute 90% of the proteins in lens fibers [51], and were discovered and named nearly 125 years ago by Morner as the main structural proteins of the ocular lens [52]. The lens fibers are a long-lived, ever-growing avascular capsulated organ and the crystallin protein is essential for maintaining transparency [53–56]. To maintain its life-long transparency and optical function crystallin organization in the lens is critically important. Mutations in the crystallin genes may affect the stability, solubility, and oligomerize feature of these proteins, disrupt the ordered arrangement, and result in lens opacity [57].

Crystallin proteins are divided into Alpha α, Beta β, and Gamma γ proteins. The α-crystallins constitute approximately 35% of the lens. They are heat shock proteins that contribute to the refractive power of the lens and act as a molecular chaperone [52, 56]. α-crystallins are the most abundant water-soluble proteins in the lens and their specific, closely packed arrangements play an important role in maintaining the lens transparency [56]. β and γ crystallins are very similar in structure, and together form a superfamily, called βγ-crystallins that share a common polypeptide chain fold [58].

Major intrinsic protein (MIP) is also known as aquaporin-0 due to its function as a voltage-dependent water channel and adhesion molecule [59]. It is only expressed in terminally differentiated fiber cells and is the most abundant integral membrane protein in the lens. They provide nutrients to central fiber cells and maintain homeostasis [60]. Genetic studies reveal mutations inherited in an autosomal dominant fashion.

Connexins also known as hemichannel are hydrophilic gap junctions that provide the transfer of small molecules and maintain lens transparency [61]. Three connexins have been identified in the lens: connexin 43,46, and 50. They are also critical in eye development and the lens growth process and have been identified in nuclear CC and CC with microcornea [62, 63].

Cytoskeleton proteins interact with crystallins in the lens cells to define the structural framework of the cell [64]. Cytoskeletal proteins include actin filaments, microtubules, and intermediate filaments and provide the structure for lens fiber cells [65]. Beaded filament structural protein interacts with crystallin α and currently 14 mutations have been described contributing to inherited cataract [5].

Transcription factors regulate embryonic lens development. Mutations in the *HSF4, PITX3, MAF, and FOXE3* genes lead to cataracts, anterior chamber dysgenesis, and developmental ocular anomalies. Currently, mutations in transcription factors are associated with 19% of CC [45, 47].

Congenital cataracts universally occur in an isolated pattern but can also be a part of syndromes affecting other systemic tissues. Genes responsible for major syndromic cataracts include GLA (Fabry's disease) [66], OCRL (Lowe syndrome) [67], GALK117q (galactosemia) [68], NHS (Nance–Horan cataract–dental syndrome) [69], and PAX6 (aniridia) [70, 71]. Besides, pediatric cataract may also be one component of syndromes related to chromosomal disorder or DNA repair defects, such as Down syndrome, WAGR syndrome, Cockayne Syndrome, and Prader-Willi syndrome [72–74].

11.4 Treatment

11.4.1 Goals

The principle of treatment for congenital cataract is to preserve and restore vision, prevent permanent vision loss or blindness, and reduce the incidence of amblyopia and maximize vision potential. It is well-established that there is a "critical period" for the development of vision and that without early treatment (in many cases 6 weeks of age) permanent damage begins to accrue to the developing visual system. This critical period requiring treatment before the onset of the beginning of permanent visual deprivation has been categorized as a bilinear/plateau model [75]. During the first 14 weeks after birth vision recovery is reduced by one line for every 3 weeks in delayed treatment, from 14 to 40 weeks of age, vision recovery reaches a plateau. It should be understood that delayed treatment may result in irreversible vision loss.

While complete CC requires emergent pediatric ophthalmologic care, some morphologic types of partial CC, that have less potential damage to the developing visual system, such as anterior polar, or punctate cataract, may not require immediate surgery [18, 76].

11.4.2 Early Detection

The most critical factor in the successful treatment of CC remains early detection and early treatment [77]. Untreated dense CC (Fig. 11.1) leads to irreversible neurophysiological changes and sensory deprivation amblyopia. Associated adverse outcomes such as nystagmus and strabismus commonly coexist [17]. Therefore, it is imperative that affected infants are referred promptly to centers able to manage them appropriately. Optimal surgical results require a very early referral and intervention. The best outcomes in dense unilateral CC follow surgery and optical correction before 6–8 weeks of age [16]. More recent studies of dense bilateral CC suggest that visual outcomes follow a linear model, correlating to the length of visual deprivation, but that best results occur in those infants operated on by 8 weeks of (corrected) age [78–80]. By 8–10 months of age a child with a complete CC may no longer be capable of recovery of visual function due to irreversible changes in brain development.

Delayed detection occurs in all communities; however, it is probably highest in the developing world. The mean delay to an appropriate treatment center, 39–49 months, is often far too late for effective treatment and restoration of vision [81–83].

Community education and training of primary health care providers may be the single most critical factor in reducing worldwide childhood blindness from CC. Effective screening should be performed within the first 72 h of birth and again prior to 6 weeks of age with a direct ophthalmoscope and the "red reflex test." [3, 77] It is important for health care providers to have resources for detection, recognize the urgency of treatment for CC, and be provided with tertiary centers capable of treatment. Additionally, community education is necessary for families to reduce educational barriers, cultural barriers, and provide access to care.

Finally, advances in 3D ultrasound have recently made it possible to diagnose CC in utero [84]. For families at risk, prenatal genetic testing of fetal DNA is possible to diagnose the likelihood of CC [85].

11.4.3 Evaluation

While identification and timely surgical intervention in infants and children are crucial for the preservation of sight, precise diagnosis is also important. CC is a highly heterogeneous disorder associated with a number of systemic diseases. Etiologies may include trauma, maternal infection, intrauterine chemical or drug exposure, biochemical disturbance, and genetic variation (chromosomal abnormalities or single-gene mutation-associated disorders). Pinpointing a diagnosis, even with the use of clinical algorithms, is complicated, and often protracted [17, 18].

A comprehensive history, including extended family history, is important. Examination of family members can be of critical importance because autosomal dominant cataract with significant phenotypic heterogeneity is responsible for a vast majority of inherited CC. Historically clinicians have pursued biochemical, genetic, clinical, and imaging tests either simultaneously or consecutively and iteratively [77]. Investigations performed will typically include chromosomal analysis and a "TORCH" screen to look for evidence of intrauterine infection with toxoplasmosis, rubella, cytomegalovirus, and herpes. Biochemical tests including urinary assays of amino acid profile, oligosaccharides, organic acids, and reducing substances together with blood tests for plasma amino acid profile, liver function tests, renal profile, and assay of Gal-1-P-uridyl transferase are often performed [4].

11.4.4 Morphology

In the management of CC, the morphology of the cataract is very useful because quantification of visual acuity in a preverbal child is often not possible and is associated with a significant overlay of amblyopia or associated neurodevelopmental impairment. The phenotypic classification is based on location of the opacity and size and can be categorized into eight subtypes including (1) total, (2) anterior polar, (3) cortical lamellar, (4) Fetal nuclear, (5) posterior polar, (6) posterior lentiglobus/lenticonus, (7) subcapsular, and (8) persistent fetal vasculature (PFV) [18]. Many CC, if left untreated will slowly become diffuse, total cataracts.

In the Toddler Aphakia and Pseudophakia study (TAPS), the cataract morphologic characteristics for bilateral CC were classified as nuclear (43%), cortical and lamellar (32%), total white or mature (4%), posterior capsular or subcapsular (4%), posterior lenticonus (4%), anterior capsular or subcapsular (1%), ectopia lentis et pupillae (1%), and unknown (11%). Microphthalmia was detected in 117 eyes (50%). Microcornea was present in 19 eyes (11%), and other anterior segment abnormalities were present in 12 eyes (7%) [86].

Twenty-four children (25%) in this series demonstrated bilateral cataracts associated with chromosomal and neurodevelopmental anomalies. The IoLunder2 study reported a systemic disorder or neurodevelopmental impairment in 55% of children with bilateral cataracts [78]. These studies suggest a higher rate of ocular and systemic comorbidity than is present in the epidemiologic literature [13].

11.4.5 Surgical Treatment

Assuming the CC is identified through early detection and appropriate timely referral is achieved, the successful management of CC is one of the most time-intensive and resource-demanding treatments. Currently, even though a high percentage of CC has a monogenetic etiology, there is no theoretical treatment paradigm that would allow for the restoration of lenticular clarity through gene replacement. Treatment for the foreseeable future relies on surgical management to (1) restore clarity to the optical media, (2) manage optical (refractive) rehabilitation, (3) Prevent and treat amblyopia, and (4) constant surveillance for secondary complications.

Age at surgery is a known determinant of successful visual outcome. Consensus in the literature recommends surgery at less than 6–8 weeks of age for unilateral cataract and 6–10 weeks of age for bilateral cataract surgery with less than 2 weeks between operations [18, 77, 87]. In an attempt to improve visual outcomes in this visually handicapping condition, the IOLunder2 study* and Infantile Aphakia Treatment Study (IATS) have confirmed and refined the management strategy for treatment of children with this condition [78, 88].

Modern surgical management relies on the vitrectomy machine to perform the major components of the surgical procedure. The vitrector can be used to perform the capsulorhexis (vitrectorhexis), lensectomy, posterior capsulotomy, and core vitrectomy of the anterior hyaloid face. Since secondary opacification of the capsule and anterior hyaloid occurs with a rate of essentially 100% in cases of congenital cataract, removal at the time of primary surgery is the standard of care [89, 90]. Standard vitrectomy instrumentation has relied on a 20-gauge system. Due to low scleral rigidity in children, surgical wounds tend to leak, creating an unstable anterior chamber during surgery. Advances in surgical vitrectomy intervention have recently been refined to smaller gauge systems with recent addition of 23-, 25- and 27-gauge instrumentation [91, 92]. Smaller surgical wounds, accompanying the smaller instrumentation, have allowed for increased stability of surgical intervention.

Anterior capsulotomy is generally performed by curvilinear capsulorhexis using a 20- or 23-gauge microfixation forceps, or by vitrectorhexis [18]. Femtosecond laser-assisted capsulorhexis has been used in pediatric cataract surgery but is associated with the negative consequences of posttreatment enlargement of the capsule opening and the necessity for cantholysis to accommodate the laser equipment [93].

Determination of the use (or not) of an intraocular lens (IOL) has received considerable study. In children with a normal-sized eye under 7 months of age, the capsule measurement is approximately 7 mm in diameter [77]. Primary IOL implantation in children under 7 months of age is therefore not only challenging but did not confer any improvement in visual outcome and was associated with a higher rate of adverse events and need for additional surgery in the IATS [88, 94, 95]. These findings were supported by the IOLunder2 study [78]. However, IOL implantation in children over 7 months of age has been shown to confer a decreased risk of adverse events that is equivalent to IOL implantation in children over 2 years of age [96, 97].

Visual Axis obscuration (VAO) is a known common adverse event following pediatric cataract surgery, which increases in rate inverse to age at surgery. This effect is explained by a "scaffold effect" of the implanted IOL in the child's eye [77]. Thus, the use of primary IOL implantation in children under 2 should be accompanied by an informed consent process of the potential need for additional surgical intervention.

Determination of the power of the IOL implantation is additionally a more complex process. Growth of the eye and changes in the corneal curvature during childhood will change the refractive outcome as the child matures. The elements that are crucial in selecting the initial postoperative refractive goal are IOL calculation, amblyopia management, anisometropia management, and the logarithmic growth of the eye [98]. Biometry in CC is typically performed in the operating room. IOL calculations in children are of lesser accuracy than in adults, influenced by greater errors of biometry and the lack of an IOL formula for children. The IOL formulas shown to have the least error and greatest reproducibility in children have been the SRK/T and Holliday 2 formulas [99–101].

Anisometropia is of great concern in children who have unilateral cataract surgery. Optical correction with spectacles in this situation is generally not acceptable due to induced aniseikonia. Aphakic contact lenses are therefore relied on when IOL implantation is not advised. While there are several options for aphakic lens correction, many pediatric ophthalmologists rely on the extended wear "Silsoft" soft silicone lens (Bausch and Lomb) because of the high tolerance and oxygen permeability characteristics [102, 103].

From infancy, the growth of the eye follows a logarithmic curve [104]. This growth results in a myopic shift of the refraction over the first 20 years of life. Predicting the refractive trajectory of the eye is therefore troublesome, leading to the need in some children who undergo primary IOL placement in infancy, for IOL exchange later [88]. Another potential option is an investigational IOL which involves a two-part IOL that includes an exchangeable optic for refractive management without the need to explant the entire lens [105]. A pediatric IOL selection computer program has been published that allows surgeons to calculate the relative myopic shift in a child who has IOL implantation [106].

11.4.6 Complications

The complications of visual deprivation and secondary amblyopia have been discussed, but despite the relative ability to treat these complications given timely referral, they remain the most visually disabling. Secondary visual axis opacification (VAO) has also been discussed and can occur with or without IOL implantation, but the rate is higher in CC with IOL implantation.

Postoperative open-angle glaucoma is emerging as potentially the most important visually disabling consequence of surgery for congenital or infantile cataract. It has been reported to occur in between 6% and 58.7% of children after cataract extraction, depending on the population studied and the length of follow-up [107–110]. It is insidious, can be difficult to detect, and may occur many years after surgery.

Many factors have been reported to increase the risk of postoperative glaucoma including age at detection of cataract, age at cataract surgery, primary intraocular lens implantation, significant postoperative uveitis, conspicuous family history, and associated ocular malformations, such as microphthalmos or persistent fetal vasculature (PFV) [86, 107, 108, 111, 112]. Despite speculation, IOL implantation has not conferred protection from the risk of secondary glaucoma, with multiple studies showing no associated risk or benefit [77, 113, 114].

Cataract surgery during early infancy is well-established to be the most important factor for the formation of postoperative secondary glaucoma. It should be considered that although younger age at the time of cataract removal can provide better prerequisites for prophylaxis of amblyopia, it also confers a higher risk of the development of glaucoma.

In one study, younger age at surgery and smaller (<9.5 mm) corneal diameter at surgery conferred an increased risk for glaucoma or glaucoma suspect designation (younger age: odds ratio [OR], 1.44; and smaller cornea: OR, 3.95). Multivariate analysis in this bilateral cohort also revealed that younger age at surgery conferred an increased risk of glaucoma. The OR analysis suggested that each month of reduced age increased the risk of glaucoma by approximately 40% [86].

The incidence of secondary glaucoma is unpredictable but constant, the risks include the age at the time of surgery, on the ocular anatomy, and on the follow-up duration. It is advisable that all children should be considered at risk for the remainder of their lives [114].

Strabismus is also a complication of CC. In the IATS trial, strabismus surgery was performed in approximately 50% (with or without IOL) of patients with strabismus by 5 years of age; esotropia surgery was twice as common as exotropia surgery [115]. Additionally, children without strabismus had better visual acuity than those with strabismus. It has not been known whether better acuity in the treated eye is protective for the development of strabismus or whether straighter alignment improves amblyopia treatment after cataract surgery. In the present study, visual acuity was better in children who did not undergo strabismus surgery than in those who did (0.70/1.10 log MAR, $P = 0.097$).

Anisometropia is a constant postoperative challenge in the optical rehabilitation of children with unilateral CC. In the IATS study, infants that underwent unilateral IOL implantation at primary surgery were noted to have significant postoperative anisometropia, with the treated eye more myopic than the fellow eye in almost all cases. Anisometropia is likely one of the factors that contribute to both amblyopia and decreased binocular function in children with unilateral pseudophakia [116]. It is known that 2 diopters or more of spherical myopic anisometropia and 1 diopter or more of spherical hypermetropic anisometropia significantly increase the incidence of amblyopia and decreased binocular function [117].

Numerous encouraging advances in the recent science behind congenital cataract affords a new window into our management and understanding of this condition, with new insights into the risk factors, pathophysiology, and potential therapeutic strategies. Congenital cataract will remain a challenge for epidemiology, preventability, early diagnosis, heritable etiology, and technical therapeutic management.

The primary goal of preventing or reducing the incidence of congenital cataract development through congenital Rubella and Herpes reduction programs and genetic heritability studies is encouraging. The development of early detection, referral, and treatment programs are critical to the success of the elimination of blindness from CC. Finally, technical advances have made the goal to preserve and restore vision, prevent permanent vision loss or blindness, reduce the incidence of amblyopia, and maximize vision potential, achievable.

References

1. Gilbert C, Foster A. Childhood blindness in the context of VISION 2020—the right to sight. Bull World Health Organ. 2001;79(3):227–32.
2. Jain IS, et al. Congenital cataract: etiology and morphology. J Pediatr Ophthalmol Strabismus. 1983;20(6):238–42.
3. Gogate P, Kalua K, Courtright P. Blindness in childhood in developing countries: time for a reassessment? PLoS Med. 2009;6(12):e1000177.
4. Gillespie RL, et al. Personalized diagnosis and management of congenital cataract by next-generation sequencing. Ophthalmology. 2014;121(11):2124–37.e1–2.
5. Li J, et al. Molecular genetics of congenital cataracts. Exp Eye Res. 2020;191:107872.
6. Berry V, et al. Inherited cataracts: molecular genetics, clinical features, disease mechanisms and novel therapeutic approaches. Br J Ophthalmol. 2020;104(10):1331–7.
7. Foster A, Gilbert C, Rahi J. Epidemiology of cataract in childhood: a global perspective. J Cataract Refract Surg. 1997;23(Suppl 1):601–4.
8. Rahi JS, et al. Measuring the burden of childhood blindness. Br J Ophthalmol. 1999;83(4):387–8.
9. Ozturk T, et al. Changing trends over the last decade in the aetiology of childhood blindness: a study from a tertiary referral centre. Br J Ophthalmol. 2016;100(2):166–71.

10. Kemmanu V, et al. Prevalence of childhood blindness and ocular morbidity in a rural pediatric population in southern India: the Pavagada pediatric eye disease study-1. Ophthalmic Epidemiol. 2016;23(3):185–92.
11. Aghaji A, Okoye O, Bowman R. Causes and emerging trends of childhood blindness: findings from schools for the blind in Southeast Nigeria. Br J Ophthalmol. 2015;99(6):727–31.
12. Kong L, et al. An update on progress and the changing epidemiology of causes of childhood blindness worldwide. J AAPOS. 2012;16(6):501–7.
13. Wu X, et al. Prevalence and epidemiological characteristics of congenital cataract: a systematic review and meta-analysis. Sci Rep. 2016;6:28564.
14. Wirth MG, et al. Aetiology of congenital and paediatric cataract in an Australian population. Br J Ophthalmol. 2002;86(7):782–6.
15. Rahi JS, Dezateux C, British Congenital Cataract Interest Group. Measuring and interpreting the incidence of congenital ocular anomalies: lessons from a national study of congenital cataract in the UK. Invest Ophthalmol Vis Sci. 2001;42(7):1444–8.
16. Birch EE, Stager DR. The critical period for surgical treatment of dense congenital unilateral cataract. Invest Ophthalmol Vis Sci. 1996;37(8):1532–8.
17. Lloyd IC, et al. Advances in the management of congenital and infantile cataract. Eye (Lond). 2007;21(10):1301–9.
18. Wilson ME, Trivedi RH, editors. Pediatric cataract surgery. 1st ed. Philadelphia, PA: Lippincott Williams & Wilkins; 2014.
19. Gillespie RL, et al. Next-generation sequencing in the diagnosis of metabolic disease marked by pediatric cataract. Ophthalmology. 2016;123(1):217–20.
20. Rahi JS, Dezateux C. Congenital and infantile cataract in the United Kingdom: underlying or associated factors. British congenital cataract interest group. Invest Ophthalmol Vis Sci. 2000;41(8):2108–14.
21. Mehta A, et al. Persistent fetal vasculature - clinical spectrum. Indian J Ophthalmol. 2018;66(12):1860.
22. Zahavi A, et al. Management of severe persistent fetal vasculature: case series and review of the literature. Int Ophthalmol. 2019;39(3):579–87.
23. Traboulsi EI, et al. Associated systemic and ocular disorders in patients with congenital unilateral cataracts: the infant aphakia treatment study experience. Eye (Lond). 2016;30(9):1170–4.
24. Solebo AL, et al. Congenital cataract associated with persistent fetal vasculature: findings from IoLunder2. Eye (Lond). 2016;30(9):1204–9.
25. Grahn BH, Storey ES, McMillan C. Inherited retinal dysplasia and persistent hyperplastic primary vitreous in miniature schnauzer dogs. Vet Ophthalmol. 2004;7(3):151–8.
26. Zigler JS, et al. βA3/A1-crystallin and persistent fetal vasculature (PFV) disease of the eye. Biochim Biophys Acta. 2016;1860(1 Pt B):287–98.
27. Zhang J, Fuhrmann S, Vetter ML. A nonautonomous role for retinal frizzled-5 in regulating hyaloid vitreous vasculature development. Invest Ophthalmol Vis Sci. 2008;49(12):5561–7.
28. Bell S, et al. Clinical spectrum and genetic diagnosis of 54 consecutive patients aged 0-25 with bilateral cataracts. Genes (Basel). 2021;12(2)
29. Khokhar S, Pillay G, Agarwal E. Pediatric cataract - importance of early detection and management. Indian J Pediatr. 2018;85(3):209–16.
30. Singh MP, et al. Infectious agents in congenital cataract in a tertiary care referral center in North India. Diagn Microbiol Infect Dis. 2016;85(4):477–81.
31. Robertson SE, et al. Rubella and congenital rubella syndrome: global update. Rev Panam Salud Publica. 2003;14(5):306–15.
32. PAHO. Americas region is declared the world's first to eliminate rubella. Washington, DC: PAHO; 2015.
33. WHO. Rubella and congenital rubella syndrome control and elimination -- global progress 2000–2014. Wkly Epidemiol Rec. 2015;90(39):6.
34. Edwards AO. Clinical features of the congenital vitreoretinopathies. Eye (Lond). 2008;22(10):1233–42.

35. Li J, et al. Screening, genetics, risk factors, and treatment of neonatal cataracts. Birth Defects Res. 2017;109(10):734–43.
36. Shiels A, Hejtmancik JF. Mutations and mechanisms in congenital and age-related cataracts. Exp Eye Res. 2017;156:95–102.
37. Santana A, Waiswo M. The genetic and molecular basis of congenital cataract. Arq Bras Oftalmol. 2011;74(2):136–42.
38. Hejtmancik JF. Congenital cataracts and their molecular genetics. Semin Cell Dev Biol. 2008;19(2):134–49.
39. Long E, et al. Monitoring and morphologic classification of Pediatric cataract using slit-lamp-adapted photography. Transl Vis Sci Technol. 2017;6(6):2.
40. Patel N, et al. Novel phenotypes and loci identified through clinical genomics approaches to pediatric cataract. Hum Genet. 2017;136(2):205–25.
41. Medsinge A, Nischal KK. Pediatric cataract: challenges and future directions. Clin Ophthalmol. 2015;9:77–90.
42. Liu H, et al. Whole exome sequencing identifies a novel mutation in the. Ann Clin Lab Sci. 2017;47(1):92–5.
43. Musleh M, et al. Improving diagnosis for congenital cataract by introducing NGS genetic testing. BMJ Qual Improv Rep. 2016;5(1)
44. Zhai Y, et al. Targeted exome sequencing of congenital cataracts related genes: broadening the mutation spectrum and genotype-phenotype correlations in 27 Chinese Han families. Sci Rep. 2017;7(1):1219.
45. Ma AS, et al. Sporadic and familial congenital cataracts: mutational Spectrum and new diagnoses using next-generation sequencing. Hum Mutat. 2016;37(4):371–84.
46. Astiazarán MC, et al. Next generation sequencing-based molecular diagnosis in familial congenital cataract expands the mutational spectrum in known congenital cataract genes. Am J Med Genet A. 2018;176(12):2637–45.
47. Ma A, et al. Genome sequencing in congenital cataracts improves diagnostic yield. Hum Mutat. 2021;42(9):1173–83.
48. Shiels A, Bennett TM, Hejtmancik JF. Cat-map: putting cataract on the map. Mol Vis. 2010;16:2007–15.
49. Kakrana A, et al. iSyTE 2.0: a database for expression-based gene discovery in the eye. Nucleic Acids Res. 2018;46(D1):D875–85.
50. Lachke SA, et al. iSyTE: integrated systems tool for eye gene discovery. Invest Ophthalmol Vis Sci. 2012;53(3):1617–27.
51. Shiels A, Hejtmancik JF. Genetic origins of cataract. Arch Ophthalmol. 2007;125(2):165–73.
52. Horwitz J. Alpha-crystallin. Exp Eye Res. 2003;76(2):145–53.
53. Riazuddin SA, et al. Mutations in betaB3-crystallin associated with autosomal recessive cataract in two Pakistani families. Invest Ophthalmol Vis Sci. 2005;46(6):2100–6.
54. Bassnett S, Shi Y, Vrensen GF. Biological glass: structural determinants of eye lens transparency. Philos Trans R Soc Lond Ser B Biol Sci. 2011;366(1568):1250–64.
55. Kuszak JR, Zoltoski RK, Sivertson C. Fibre cell organization in crystalline lenses. Exp Eye Res. 2004;78(3):673–87.
56. Hejtmancik JF, et al. Lens biology and biochemistry. Prog Mol Biol Transl Sci. 2015;134:169–201.
57. Wistow G. The human crystallin gene families. Hum Genomics. 2012;6:26.
58. Hejtmancik JF, Wingfield PT, Sergeev YV. Beta-crystallin association. Exp Eye Res. 2004;79(6):377–83.
59. Huang B, He W. Molecular characteristics of inherited congenital cataracts. Eur J Med Genet. 2010;53(6):347–57.
60. Geyer DD, et al. Novel single-base deletional mutation in major intrinsic protein (MIP) in autosomal dominant cataract. Am J Ophthalmol. 2006;141(4):761–3.
61. Berthoud VM, Ngezahayo A. Focus on lens connexins. BMC Cell Biol. 2017;18(Suppl 1):6.
62. Devi RR, Vijayalakshmi P. Novel mutations in GJA8 associated with autosomal dominant congenital cataract and microcornea. Mol Vis. 2006;12:190–5.

63. Hu S, et al. A novel mutation in GJA8 causing congenital cataract-microcornea syndrome in a Chinese pedigree. Mol Vis. 2010;16:1585–92.
64. Reddy MA, et al. Molecular genetic basis of inherited cataract and associated phenotypes. Surv Ophthalmol. 2004;49(3):300–15.
65. Cheng C, Nowak RB, Fowler VM. The lens actin filament cytoskeleton: diverse structures for complex functions. Exp Eye Res. 2017;156:58–71.
66. Li P, et al. Functional evaluation of a novel GLA causative mutation in Fabry disease. Mol Genet Genomic Med. 2019;7(9):e864.
67. De Matteis MA, et al. The 5-phosphatase OCRL in Lowe syndrome and dent disease 2. Nat Rev Nephrol. 2017;13(8):455–70.
68. Nema N, et al. Association of presenile cataract with galactose-1-phosphate uridyl transferase gene mutations. Natl Med J India. 2017;30(2):73–5.
69. Ling C, et al. Whole exome sequencing identified a novel truncation mutation in the NHS gene associated with Nance-Horan syndrome. BMC Med Genet. 2019;20(1):14.
70. Jin C, et al. A recurrent PAX6 mutation is associated with aniridia and congenital progressive cataract in a Chinese family. Mol Vis. 2012;18:465–70.
71. Zhang R, et al. Novel variants in PAX6 gene caused congenital aniridia in two Chinese families. Eye (Lond). 2017;31(6):956–61.
72. Ferreira MAT, et al. WAGRO syndrome: a rare genetic condition associated with aniridia and additional ophthalmologic abnormalities. Arq Bras Oftalmol. 2019;82(4):336–8.
73. Hamid MA, Mehta MC, Kuppermann BD. Multimodal imaging in a patient with Prader-Willi syndrome. Int J Retina Vitreous. 2018;4:45.
74. Sanchez-Roman I, et al. Two Cockayne syndrome patients with a novel splice site mutation - clinical and metabolic analyses. Mech Ageing Dev. 2018;175:7–16.
75. Birch EE, et al. The critical period for surgical treatment of dense congenital bilateral cataracts. J AAPOS. 2009;13(1):67–71.
76. Forster JE, et al. Grading infantile cataracts. Ophthalmic Physiol Opt. 2006;26(4):372–9.
77. Self JE, et al. Cataract management in children: a review of the literature and current practice across five large UK centres. Eye (Lond). 2020;34(12):2197–218.
78. Solebo AL, et al. 5-year outcomes after primary intraocular lens implantation in children aged 2 years or younger with congenital or infantile cataract: findings from the IoLunder2 prospective inception cohort study. Lancet Child Adolesc Health. 2018;2(12):863–71.
79. Jain S, et al. Duration of form deprivation and visual outcome in infants with bilateral congenital cataracts. J AAPOS. 2010;14(1):31–4.
80. Abadi RV, Forster JE, Lloyd IC. Ocular motor outcomes after bilateral and unilateral infantile cataracts. Vis Res. 2006;46(6–7):940–52.
81. Mwende J, et al. Delay in presentation to hospital for surgery for congenital and developmental cataract in Tanzania. Br J Ophthalmol. 2005;89(11):1478–82.
82. You C, et al. Visual impairment and delay in presentation for surgery in Chinese pediatric patients with cataract. Ophthalmology. 2011;118(1):17–23.
83. Bowman RJ, et al. Outcomes of bilateral cataract surgery in Tanzanian children. Ophthalmology. 2007;114(12):2287–92.
84. Ashwal E, et al. Prenatal ultrasonographic diagnosis of cataract: in utero manifestations of cryptic disease. Ultraschall Med. 2018;39(2):213–8.
85. Hartwig TS, et al. Discordant non-invasive prenatal testing (NIPT) - a systematic review. Prenat Diagn. 2017;37(6):527–39.
86. Bothun ED, et al. Outcomes of bilateral cataracts removed in infants 1 to 7 months of age using the toddler aphakia and pseudophakia treatment study registry. Ophthalmology. 2020;127(4):501–10.
87. Lim ME, Buckley EG, Prakalapakorn SG. Update on congenital cataract surgery management. Curr Opin Ophthalmol. 2017;28(1):87–92.
88. Lambert SR, et al. Comparison of contact lens and intraocular lens correction of monocular aphakia during infancy: a randomized clinical trial of HOTV optotype acuity at age 4.5 years and clinical findings at age 5 years. JAMA Ophthalmol. 2014;132(6):676–82.

89. Zwaan J, et al. Pediatric intraocular lens implantation. Surgical results and complications in more than 300 patients. Ophthalmology. 1998;105(1):112–8; discussion 118–9
90. Brady KM, et al. Cataract surgery and intraocular lens implantation in children. Am J Ophthalmol. 1995;120(1):1–9.
91. Charles S, et al. Clinical comparison of 27-gauge and 23-gauge instruments on the outcomes of pars plana vitrectomy surgery for the treatment of vitreoretinal diseases. Curr Opin Ophthalmol. 2020;31(3):185–91.
92. Ma F, Wang Q, Wang L. Advances in the management of the surgical complications for congenital cataract. Front Med. 2012;6(4):360–5.
93. Dick HB, Schelenz D, Schultz T. Femtosecond laser-assisted pediatric cataract surgery: Bochum formula. J Cataract Refract Surg. 2015;41(4):821–6.
94. Lambert SR, Bothun ED, Plager DA. Five-year postoperative outcomes of bilateral aphakia and pseudophakia in children up to 2 years of age: a randomized clinical trial. Am J Ophthalmol. 2019;199:263–4.
95. Plager DA, et al. Complications in the first 5 years following cataract surgery in infants with and without intraocular lens implantation in the infant aphakia treatment study. Am J Ophthalmol. 2014;158(5):892–8.
96. Struck MC. Long-term results of pediatric cataract surgery and primary intraocular lens implantation from 7 to 22 months of life. JAMA Ophthalmol. 2015;133(10):1180–3.
97. Bothun ED, et al. Outcomes of unilateral cataracts in infants and toddlers 7 to 24 months of age: toddler aphakia and pseudophakia study (TAPS). Ophthalmology. 2019;126(8):1189–95.
98. McClatchey S, Hofmeister E. Calculation and selection of intraocular lens power for children. In: Wilson M, Trivedi R, editors. Pediatric cataract surgery. 1st ed. Philadelphia, PA: Lippincott Williams & Wilkins; 2014. p. 6.
99. Trivedi RH, Wilson ME, Reardon W. Accuracy of the Holladay 2 intraocular lens formula for pediatric eyes in the absence of preoperative refraction. J Cataract Refract Surg. 2011;37(7):1239–43.
100. Joshi P, Mehta R, Ganesh S. Accuracy of intraocular lens power calculation in pediatric cataracts with less than a 20 mm axial length of the eye. Nepal J Ophthalmol. 2014;6(11):56–64.
101. Vanderveen DK, et al. Predictability of intraocular lens power calculation formulae in infantile eyes with unilateral congenital cataract: results from the infant aphakia treatment study. Am J Ophthalmol. 2013;156(6):1252–1260.e2.
102. Aasuri MK, et al. Management of pediatric aphakia with silsoft contact lenses. CLAO J. 1999;25(4):209–12.
103. Trivedi RH, Wilson ME. Selection of an initial contact lens power for infantile cataract surgery without primary intraocular lens implantation. Ophthalmology. 2013;120(10):1973–6.
104. McClatchey SK, Parks MM. Myopic shift after cataract removal in childhood. J Pediatr Ophthalmol Strabismus. 1997;34(2):88–95.
105. Medical C, A Clinical Investigation of the ClarVista HARMONI™ Modular Intraocular Lens Implant Following Cataract Surgery.
106. McClatchey SK. Intraocular lens calculator for childhood cataract. J Cataract Refract Surg. 1998;24(8):1125–9.
107. Egbert JE, et al. A prospective study of ocular hypertension and glaucoma after pediatric cataract surgery. Ophthalmology. 1995;102(7):1098–101.
108. Magnusson G, Abrahamsson M, Sjöstrand J. Glaucoma following congenital cataract surgery: an 18-year longitudinal follow-up. Acta Ophthalmol Scand. 2000;78(1):65–70.
109. Keech RV, Tongue AC, Scott WE. Complications after surgery for congenital and infantile cataracts. Am J Ophthalmol. 1989;108(2):136–41.
110. Asrani SG, Wilensky JT. Glaucoma after congenital cataract surgery. Ophthalmology. 1995;102(6):863–7.
111. Chen TC, et al. Risk factors for the development of aphakic glaucoma after congenital cataract surgery. Trans Am Ophthalmol Soc. 2006;104:241–51.
112. Vishwanath M, et al. Is early surgery for congenital cataract a risk factor for glaucoma? Br J Ophthalmol. 2004;88(7):905–10.

113. Bothun ED, et al. Outcomes of bilateral cataract surgery in infants 7 to 24 months of age using the toddler aphakia and pseudophakia treatment study registry. Ophthalmology. 2021;128(2):302–8.
114. Freedman SF, et al. Glaucoma-related adverse events in the first 5 years after unilateral cataract removal in the infant aphakia treatment study. JAMA Ophthalmol. 2015;133(8):907–14.
115. Bothun ED, et al. Strabismus surgery outcomes in the infant aphakia treatment study (IATS) at age 5 years. J AAPOS. 2016;20(6):501–5.
116. Weakley D, et al. Anisometropia at age 5 years after unilateral intraocular lens implantation during infancy in the infant aphakia treatment study. Am J Ophthalmol. 2017;180:1–7.
117. Weakley DR. The association between nonstrabismic anisometropia, amblyopia, and subnormal binocularity. Ophthalmology. 2001;108(1):163–71.

Pediatric Corneal Transplantation 12

Ramez Borbara, Asim Ali, and Kamiar Mireskandari

12.1 Introduction

Corneal diseases remain a major cause of pediatric blindness. Etiologies can be divided into three main categories: congenital corneal opacities (CCOs), acquired traumatic corneal disorders, and acquired nontraumatic corneal disorders, with the prevalence and incidence varying in different geographic areas. Congenital corneal opacities such as Peters anomaly (PA), sclerocornea, and limbal dermoids present at birth. While corneal endothelial dystrophies and glaucoma with corneal edema can present at birth or soon after, congenital hereditary stromal dystrophy and metabolic storage disease present in early or late childhood. Acquired, nontraumatic causes such as keratoconus typically present in late childhood. Infectious and noninfectious corneal scars as well as penetrating and non-penetrating corneal injuries may present at any age.

The success of corneal transplantation varies across etiologies. For instance, the CCOs carry a lower graft survival rate compared to acquired causes, 35% vs 84% at 1 year respectively [1]. Heterogeneous conditions within the CCO group, such as PA, have a variable graft survival rate [2, 3].

Pediatric corneal transplants carry unique intraoperative and postoperative challenges and corneal transplant surgery is primarily reserved for specialized quaternary referral centers [4]. Here we discuss the indications for and types of pediatric corneal transplant, pre- and postoperative management, and will highlight the challenges, complications, and outcomes of surgery.

R. Borbara · A. Ali · K. Mireskandari (✉)
Department of Ophthalmology and Vision Sciences, Hospital for Sick Children and University of Toronto, Toronto, ON, Canada
e-mail: ramez.borbara@sickkids.ca; asim.ali@sickkids.ca; kamiar.mireskandari@sickkids.ca

A. Ramasubramanian (ed.), *Pediatric Ophthalmology*, Current Practices in Ophthalmology, https://doi.org/10.1007/978-981-19-4963-0_12

12.2 Preoperative Consideration

A holistic approach is required when managing pediatric patients with corneal opacity. Corneal transplant in the pediatric age group is challenging at many levels and considerations should be given to the following main factors; (1) systemic comorbidities and anesthetic risk and (2) ocular comorbidities and prognosis for vision.

12.2.1 Systemic Considerations

It is not unusual that children have other coexisting systemic comorbidities which may be linked to the primary ocular condition. Cardiopulmonary, neurological, and genitourinary abnormalities may limit the child's fitness for general anesthesia (GA) and surgery. Often, these conditions take precedence and may necessitate life-saving surgery, which in turn delays ocular surgery and increases the risk of amblyopia.

Anesthesiologists specializing in pediatric care are ideal for these cases [5]. General anesthesia carries an increased risk of cardiac arrest in children under the age of 1 year of age, and corneal transplant patients require prolonged anesthetic time and multiple GAs [6]. The FDA issued a warning on the neurodevelopmental effects of anesthesia in 2017 for surgeries longer than 3 h or if multiple procedures are required in children under the age of 3 [7]. An experienced pediatric anesthetist is pivotal to consider the use of agents with limited or low neurotoxicity such as short-acting opioids and alpha agonists [6].

Given the potential risks of anesthesia and need for repeated GA, preoperative planning should be taken into consideration if nonsurgical options, including no intervention, are in the child's best interest. Alternatively, a less invasive procedure than a corneal transplant, such as an optical iridectomy, can be considered (see below). Family engagement in the decision-making is crucial when balancing the potential benefits of improving vision with the risks to the overall well-being of the child.

12.2.2 Ocular Considerations, Examination, and Imaging Modalities

A thorough and detailed preoperative examination is necessary to:

1. Establish a diagnosis and identify affected corneal layers so that surgery is planned accordingly.
2. Detect preexisting ocular comorbidities such as glaucoma, retinal detachment, and cataract. This information helps determine visual potential, guides surgical planning, and helps counsel patients and family.

At times, ocular examination needs to be carried out under GA or sedation due to lack of cooperation with an awake exam. Examination should include corneal diameter, intraocular pressure, corneal thickness, assessment of anterior chamber (AC) depth, lens position and presence of cataract, axial length measurement, and fundus examination if possible. B-scan ultrasonography to exclude posterior segment abnormalities is mandatory when fundus view is limited. In CCOs, imaging is often required as the corneal opacity prohibits view of the anterior segment structures [8, 9]. Ultrasound biomicroscopy (UBM) and anterior segment optical coherence tomography (AS-OCT) can identify characteristic diagnostic and prognostic features of anterior segment dysgenesis including the corneal layers involved, iris abnormalities, and state of the lens (Fig. 12.1).

12.2.3 Surgical Planning

The surgical approach of choice varies according to the etiology and the affected corneal layer (Table 12.1). The evolution of pediatric corneal transplant from full thickness to lamellar surgery, where selective removal of the affected corneal tissue is performed, has resulted in favorable visual outcome with reduced graft rejection rates [10, 11]. In general, surgical intervention is performed when opacity is affecting an area greater than the central 3 mm of the visual axis. Conditions partially involving the visual axis with clear corneal periphery can be treated with pupillary dilation, either pharmacologically or via surgical optical iridectomy.

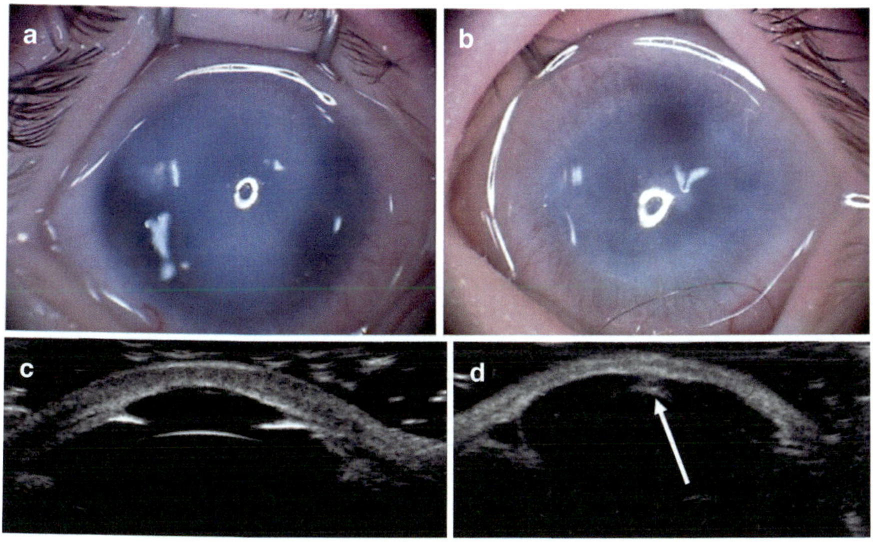

Fig. 12.1 3 months old child with bilateral congenital corneal opacities. Slit-lamp images (**a**) and (**b**) show the right and the left eye, respectively. Due to the corneal opacities, anterior segment evaluation is limited and it is not possible to establish whether the iris and/or the lens are involved. UBM images (**c**) and (**d**) from the right and left eye respectively show iridocorneal involvement but no keratolenticular touch in the right eye (Peters type 1) while evidence of lenticular involvement in the left eye (white arrow) (Peters type 2)

Table 12.1 Common indications for pediatric keratoplasty

Indications		Age at presentation	Procedure of choice
Category	Etiology		
Congenital	Peters anomaly	At birth	PK/optical iridectomy
	Sclerocornea	At birth	PK
	Dermoids	At birth	PK/ALK
	Corneal endothelial dystrophies	Any age	PK/EK
	Glaucoma with corneal edema	Any age	PK/EK
	Congenital hereditary stromal dystrophy	Early/late childhood	PK/ALK
	Metabolic storage diseases	Early/late childhood	PK/ALK
Acquired, nontraumatic	Keratoconus	Late childhood	PK/ALK
	Infectious keratitis	Any age	PK/ALK
	Noninfectious corneal scars	Any age	PK/ALK
Acquired, traumatic	Penetrating corneal or corneoscleral laceration	Any age	PK
	Non-penetrating corneal laceration with scar	Any age	PK/ALK

PK penetrating keratoplasty, *EK* endothelial keratoplasty, *ALK* anterior lamellar keratoplasty (can be deep at pre-Descemet level referred to in the text also as DALK)

12.2.4 Timing of Surgery

Timely intervention is crucial to allow adequate visual development. We aim to perform surgery by 3 months of age to allow for early visual rehabilitation and reduce the risk of amblyopia (bearing in mind that unilateral CCOs carry the worst outcome), yet balancing the anesthetic risk of early intervention, technical challenges of operating on a small eye, and risk of glaucoma and graft rejection. If second eye surgery is required, 1-week interval between the operated eyes is appropriate as this will reduce the risk of amblyopia and simplify the postoperative care in terms of follow-up visits, suture removal, examination under anesthesia (EUAs), and drop regimen at home. The eye with better vision is operated first to reduce amblyopia in the better eye.

An alternate viewpoint advocates for delayed corneal transplant surgery as corneal graft survival might be better. Other benefits of this approach include increased scleral rigidity, reduced risk of expulsion of intraocular contents, and collapse of the eye during the "open sky" stage of surgery, especially when intraoperative mannitol cannot be used due to systemic comorbidities. When coexisting glaucoma mandates drainage implant surgery to control intraocular pressure, the sequence of ocular surgery may delay corneal transplantation. Given all that, the decision should also be balanced against the anesthetic risk and the risk of developing amblyopia and nystagmus when possible.

12.2.5 Counseling and Expectations

It is pertinent to counsel parents, to get them on board and committed to the postoperative follow ups and engaged with the amblyopia treatment and intensive drop regimen. It is best to manage their expectations and acknowledge the emotional, psychological, social, and financial impact this may have on the family. Allow timely discussion, outlining a road map, detailing risks, and benefits of intervention as well as the risk of failure and needing multiple or further surgeries. If full thickness corneal transplant is offered, children should be cautious with contact sports for life, they may need to wear eye or head protection, again, this may have huge repercussions on the child therefore counseling older children at some stage may be required. Lastly, offer an introduction to support groups and other families with similar experiences. The long-term relationship and rapport that you build with children and their families is an essential part of surgical success and aids visual rehabilitation.

12.3 General Surgical Considerations

Pediatric eyes pose intraoperative challenges which must be anticipated and addressed ahead of surgery. Notably, intraoperative increased positive vitreous pressure may cause expulsion of intraocular contents with devastating outcomes. A discussion with an experienced pediatric anesthetist to reduce such risk is needed. Appropriate measures to reduce vitreous pressure may include deep anesthesia, muscle relaxants, hyperventilation, intravenous 20% mannitol (0.5 g/kg), and digital massage [12]. The safety of some of these measures need to be balanced against the patient's systemic comorbidities.

The "open sky" part of a penetrating keratoplasty (PK) procedure carries a considerable risk of expulsion of intraocular contents from positive posterior pressure exerted by the vitreous. However, this posterior pressure is also problematic in non-open sky scenarios such as when the anterior chamber (AC) collapses during Descemet membrane stripping and insertion of donor tissue in endothelial keratoplasty. Not only is there a risk of damaging the crystalline lens, but also increased trauma to the iris, trabecular meshwork and the donor cornea. Alongside the above-mentioned maneuvers and modifications to reduce the vitreous pressure, the following surgical adjustments will help mitigate such risks.

A suitably sized speculum is used to reduce pressure on the globe while providing adequate exposure. When exposure is still not adequate, lateral canthotomy can be performed. The use of a Flieringa ring counters the increased elasticity and low rigidity of the sclera in pediatric eyes, giving the surgeon better scleral support and globe stability and integrity to counter the posterior pressure. For "open sky" scenarios, preplacement of overlay suture to secure the corneal donor tissues quickly, or using a "sandwich donor" technique (will be discussed in the next section) to minimize the time an eye is at risk of expulsive events, is utilized.

In general, when case selection permits, lamellar keratoplasty is preferred to full thickness surgery as it minimizes the risk of intraocular content expulsion and suprachoroidal hemorrhage [13]. This advantage is not limited to the perioperative period. Lamellar surgery provides better tectonic strength for the child's entire life. Children are prone to ocular trauma and ocular loss in full thickness graft rupture. Similar to adults, deep anterior lamellar keratoplasty also preserves the patient's own corneal endothelium avoiding the risk of endothelial rejection. Reduced rejection rates, astigmatism, and faster visual rehabilitation are also seen when endothelial keratoplasty is performed instead of PK.

Corneal neovascularization may increase the risk of graft rejection. In such cases, treatment with fine needle diathermy before or after transplantation with or without intrastromal and subconjunctival bevacizumab can be considered [14].

12.4 Penetrating Keratoplasty

12.4.1 Indications

Penetrating keratoplasty is a full thickness replacement of the affected cornea with a donor tissue. It treats all causes of corneal blindness and is the surgery of choice when corneal pathology affects the full thickness of the cornea and the endothelium is unhealthy as well. Table 12.1 demonstrates the types of keratoplasty which can be performed for various etiologies. Peters anomaly, sclerocornea, and acquired conditions such as traumatic full thickness corneal scarring are some of the common indications for PK [15].

12.4.2 Surgical Technique

While the concept of PK is similar between adults and pediatric patients, the aforementioned general considerations with anesthesia, speculum, and use of Flieringa rings are essential in children. Further specific surgical issues and caveats and ways to manage them are discussed below.

In some cases of CCOs, notable PA, there is an anterior insertion of the conjunctiva onto the cornea. Peritomy and conjunctival recession are performed to allow adequate corneal exposure and accurate measurement of corneal diameter prior to deciding on corneal trephination and donor tissue size. Donor tissue size influences wound closure, refractive outcome, risk of graft rejection, and transfer of sufficient endothelial cells. In our practice, we tend to oversize by 0.5 mm. Evidence suggests that oversizing the donor tissue by 0.5–0.75 mm in phakic eyes and 0.75–1 mm in aphakic eyes facilitates wound closure while achieving a good refractive outcome [16]. This is balanced against the higher risk of excessive corneal steepening, high myopia, and postoperative corneal protrusion [2]. Donor size of 8 mm and more carries higher risk of rejection due to the proximity to limbal and conjunctival blood vessels [17].

During the trephination stage, caution is required as the cornea can be thin in areas in CCOs. These thin areas are clinically apparent as "more translucent" within the corneal opacity and should ideally have been identified preoperatively when AS-OCT or UBM imaging was performed. Judicious use of ophthalmic viscoelastic devices (OVDs) can help prevent iridolenticular injury. OVD cannula can also be used to bluntly divide iridocorneal and keratolenticular adhesions (if present) by gently sweeping the cannula across the anterior chamber avoiding endothelial and lenticular touch.

Post trephination, a staged corneal host dissection is recommended to reduce open sky time. The corneal incision is gradually extended along the trephined groove for 6 clock hours and the host cornea is sutured back using a single 9–0 nylon bite half way through the groove, creating an anchor point maintaining ocular integrity. The corneal incision is further extended by 2 clock hours on each side of the groove leaving the host corneal attached opposite to the anchoring suture in the host cornea. The host cornea is then covered with a generous layer of OVD, and the donor tissue is laid on top of it. The donor is then sutured to the host rim 90° from the host anchoring suture using 9–0 nylon. One of these sutures is tightened and the other remains a pre-placed suture to be tied later. Effectively, the donor is now a flap ready to be closed as soon as the host cornea is removed. The remaining attached part of the host cornea and anchoring suture are then cut and the host cornea can slide out from under the donor cornea, following which the donor cornea is secured by tying the pre-placed suture. This maneuver ensures that at least two strongly secured areas of the cornea are in place for all but a few seconds during the procedure and expulsive risk is minimized [18].

Corneal suturing is then completed using interrupted 10–0 nylon sutures. Depending on the donor size, 16–24 interrupted 10–0 nylon sutures using slipknot technique are used to close the eye and adjust tension as needed. The cardinal sutures are replaced with 10–0 nylon and knots buried in the host cornea.

12.4.3 Postoperative Management

Postoperative drop regimen involves intensive topical corticosteroids tapered slowly over a few months to once daily or alternate days and maintained long term to reduce the risk of rejection. Some studies have considered the use of steroid sparing agents such as topical cyclosporine; however, there is a lack of evidence to whether such agents reduce the rejection rate [19]. Antibiotic drops are used until complete suture removal.

During the frequent postoperative follow up visits the cornea is assessed for signs of infection and rejection and loose or broken sutures are removed. Evaluation is performed when needed under GA to allow for accurate assessment or when patient cooperation is limited. As a rough guide, we aim for suture removal under GA at 6 weeks postoperatively in infants and this interval increases with increasing age. Refractive correction is commenced soon after suture removal to optimize amblyopia therapy and aid visual rehabilitation.

12.4.4 Complications

Postoperative complications are common and 75% of eyes experience at least one complication during the rehabilitation period [20]. Loose or broken sutures are a common occurrence in pediatric penetrating keratoplasty as children have rapid graft healing. Loose and broken sutures account for most early graft-related infections and subsequent rejection. When identified, sutures are removed as soon as possible and intensive antibiotic therapy is initiated if there are signs of infection. Other than infection, secondary glaucoma and graft rejection/failure are the most frequent complications [20]. Less common complications include wound leak and dehiscence, cataract formation, endophthalmitis, retinal detachment, and phthisis bulbi [21].

Corneal graft rejections occur more frequently in children compared to adults (22–43%) and are less likely to resolve [21]. Furthermore, children may not report symptoms early therefore prevention using an intensive postoperative topical corticosteroid regimen with gradual taper and lifelong low-dose steroids are important. The incidence of secondary glaucoma varies between 5 and 16% [21]. Some may have preexisting glaucoma as part of their primary condition; therefore, evaluation is performed at every postoperative visit and treatment is initiated early when required to help maintain corneal clarity and reduce the risk of retinal nerve fiber layer loss.

12.4.5 Outcomes

Reported graft survival and visual outcomes following PK depend on many factors including length of follow up and the etiology of initial corneal disease. Generally, children at an older age with traumatic corneal injuries have completed their visual development prior to the injury. Therefore, they have a better visual prognosis post PK compared to younger children with anterior segment dysgenesis who may have dense amblyopia.

Congenital endothelial dystrophies such as congenital hereditary endothelial dystrophy (CHED) and posterior polymorphous corneal dystrophy (PPCD) were found to have the highest rate of graft survival (92–100% at 1 year) nevertheless visual improvement can be limited by the degree of amblyopia [22]. Peters anomaly carries a worse graft survival rate compared to endothelial dystrophies. Type 2 PA, the more severe form involving the lens, carries worst prognosis (38%) compared to type 1 (74%) at 10 years follow up [3]. Visual outcomes in PA vary considerably and range between 20/25 to no light perception with 56% of eyes post PK achieving 20/200 or better at 10 years follow up [3]. Therefore, outcomes need to be discussed with families during the counseling process, and put in context given the visual potential of the fellow eye.

A study on long-term endothelial cell loss in pediatric corneal transplants, largely for Peters anomaly, showed favorable cell densities in surviving grafts compared to that seen in the Corneal Donor Study which reported outcomes in adults largely with Fuchs endothelial corneal dystrophy [23, 24].

12.5 Anterior Lamellar Keratoplasty

In this section, we refer to both superficial lamellar keratoplasty and deep anterior lamellar keratoplasty (DALK) as anterior lamellar keratoplasty (ALK).

12.5.1 Indications

ALK is the selective replacement of affected stromal tissues, where the endothelial and Descemet layers are functional. Such conditions include limbal dermoids, congenital hereditary stromal dystrophy, corneal clouding due to metabolic storage disease, keratoconus, infective keratitis, and traumatic anterior stromal scarring (see Table 12.1) [25].

This approach has gained popularity over the past two decades as it has many intraoperative and postoperative advantages [13]. Maintaining globe integrity during surgery eliminates the risk of expulsion of intraocular contents and reduces the risk of intraocular infection. ALK preserves a patient's own endothelium and eliminates the risk of endothelial graft rejection, the most common form of corneal graft rejection, and consequently less immunosuppression is needed postoperatively. Nevertheless, surgery can be challenging and conversion to penetrating keratoplasty can occur so preoperative preparation would be identical to that of PK as outlined above. Furthermore, parents must be counseled and consented for conversion to penetrating keratoplasty.

12.5.2 Surgical Technique

The surgical method of choice varies according to the etiology, the surgeon's preference, and the desired depth of dissection. Superficial dermoids are treated by simple excision. For dermoids that have deeper involvement of the cornea, the defect following excision is replaced with corneal tissue and secured with 10–0 nylon sutures.

Conditions which involve deeper stromal involvement and conditions such as keratoconus would generally benefit from DALK. Two main approaches for DALK exist; manual dissection with various techniques to visualize the depth of stromal dissection or the big bubble technique which aims to dissect the corneal layers along pre-Descemet's layer using air or ophthalmic viscoelastic devices injected in the deep cornea.

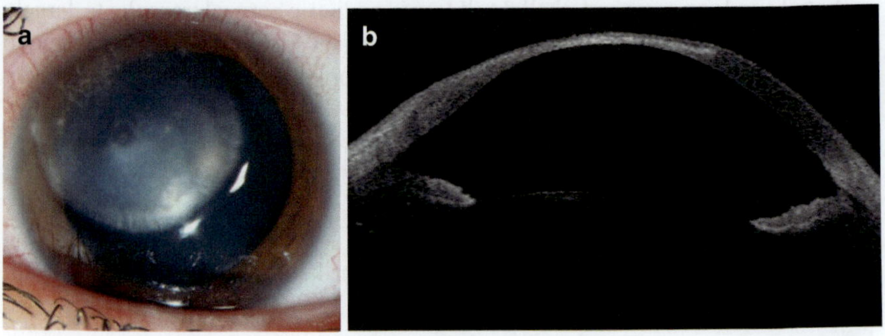

Fig. 12.2 (**a**) Color image of corneal scar and corresponding anterior segment OCT (**b**) showing superior corneal thinning due to previous microbial keratitis. Identifying areas of corneal thinning is essential for surgical planning, making a decision about dissection depth, and corneal graft suturing

In our practice, we perform manual dissection as the big bubble technique has a higher risk of perforation due to stronger attachment of the Descemet membrane (DM) to the stroma in pediatric corneas [10]. A Flieringa ring is used as described for PK. A partial thickness trephination of appropriate depth is performed based on preoperative AS-OCT measurements (Fig. 12.2) and a stromal pocket is created with a lamellar dissector. The dissection depth can be deepened as required to be as close to the Descemet layer as needed. Intraoperative OCT can aid surgical accuracy. A residual stromal thickness of up to 80 μm is typically not visually significant. Microperforation can be managed with air injection into the anterior chamber and adjustment of the dissection level. The dissection plane should be extended beyond the trephination margin on the host side to allow better tissue apposition and facilitate graft suturing. Suitably sized donor tissue (oversized by 0.25–0.5 mm) is sutured with 16 interrupted 10–0 nylon sutures.

12.5.3 Complications

Similar to PK, suture-related complications of loosening, keratitis, and neovascularization are the most common. Other complications include persistent epithelial defect, graft failure, and glaucoma. Descemet membrane detachment may rarely occur and be managed with air injections into the anterior chamber [26]. As in adults, graft rejection is rare and only involves the donor stroma [26, 27].

12.5.4 Outcomes

Much of the literature is focused on ALK in the management of limbal dermoid with visual outcomes primarily affected by whether preexisting amblyopia is present [28]. Watts et al. demonstrated corrected distant visual acuity (CDVA) of 20/40 or better in 86.7% at 12 months postsurgery. Smaller grafts and older age are associated with better visual acuity [25]. Ashar et al. reported on 26 cases of DALK with 62% achieving CDVA of 20/80 of better at 1.3 years of follow up [27].

Recent study demonstrated no significant difference in visual acuity and graft survival outcomes between DALK and PK in the treatment of pediatric keratoconus at 5 years follow up [29]. Elbaz et al. published outcomes on 51 eyes of 42 cases who underwent manual dissection DALK, the most common indications for surgery were mucopolysaccharidosis (29.4%) and keratoconus (23.5%). In this series, 2% had conversion to PK and 9.8% experienced stromal rejection of which one eye failed as a result. Visual acuity of 20/80 or better was achieved in 75% of eyes at a mean of 3 years follow up [10].

12.6 Endothelial Keratoplasty

Endothelial keratoplasty (EK) involves the selective replacement of the posterior corneal layers (DM and endothelium complex). Commonly performed types of EK include Descemet Stripping Automated Endothelial Keratoplasty (DSAEK), in which a microkeratome is used to cut the donor DM-endothelial complex with stromal tissue. Descemet Membrane Endothelial Keratoplasty (DMEK) only transplants DM-endothelial complex without donor stroma. EK has the advantage of maintaining the globe's tectonic strength, rapid visual recovery and avoiding the open sky step of PK and suture-related complications.

12.6.1 Indications

The most common indications for EK are disease processes affecting the endothelial layer that cause localized or generalized corneal edema. These include CHED (Fig. 12.3), PPCD, aphakic bullous keratopathy, and birth trauma [30, 31] [32]. Persistent stromal edema secondary to endothelial dysfunction may cause stromal haze and scarring which can be difficult to clear despite successful anatomical EK. In such cases, a PK may be indicated despite the primary pathology being at the endothelium.

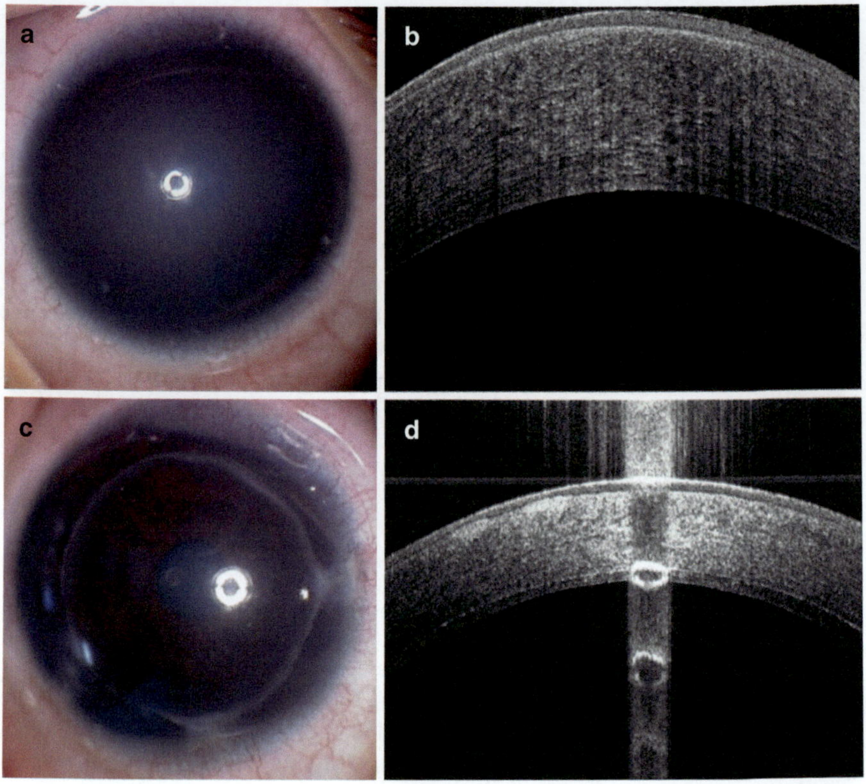

Fig. 12.3 Image of a child with CHED. Color Image (**a**) demonstrates corneal edema and haze which corresponds to epithelial and stromal edema on OCT (**b**). Color image (**c**) post endothelial keratoplasty with corresponding OCT image (**d**) showing thin endothelial graft with resolution of stromal edema

12.6.2 Surgical Techniques and Challenges

Pediatric EK is more challenging compared to adult EK. Severe corneal edema may limit AC view during DM stripping and unfolding of the graft. Manipulations within the eye can be tricky due to shallow anterior chamber with a tendency to collapse, positive vitreous pressure and anteriorly positioned crystalline lens. Furthermore, posterior and/or peripheral anterior synechiae may exist as part of the ocular disease which may limit AC depth. All the above factors can lead to prolonged surgery and maneuvering in the AC causing fibrinous inflammatory reaction. This fibrin can be problematic for the unfolding of a DMEK graft in particular, which is very thin. Bleeding from an inferior peripheral iridectomy required for surgery may exacerbate fibrin production, further complicating the procedure.

The basic technique for DSAEK and DMEK procedures in children are similar to those in adults. We highlight the following steps when performing EK to counter some of the challenges described above. A temporal scleral tunnel and an AC maintainer help prevent AC collapse or fluctuations during the procedure. Intracameral air or trypan blue dye may aid visualization of the Descemet membrane to ensure complete stripping from the host cornea. Pupil constriction with acetylcholine chloride helps avoid intraoperative lenticular trauma or loss of donor tissue behind the iris. Since a preoperative YAG laser peripheral iridotomy is not possible in children, an inferiorly placed surgical iridectomy is required to prevent pupillary block. This can be performed using a vitrector just before EK insertion. We favor a pull-through technique using forceps for graft insertion into the anterior chamber. This ensures that the tissue is held in place before unfolding and a little air is then injected to hold the graft in position. Following wound suturing, the graft is centered and non-expansile gas is injected achieving intraoperative tamponade for 20 mins. The use of intraoperative OCT can aid visualization and confirmation of graft apposition to the cornea. Any residual interface fluid can be massaged out or released through venting incisions. A limited air-fluid exchange is performed to avoid high postoperative IOP after all paracenteses are secured.

12.6.3 Postoperative Management

Postoperative drops regimen is similar to PK with intensive corticosteroid drops, tapered gradually and maintained long term. Parents are advised about the importance of posturing and against eye rubbing which one may appreciate can be difficult to achieve in the pediatric age group resulting in an increased risk of graft detachment. When AS-OCT cannot be performed awake after surgery, EUA should be performed 1 week postoperatively to ensure graft attachment.

12.6.4 Outcomes

Most outcomes in the literature focus on endothelial keratoplasty for the treatment of CHED. Unlike other endothelial dystrophies, CHED is associated with variable postoperative outcomes with eyes undergoing DSAEK generally having poorer visual outcomes when compared to PK despite anatomical attachment and good endothelial function. It is thought that persistent corneal scarring secondary to corneal edema is the cause of such difference; therefore, we advocate for meticulous case selection and still consider PK as an alternative [33]. Ashar et al. conducted paired eye comparison with one eye undergoing DSAEK and the other PK for the treatment of CHED. The DSAEK eyes had faster visual rehabilitation, earlier stabilization of refraction, and less astigmatism compared to PK at 1 year follow up. Visual acuity was not statistically different nevertheless corneal clarity in DSAEK eyes never reached the same level as PK eyes [34]. Yang et al. reported the outcome of DSAEK in CHED in two pediatric groups; infants and older children. The group with older children achieve postoperative BCVA of 0.4 logMAR or better at 4 years follow up in 30% of cases compared to 86% in the infant group [35]. Belliveau et al. reported on a 12-year old with PPCD undergoing DSEK with visual improvement from 20/200 OU to 20/80 and 20/30 in the right and left eye, respectively [32].

As in adults, pediatric DMEK although challenging could potentially provide superior and faster visual rehabilitation and reduced graft rejection rate compared to DSAEK. Srinivasan et al. have reported the outcome of DMEK surgery on 5 eyes (4 with CHED and 1 failed PK) with improvement in vision from 1.93 to 0.98 logMAR over 13 months follow up. Two eyes (40%) required rebubbling and one eye had primary graft failure [36]. Overall, this study provides encouraging results.

12.7 What Does the Future Hold?

Despite the abovementioned advances in pediatric corneal transplant, certain issues still remain and need addressing. Global shortages in graft material make pediatric corneal transplant inaccessible to everyone and high graft failure and rejection rates remain a concern, especially in the pediatric age group.

With the emergence of new innovations in the field of cellular culture, regeneration, and biocompatible microstructural scaffolds enhancing cellular growth, there is anticipation that these will be utilized for the treatment of corneal blindness.

Rho kinase is an important regulator of cellular function; growth, migration, metabolism, and apoptosis and its activity were found to increase in various pathological conditions. Rho kinase inhibitors are hypothesized to play a part in endothelial cell proliferation and are showing promising results in promoting endothelial cell regeneration and reducing corneal edema [37].

There is an ongoing research in the field of cultivating human corneal endothelial cells; however, difficulty in maintaining endothelial function remains a concern [38]. In the future, we may see less invasive and more accessible methods to treat corneal pathologies which will transform the way we manage corneal blindness.

12.8 Conclusion

Pediatric corneal transplant in children is challenging compared to adults and surgical adjustments are required when transferring such techniques to the pediatric setting. Patient selection, timing of surgery, and a holistic and multidisciplinary team approach are essential for surgical success and optimal visual outcome. Lamellar surgery has transformed the way we manage corneal pathologies, and despite gaining popularity, to this date, penetrating keratoplasty remains the most commonly performed corneal transplant in children.

Our understanding of disease processes is constantly evolving and with the emergence of new imaging and surgical technologies, we look forward to improvements in surgical and visual outcomes. The prospect of endothelial cell regeneration and culture using tissue engineering techniques holds promise and we anticipate significant advances in the near future (Fig. 12.3).

Key Points

1. A holistic approach is required when managing children with corneal pathologies and family counseling and engagement with treatment are crucial for optimal visual rehabilitation.
2. Pediatric corneal transplant is challenging and therefore requires preoperative surgical planning, anesthetic adjustments, and intraoperative modification to enhance the success of surgery. These are best managed in specialized centers.
3. Case selection is crucial and at times a nonsurgical approach or minimally invasive surgery rather than corneal transplantation may prove sufficient to achieve optimal visual rehabilitation.
4. Lamellar surgery is gaining popularity and surgical techniques are constantly evolving.

Acknowledgments We thank Ms. Cynthia VandenHoven (CRA FOPS) imaging specialist for her assistance with the figures in this chapter.

References

1. Al-Ghamdi A, Al-Rajhi A, Wagoner MD. Primary pediatric keratoplasty: indications, graft survival, and visual outcome. J AAPOS. 2007;11(1):41–7.
2. Zaidman GW, Flanagan JK, Furey CC. Long-term visual prognosis in children after corneal transplant surgery for peters anomaly type I. Am J Ophthalmol. 2007;144(1):104–8.
3. Elbaz U, Strungaru H, Mireskandari K, Stephens D, Ali A. Long-term visual outcomes and clinical course of patients with peters anomaly. cornea. 2021;40(7):822–30.
4. fung s, ali a, mireskandari k. Pediatric corneal transplantation—where are we heading? Curr Ophthalmol Rep. 2017;5(1):23–37.
5. Paterson N, Waterhouse P. Risk in pediatric anesthesia. Paediatr Anaesth. 2011;21(8):848–57.
6. Bartels DD, McCann ME, Davidson AJ, Polaner DM, Whitlock EL, Bateman BT. Estimating pediatric general anesthesia exposure: quantifying duration and risk. Paediatr Anaesth. 2018;28(6):520–7.
7. FDA Drug Safety Communication: FDA approves label changes for use of general anesthetic and sedation drugs in young children [Internet]; 2017. https://www.fda.gov/drugs/drug-safety-and-availability/fda-drug-safety-communication-fda-approves-label-changes-use-general-anesthetic-and-sedation-drugs.
8. Elbaz U, Ali A, Strungaru H, Mireskandari K. Phenotypic spectrum of peters anomaly: implications for management. Cornea. 2022;41(2):192–200. PMID: 34176915.
9. Mireskandari K, Tehrani NN, Vandenhoven C, Ali A. Anterior segment imaging in pediatric ophthalmology. J Cataract Refract Surg. 2011;37(12):2201–10.
10. Elbaz U, Kirwan C, Shen C, Ali A. Avoiding big bubble complications: outcomes of layer-by-layer deep anterior lamellar keratoplasty in children. Br J Ophthalmol. 2018;102(8):1103–8.
11. Hong Y, Peng RM, Wang M, Qu HQ, Hong J. Suture pull-through insertion techniques for Descemet stripping automated endothelial keratoplasty in Chinese phakic eyes: outcomes and complications. PLoS One. 2013;8(4):e61929.

12. Javadi MA, Baradaran-Rafii AR, Zamani M, Karimian F, Zare M, Einollahi B, et al. Penetrating keratoplasty in young children with congenital hereditary endothelial dystrophy. Cornea. 2003;22(5):420–3.
13. Tan DT, Mehta JS. Future directions in lamellar corneal transplantation. Cornea. 2007;26(9 Suppl 1):S21–8.
14. Elbaz U, Mireskandari K, Shen C, Ali A. Corneal fine needle diathermy with adjuvant bevacizumab to treat corneal neovascularization in children. Cornea. 2015;34(7):773–7.
15. Harissi-Dagher M, Colby K. Anterior segment dysgenesis: peters anomaly and sclerocornea. Int Ophthalmol Clin. 2008;48(2):35–42.
16. Vajpayee RB, Ramu M, Panda A, Sharma N, Tabin GC, Anand JR. Oversized grafts in children. Ophthalmology. 1999;106(4):829–32.
17. Yang LL, Lambert SR, Lynn MJ, Stulting RD. Long-term results of corneal graft survival in infants and children with peters anomaly. Ophthalmology. 1999;106(4):833–48.
18. Arslan OS, Unal M, Arici C, Cicik E, Mangan S, Atalay E. Novel method to avoid the open-sky condition in penetrating keratoplasty: covered cornea technique. Cornea. 2014;33(9):994–8.
19. Abudou M, Wu T, Evans JR, Chen X. Immunosuppressants for the prophylaxis of corneal graft rejection after penetrating keratoplasty. Cochrane Database Syst Rev. 2015;8:CD007603.
20. Dana MR, Schaumberg DA, Moyes AL, Gomes JA. Corneal transplantation in children with Peters anomaly and mesenchymal dysgenesis. Multicenter Pediatric Keratoplasty Study. Ophthalmology. 1997;104(10):1580–6.
21. Vanathi M, Panda A, Vengayil S, Chaudhuri Z, Dada T. Pediatric keratoplasty. Surv Ophthalmol. 2009;54(2):245–71.
22. Michaeli A, Markovich A, Rootman DS. Corneal transplants for the treatment of congenital corneal opacities. J Pediatr Ophthalmol Strabismus. 2005;42(1):34–44.
23. Elbaz U, Ali A, Mireskandari K. Long-term corneal endothelial cell counts after penetrating keratoplasty in infants. Cornea. 2016;35(6):784–8.
24. Cornea Donor Study Investigator G, Lass JH, Gal RL, Dontchev M, Beck RW, Kollman C, et al. Donor age and corneal endothelial cell loss 5 years after successful corneal transplantation. Specular microscopy ancillary study results. Ophthalmology. 2008;115(4):627–32 e8.
25. Watts P, Michaeli-Cohen A, Abdolell M, Rootman D. Outcome of lamellar keratoplasty for limbal dermoids in children. J AAPOS. 2002;6(4):209–15.
26. Low JR, Anshu A, Tan AC, Htoon HM, Tan DT. The outcomes of primary pediatric keratoplasty in Singapore. Am J Ophthalmol. 2014;158(3):496–502.
27. Ashar JN, Pahuja S, Ramappa M, Vaddavalli PK, Chaurasia S, Garg P. Deep anterior lamellar keratoplasty in children. Am J Ophthalmol. 2013;155(3):570–4. e1
28. Pirouzian A. Management of pediatric corneal limbal dermoids. Clin Ophthalmol. 2013;7:607–14.
29. Feizi S, Javadi MA, Karimian F, Abolhosseini M, Moshtaghion SM, Naderi A, et al. Penetrating keratoplasty versus deep anterior lamellar keratoplasty in children and adolescents with keratoconus. Am J Ophthalmol. 2021;226:13–21.
30. Jeng BH, Marcotty A, Traboulsi EI. Descemet stripping automated endothelial keratoplasty in a 2-year-old child. J AAPOS. 2008;12(3):317–8.
31. Ponchel C, Malecaze F, Arne JL, Fournie P. Descemet stripping automated endothelial keratoplasty in a child with Descemet membrane breaks after forceps delivery. Cornea. 2009;28(3):338–41.
32. Belliveau MJ, Rocha G, Manchur A, Brownstein S. Bilateral Descemet's stripping with endothelial keratoplasy for posterior polymorphous corneal dystrophy in a young phakic patient. Can J Ophthalmol. 2010;45(2):180–1.
33. Medsinge A, Nischal KK. Paediatric keratoplasty: choices and conundrums. Br J Ophthalmol. 2013;97(10):1225–7.

34. Ashar JN, Ramappa M, Vaddavalli PK. Paired-eye comparison of Descemet's stripping endothelial keratoplasty and penetrating keratoplasty in children with congenital hereditary endothelial dystrophy. Br J Ophthalmol. 2013;97(10):1247–9.
35. Yang F, Hong J, Xiao G, Feng Y, Peng R, Wang M, et al. Descemet stripping endothelial keratoplasty in pediatric patients with congenital hereditary endothelial dystrophy. Am J Ophthalmol. 2020;209:132–40.
36. Srinivasan B, Agarwal M, Iyer G, Agarwal S, Padmanabhan P. Pediatric Descemet membrane endothelial keratoplasty. Am J Ophthalmol. 2021;227:12–7.
37. Koizumi N, Okumura N, Ueno M, Nakagawa H, Hamuro J, Kinoshita S. Rho-associated kinase inhibitor eye drop treatment as a possible medical treatment for Fuchs corneal dystrophy. Cornea. 2013;32(8):1167–70.
38. Okumura N, Koizumi N. Regeneration of the corneal endothelium. Curr Eye Res. 2020;45(3):303–12.

Current Management of Optic Pathway Glioma

13

Alyson Tukan, Lindsey M. Hoffman,
and Aparna Ramasubramanian

13.1 Introduction

Optic pathway gliomas (OPGs) are low-grade neoplasms arising from the optic nerve, chiasm, tracts, or radiations. Although they can arise sporadically, they are commonly associated with neurofibromatosis type 1 (NF-1). The clinical course of OPGs is variable and unpredictable, which has limited the development of standardized treatment protocols. This chapter reviews the clinical presentation of OPGs, screening recommendations, diagnostic tools, current treatment options, and future directions for management.

13.2 Defining Optic Pathway Gliomas

OPGs are low-grade tumors that can arise anywhere along the optic pathway, including the optic nerve, optic chiasm, optic tracts, and optic radiations [1–3], and most commonly present in the first decade of life [4]. OPGs account for 2–5% of pediatric central nervous system tumors [1, 4–6]. While OPGs can arise sporadically, there is a strong association with NF-1, a genetic neuro-cutaneous disorder

Aparna Ramasubramanian, M.D. has had full access to all the data in the study and takes responsibility for the integrity of the data.

A. Tukan · L. M. Hoffman · A. Ramasubramanian (✉)
Phoenix Children's Hospital, Phoenix, AZ, USA
e-mail: atukan@email.arizona.edu; lhoffman1@phoenixchildrens.com; aramasubramanian@phoenixchildrens.com

A. Ramasubramanian (ed.), *Pediatric Ophthalmology*, Current Practices in Ophthalmology, https://doi.org/10.1007/978-981-19-4963-0_13

that affects 1:3000 persons annually (ref). Approximately 15–20% of patients with NF-1 will develop an OPG [1, 7–10], most commonly along the optic nerve or chiasm [7]. Because of the frequency of OPGs in NF-1, one of the seven potential diagnostic qualifications for NF-1, as defined by the NIH, is the presence of an optic glioma [6, 11]. Histologically, OPGs are most commonly classified as pilocytic astrocytoma (WHO grade I) [1, 2, 12, 13] but are less commonly classified as other, sometimes more aggressive LGG-subtypes, including pilomyxoid astrocytoma, pleomorphic xanthoastroctyoma, or diffuse fibrillary astrocytoma [1].

13.2.1 Symptoms

- Proptosis [10, 14, 15].
- Decreased visual acuity or vision loss [2, 10, 14, 15].
- Impaired color vision [15].
- Strabismus [10, 14].
- Relative afferent pupillary defect [10, 14, 15].
- Papilledema [10, 14] (Fig. 13.1a).
- Optic disc atrophy [10, 14] (Fig. 13.1b).
- Visual field defects—bitemporal hemianopia from chiasm involvement [10, 14].
- Central retinal vein occlusion [14].
- Dissociated vertical nystagmus [14].
- Precocious puberty with chiasm involvement [10, 15].

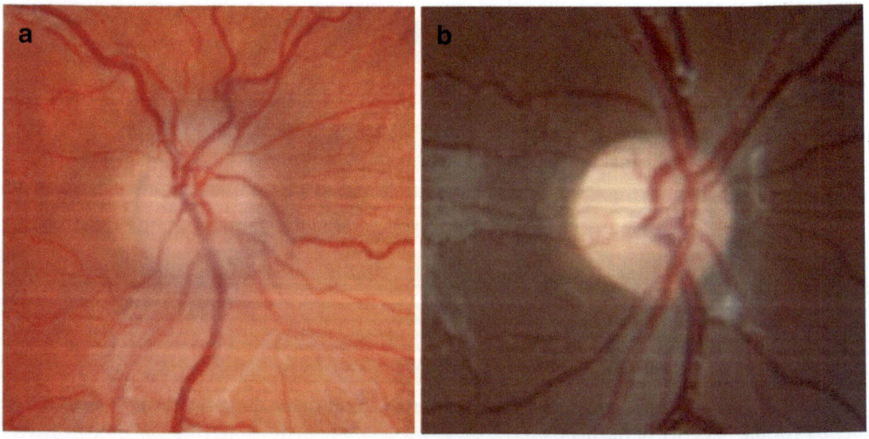

Fig. 13.1 Optic nerve glioma presenting with (**a**) disc edema and (**b**) optic nerve pallor

13.2.2 Prognostic Factors

Better prognosis	Worse prognosis
Tumor limited to optic nerve [9]	Tumor involving optic chiasm, posterior to the optic chiasm, or involving the hypothalamus [16]
NF1 association	Tumor arising in children age < 1 year [12, 17]
	Female gender: Higher rate of requiring therapy and 5–10× more likely than males to lose vision [10]
	Sporadic (non-NF1 associated) OPG [12, 17]: More aggressive course [12, 17], higher chance of causing increased intracranial pressure [8]

13.2.3 Pathophysiology of NF1-Associated OPGs

OPGs that arise in the context of NF1 are driven by biallelic silencing of the *NF1* gene silencing by mutation, methylation, or deletion [10]. The gene product normally produced by *NF1,* the protein neurofibromin, is analogous to GTPase activating proteins and plays a role in inhibiting the proto-oncogenic effects of RAS [10]. When neurofibromin is not functional, RAS activates AKT and MEK, allowing dysregulated cell growth through the mTOR complex and ERK [10]. Absent neurofibromin and unchecked RAS also decrease levels of cAMP, which leads to apoptosis of the retinal ganglion cell (RGC) layer [10]. Therefore, inhibiting RAS or increasing cAMP levels can decrease RGC loss and preserve vision for patients with NF1-OPGs. Additionally, microglia are implicated in tumor growth through the production of inflammatory cytokines like IL-1ß and IL-6 that act as neurotoxins to the RGCs and retinal nerve fiber layer (RNFL) [18]. Estradiol potentiates this effect; this may partly explain why vision loss is more severe in females [2]. Sporadic OPGs often arise from alterations to *BRAF* (most commonly BRAFV600E mutation or BRAF-KIAA1549 fusion) that activate the mitogen-activated protein kinase (MAPK) pathway [19].

13.3 Diagnosis

13.3.1 Dodge Classification

In 1958, Dodge and colleagues published a series of 46 patients with OPG divided into categories meant to distinguish management based on tumor location [20]. Type A tumors involved the optic nerve, Type B tumors involved the optic chiasm, and Type C "tractal" tumors were more diffuse [20]. Criteria derived from this series have been adapted into the Modified Dodge Classification System, also known as the PLAN score after the four centers that contributed to its development (Padua, Leeds, Augsburg, and Nottingham) [21]:

- Dodge 1—optic nerve only.
  - 1a: Single optic nerve

  - 1b: Bilateral optic nerves
  - 1c: Cisternal segment optic nerve
- Dodge 2—optic chiasm ± optic nerve.
  - 2a: Central chiasmatic
  - 2b: Asymmetric chiasmatic
- Dodge 3—anterior optic tracts.
  - 3b: Asymmetric optic tracts
- Dodge 4—posterior optic tracts ± hypothalamus.
  - 4b: Asymmetric posterior tracts
  - H±: Hypothalamic involvement.
  - LM±: Leptomeningeal dissemination.
  - NF1±: Neurofibromatosis type 1.

13.3.2 Screening

Progression of OPGs can have devastating consequences on vision emphasizing the importance of early detection. In 1997, the OPG Task Force set forth a set of recommendations for ophthalmologic screening and surveillance of NF1-OPGs, which are still in practice today (Table 13.1) [8]. A study of 51 patients with NF1-OPGs found no tumor progression beyond age 12, which supports more frequent surveillance in younger patients and advocates for the extension of annual screening up to age 12 from the current recommendation of 8 years [23]. Table 13.2 outlines tools utilized to assess visual acuity during ophthalmologic exams based on the patient's age and literacy.

Table 13.1 Screening guidelines for visually asymptomatic patients with NF1

Age	Screening modality	Frequency of screening
<1 year	No formal recommendations	N/A
<8 years[a]	Full ophthalmic exam	Yearly
8–18 years	Full ophthalmic exam	Every 2 years[b]
Adult	No screening; routine eye care	As needed

Adapted from Listernick et al. [8]
[a] French clinical guidelines recommend annual screening until at least age 13 [22]
[b] Frequency not well-established

Table 13.2 Tools for testing visual acuity

Age/literacy	Tool
Infants (~0–2 years)	Teller acuity cards
Pre-literate (~3–4 years)	Lea figures
Pre-literate (~4–6 years)	HOTV matching
Literate (>6 years)	Snellen charts

Adapted from Listernick et al. [8]

13.3.3 Additional Recommendations

- For patients with suspected OPG on ophthalmic exam, magnetic resonance imaging (MRI) brain and orbits should be obtained.
- Patients with NF1-OPG should undergo ophthalmologic evaluation every 3 months for 1–2 years after diagnosis after which the frequency should be defined by their treating ophthalmologist. If no vision exam is stable by age 18, surveillance may be discontinued.
- Routine neuroimaging is not indicated as part of a screening protocol unless a sufficient ophthalmic exam cannot be attained.
- Routine Visual Evoked Potentials are not indicated.
- Formal visual field testing is difficult for pediatric patients to complete and is prone to many fixation errors; therefore, confrontation visual fields as part of an ophthalmic exam is sufficient.
- Annual physical examination should include screening for precocious puberty.

13.3.4 Imaging and Diagnostics

13.3.4.1 MRI

MRI is the gold standard imaging modality for identifying and monitoring OPGs in pediatric patients. The recommended imaging protocol includes coronal and axial thin-section T1-weighted and fat-saturated T2-weighted images [14], plus T1 sequences with gadolinium contrast and fluid-attenuated inversion recovery [11]. T1-weighted images are best for characterizing the size of the tumor, which will appear hypo- to isodense compared to the optic pathway (Fig. 13.2a) [4, 14].

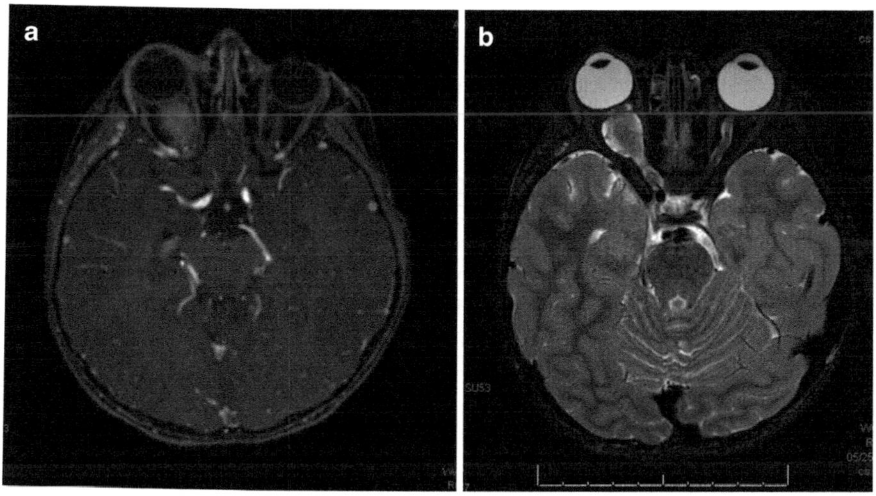

Fig. 13.2 MRI orbit showing a fusiform mass affecting the right optic nerve which is isointense on T1 imaging (**a**) and hyperintense on T2 imaging (**b**)

T2-weighted images are useful for assessing anatomical involvement, and the tumor will appear mildly hyperdense compared to surrounding structures (Fig. 13.2b) [4, 14]. Volumetric MRI is gaining popularity as an adjunctive tool for measuring tumor size since traditional measurements of these complex tumors from T1-enhanced images are limited by the two-dimensional view [4, 9]. With volumetric MRI, the complex anatomy of a tumor can be more accurately estimated [9], though it is currently limited in assessing tumors of the posterior tract [9].

13.3.4.2 DTI

Diffusion tensor imaging (DTI), another MR technique, tracks the diffusion of water along axons and can map white matter tracts like the optic tract [9]. Areas with decreased fractional anisotropy (FA) do not have coherent diffusion, representing white matter damage [9]. Decreased FA has been correlated with decreased visual acuity in patients with NF1-OPGs [9]. Interestingly, increased diffusion on DTI has also been observed as a harbinger for future tumor progression and subsequent vision loss [9]. Larger scale studies need to be conducted to determine if DTI can be consistently used as a prognostic predictor of impending vision loss.

DTI has limitations for evaluating optic nerves due to artifacts from adjacent bone, fat, and airspaces [9]. Readout-segmented multi-shot echo planar imaging (rsDTI) was found to be superior to single-shot echo planar imaging (ssDTI) for providing better resolution with less artifact of the optic nerve and optic chiasm [24].

13.3.4.3 CT

Because of the radiation exposure from computed tomography (CT) and the increased propensity for patients with NF-1 to develop cancer, CT is less commonly utilized to characterize OPGs, and MRI is the preferred method for diagnosis and serially monitoring [8].

13.3.4.4 PET

Although positron emission tomography (PET) also carries a radiation burden, it may have a role in tumor surveillance and differentiation between benign and malignant neoplasms. One study utilized fluorodeoxyglucose (FDG) as their marker of metabolic activity and found that high-grade tumor elements could be detected, which aided in risk stratification for tumor advancement given the otherwise unpredictable growth patterns of OPGs [25]. Additionally, FDG-PET was able to detect residual tumor after surgical intervention as well as tumor progression [22, 25]. Therefore, PET may have an adjunctive role in monitoring patients with OPGs, especially in postsurgical patients. Further research is needed to discern if PET is a useful prognostic tool for predicting tumor progression.

13.3.4.5 OCT

Optical coherence tomography (OCT) measures the thickness of the RNFL and inner plexiform layer/ganglion cell layer (IPL-GCL) [18]. Its use in surveillance of glaucoma demonstrated a correlation between visual field defects and peripapillary

RNFL thinning [26] which represents the underlying principle of using OCT to evaluate patients with OPG. In one study, a correlation between RNFL thickness and visual field defects was found such that patients with abnormal vision tended to have a RNFL <80 μm on Stratus OCT [27]. Another study utilized spectral-domain handheld OCT and found that RNFL was thinner in patients with abnormal visual acuity or visual field defects [26]. In this second study, the average RNFL thickness for normally seeing eyes was 125.1 μm, while patients with abnormal vision had an average RNFL thickness of 75.8 μm [26]. The disadvantage of OCT in this study was that patients had to be sedated in order to obtain quality images. The correlation between vision and RNFL thickness indicates that OCT can be a useful correlate for vision loss in patients who are unable to perform acuity or visual field screening. Cooperative children who can fixate long enough to obtain a quality scan can avoid the need for sedation, and OCT may provide additional data for analysis of disease progression and evaluation for possible treatment (Fig. 13.3).

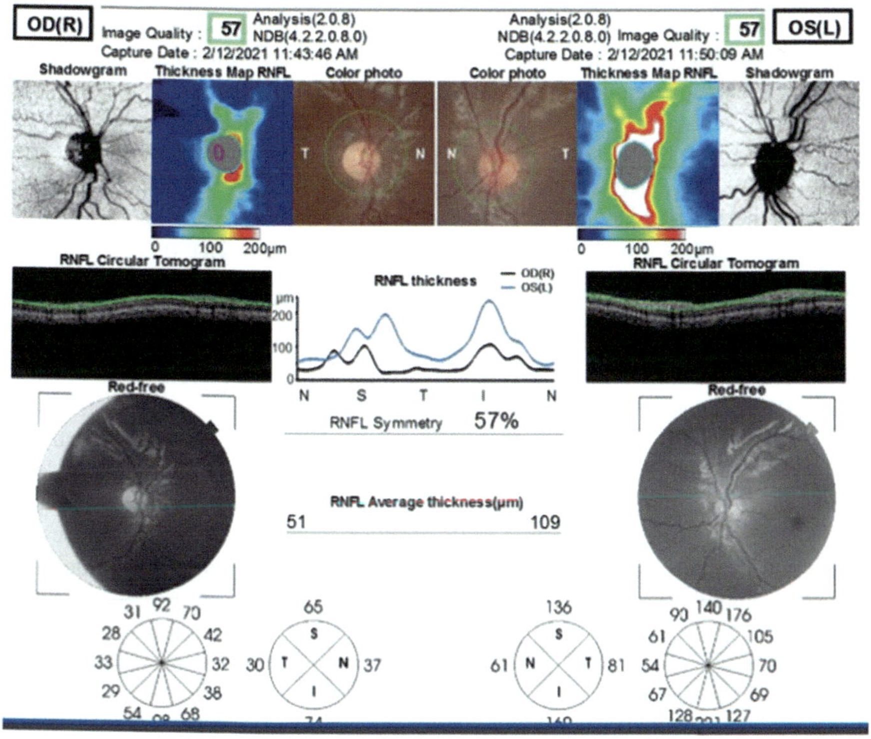

Fig. 13.3 Optical coherence tomography showing a significant difference in the average thickness of the retinal nerve fiber layer(RNFL) secondary to right optic nerve glioma. Average RNFL 51 on the right and 109 on the left

13.3.4.6 VEPs

Flash and/or pattern visual evoked potentials (VEPs), which are an electrophysiologic measure of the integrity of the visual pathway, are not recommended in screening for OPGs due to high variability in results and difficulty in making meaningful conclusions from changes on serial examinations [8]. Additionally, the test can take up to 30 min, which restricts its utility in a pediatric population with a limited attention span [4]. One study advocated for use of VEPs as a "pre-symptomatic screening tool" because it is an objective measure of visual function that may be able to demonstrate visual changes prior to neuroradiological changes [28]. However, most authors conclude that the results from VEPs are too inconsistent to warrant routine use [4]. Therefore, VEPs are not recommended as part of a routine screening protocol for NF1-OPGs [8]. VEPs may be utilized in select patients on an individualized basis, though the value they add to the diagnostic evaluation is limited.

13.3.4.7 Biopsy

Tumor biopsy is not routinely performed for pediatric patients with OPG given the risk for vision deterioration from this procedure when for most tumors, histopathology will not change the management plan [11]. However, biopsy may be informative in cases with unique tumor characteristics on MRI or ambiguous clinical presentation [4, 8]. One case study documented the increased likelihood of utilizing biopsy to confirm diagnosis in patients with sporadic OPGs compared to patients with NF1-OPGs [17]. However, for most patients, a biopsy is redundant and merely increases the risk of a negative outcome from the procedure.

13.4 Treatment

OPGs tend to be slow growing and have a low potential for malignant transformation [22]. They may even spontaneously regress or may remain stable over a long period of time with no apparent impact on vision [14]. However, OPGs can still create space-occupying symptoms, permanent vision damage [22], and rarely death [9]. Because the clinical course and progression of symptoms in OPGs are unpredictable, development of a standardized surveillance regimen has been unsuccessful thus far [13]. Some trends in treatment have emerged in the literature, while more definitive guidelines are still forthcoming.

13.4.1 Observation

Observation is a satisfactory course of action for many patients with OPG, especially those with NF1 or isolated optic nerve glioma, since spontaneous regression may occur [4, 13]. On routine screening examination, several findings that warrant increased surveillance but not necessarily treatment include change in color vision, disc pallor, optic nerve swelling, afferent pupillary defect, strabismus, and nystagmus [9]. Association with precocious puberty is also not an indication to initiate treatment for an OPG since it can be medically managed with a GnRH antagonist [9].

13.4.2 Indications for Treatment

Patients with OPG benefit from care by a multidisciplinary team consisting of an ophthalmologist, neurosurgeon, and neuro-oncologist [17]. Patients with sporadic OPG tend to have more aggressive disease and are more likely to require therapy [4]. Adolescents with OPG often present with symptomatic disease necessitating treatment [17]. To balance the risk-benefit ratio, treatment should only be considered for patients with symptomatic tumors [22], significant growth [22], and/or visual decline [14, 22]. Criteria for defining "progression" of visual deficits include the following [5]:

- Two-line change in visual acuity as measured by Snellen, HOTV, or Lea visual acuity tests, as compared to previous exams.
- Two-octave decline in Teller visual acuity.
- OR, 0.2 logMAR or greater change in visual acuity as compared to an age-matched control [9].

Although imaging may be helpful for monitoring tumor progression, it does not predict growth patterns [1] and may not correlate with actual visual acuity loss [4] or threatened visual loss [9]. Therefore, tumor growth on neuroimaging should rarely be the sole qualifier for advancing to treatment except in instances whereby a patient is unable to cooperate with vision testing and is otherwise limited in metrics other than imaging for monitoring disease progression [9]. Changes in visual fields are also an unreliable surrogate for disease progression, as patients may have worsening visual field defects without any associated decline in visual acuity [29].

Predicting timing between OPG diagnosis and onset of treatment is not well defined. Patients with NF1-OPGs tend to have a milder course and can tolerate a longer duration of observation without harmful disease progression, with suggested follow up every 3 months for the first 2 years after diagnosis [23]. Sporadic OPGs advance more rapidly and, in most cases, require treatment soon after diagnosis [23].

Though the goal of treatment is to preserve vision, a large cohort study in France found that approximately 25% of pediatric patients who underwent treatment for OPGs went on to have visual disability in adulthood [29]. Rather, treatment may halt further progression in visual decline, but evidence suggests that reversal of vision damage is unlikely.

13.4.3 Chemotherapy

Due to the unresectable nature of OPGs and the untoward effects of radiation therapy, chemotherapy is widely recognized as the current first-line treatment for OPGs [5, 10, 13, 22]. Packer and colleagues were among the first to investigate chemotherapeutic regimens for OPGs (low-grade gliomas; LGGs) with their work, published in 1993, on vincristine and carboplatin that includes a 10-week induction cycle, followed by eight 6-week maintenance cycles [30]. The overall response rate for 37 patients with newly diagnosed disease was 62%. Another commonly used chemotherapy regimen for LGG includes 6-thioguanine (6-TG), procarbazine, lomustine (CCNU), and vincristine (TPCV). This regimen was compared head-to-head with carboplatin/vincristine through the Children's Oncology Group for children with newly diagnosed LGG (including OPG); objective response rates were similar between regimens, and 5-year event-free survival was 39% and 52% for carboplatin/vincristine and TPCV, respectively [31]. Weekly vinblastine, another commonly used chemotherapeutic agent for LGG, has yielded similar rates of disease control for both newly diagnosed and relapsed/refractory low-grade gliomas [32, 33]. Dosing regimens for common chemotherapy used for OPG are outlined in Table 13.3. Of note, subjects with NF1 generally fare more favorably, both in terms of response and duration of response to chemotherapy, compared to patients with non-NF-associated LGG, including OPG.

Table 13.3 Standard chemotherapy regimens for OPG in children

Indication	Chemotherapy regimen	Adverse effects	PFS	References
1st line	Vincristine (1.5 mg/m^2) + Carboplatin (175 mg/m^2)	**Vincristine**—Peripheral nerve damage, ileus **Carboplatin**—Hypersensitivity rash [1] in up to 40% of patients [4]	5 years: 62% (Packer et al) 5 years: 39% (Ater et al)	[1, 4, 30–32]
2nd line (non-NF1)	Vinblastine (6 mg/m^2)	Bone marrow suppression	Newly diagnosed 5 years: 53% NF1—85% Non-NF1—42% (Lasssaletta et al.) Relapsed 5 years: 42% (Bouffet et al.)	[11, 32, 33]
2nd line (NF1)	MEK inhibitor (Trametinib, Selumetinib, Cobimetinib, etc.)	Rash, diarrhea, rare retinal toxicity, and cardiomyopathy		[34–39]
Other	TPCV: 6-TG (30 mg/m^2) + Procarbazine (50 mg/m^2) + CCNU (110 mg/m^2) + vincristine (1.4 mg/m^2)	Procarbazine and CCNU: Secondary leukemia (avoid alkylator therapy in patients with NF1)	5 years: 52% (Ater et al.)	[1, 4, 8, 31]
	Carboplatin (560 mg/m^2)	Bone marrow suppression, hearing loss	3 years: 64%	[40]
	Everolimus (5 mg/m^2/day)	Mucositis, bone marrow suppression	5 years: 26%	[41]
	Vinorelbine (30 mg/m^2 weekly)	Bone marrow suppression	5 years: 37%	[42]

Table 13.3 (continued)

Indication	Chemotherapy regimen	Adverse effects	PFS	References
	Temozolomide (200 mg/m^2 × 5 days)	Bone marrow suppression, secondary leukemia (avoid alkylator therapy in patients with NF1)	3 years: 57%	[43]
	Bevacizumab (10 mg/kg) Irinotecan	Bevacizumab: Hypertension, bleeding, proteinuria	2 years: 47% (Gurgurangan et al.)	[1, 10, 16, 44]

Chemotherapy is often successful in halting tumor progression or even inducing regression [10]. Despite good tumor response, full recovery of vision is rare [1, 10, 22, 33], and visual outcome is dependent on the pretreatment visual acuity [11]. The most common outcome after chemotherapy is stable vision [16]. A review study of visual outcomes found that less than 15% of patients treated with chemotherapy had improved vision and 40% had a decline in vision [33]. The authors suggest that visual changes in disease progression are irreversible regardless of the tumor's chemosensitivity [33]. Additional chemotherapy cycles are associated with either no improvement or worse visual prognosis [16, 34]. Improved visual acuity after chemotherapy was independent of any radiologic improvement in tumor size [3, 33]. Preliminary data using bevacizumab (VEGF monoclonal antibody) suggests some potential for visual improvement, though more robust longitudinal studies are needed [45, 46].

13.4.4 Radiation Therapy

Despite the efficacy of RT against OPG [1, 4, 17], the adverse effects of RT, including neurocognitive and pituitary deficits as well as vascular injury and risk of secondary malignancy, have dramatically reduced utilization of this modality for OPG. Patients with NF1 are especially susceptible to malignant transformation of low-grade glioma and development of RT-induced malignancy, such that RT should be avoided except in extreme circumstances [1, 4, 10, 22]. Patients with NF1 are also at an increased risk of the complication of moyamoya vasculopathy in which neovascularization occurs about 40 months after treatment due to ischemia of the internal carotid or cerebral arteries during radiation [5]. It is believed that the proximity of OPGs to the Circle of Willis contributes to the increased prevalence of moyamoya syndrome in this patient population [4, 10].

Because of the heavy burden of complications, radiation is typically used as salvage therapy for patients initially treated with chemotherapy [14], or as a "last resort" treatment for refractory disease or older patients [1]. It is contraindicated in patients younger than 5-years old unless disease progression occurs while undergoing chemotherapy [14]. Radiation used as salvage therapy tends to be less effective for visual outcomes than primary radiation [47].

13.4.5 Surgical Resection and Debulking

When Packer and colleagues published their work on the vincristine + carboplatin regimen for OPGs in 1993, they noted "a relative consensus that for surgically excisable lesions, gross total resection is the treatment of choice" [30]. With newer vision-preserving treatment options for OPGs, such as chemotherapy, surgery is less readily performed due to the high risk of permanent blindness and even binocular vision loss [5]. The new consensus is that surgery should only be performed on eyes with no visual potential [4, 11, 22]. In conjunction with severe visual impairment, additional indications for surgery include:

- Very large tumor [11, 22].
- Painful or cosmetically bothersome proptosis [1, 4].
- Corneal exposure keratopathy [1, 5, 8, 10].
- Hydrocephalus or other compressive symptoms [4, 8].
- Evidence of tumor growth toward chiasm [5].
  - Note: optic nerve gliomas do not typically advance toward the optic chiasm, so prophylactic surgical removal is not indicated [3, 5, 8].

Standard surgical approach is a lateral orbitotomy, with entrance to the orbital rim at the angle of the lateral canthus [1]. Resection of the entire length of the optic nerve requires a transcranial approach, which carries a higher risk of endocrinological and cerebrovascular damage [1]. New technology in computer-assisted surgery has improved surgical navigation by using a patient's neuroimaging to aid in surgical planning, simulation, and intraoperative safety near critical structures [48]. One example reported in the literature is a Medtronic Stealthstation S7® Surgical Navigation System, which utilizes an electromagnet near the surgical site to calibrate a tracker based on the patient's preoperative imaging [48]. The mirroring technique involves the projection of a patient's anatomy from the normal side onto the surgical site to allow intraoperative visualization of normal anatomy, which is another tool for minimizing damage to vital structures [48]. Although these surgical advances are streamlining the operative process for patients needing debulking or resection, other alternative treatments such as chemotherapy are still preferred.

13.4.6 Novel Treatments and Future Directions

13.4.6.1 Murine Models

Research on molecular targets for pharmaceuticals requires an animal model that can closely simulate human disease progression. The genetically engineered mouse (GEM) for NF1-OPGs has proven to be a successful model for the evaluation of the pathogenesis of OPG development and subsequent visual loss [7]. In particular, the Nf1 GEM strain ($Nf1^{flox/mut}$; GFAP-Cre, FMC mice) develops low-grade prechiasmatic and chiasmatic optic gliomas analogous to the human variants [7].

13.4.6.2 Molecular Targeting

The mitogen-activated protein kinase (MAPK) pathway plays a role in the pathogenesis of OPGs, and more recently available MAPK inhibitors are being increasingly integrated into the treatment plan for refractory or progressive OPGs (particularly if associated with NF1) [1, 19]. One such agent, selumetinib, specifically acts by inhibiting MEK-1/2 and has shown early promising results for pediatric LGG [19]. Banerjee et al. reported outcomes from the pediatric phase I clinical trial of selumetinib in children with refractory or recurrent LGG [19]. Dose levels ranged from 25 to 43 mg/m^2/dose BID, and the most common dose-limiting toxicities were elevated amylase/lipase, headache, mucositis, and rash. The recommended phase 2 dose was defined as 25 mg/m^2/dose BID, which resulted in a 2-year PFS of 69 ± SE 9.8%. Fangusaro et al. have since reported outcomes from the phase II study on which 13 patients with NF1-associated OPG and 25 with sporadic, non-NF1-associated hypothalamic/optic pathway LGG experienced 2-year PFS of 96% and 78%, respectively [35, 49]. Other clinical trials evaluating other MEK1/2 inhibitors and other targeted therapies, such as RAF, FGFR, and NTRK inhibitors, are ongoing.

Sorafenib, a multi-kinase inhibitor, was discontinued in a phase II trial due to concern for the acceleration of tumor growth [10] possibly due to resistance to BRAF inhibition causing paradoxical MAPK activation [19].

Lovastatin is a nonspecific RAS inhibitor that decreases RAS/mTOR activity implicated in tumor growth while increasing cAMP production that is protective to the RGC [7]. Lovastatin is currently utilized as a treatment for learning disabilities in children with NF-1 [7]. In an FMC mouse model, administration of lovastatin decreased microglia infiltration, increased RGC survival, and decreased RNFL thinning compared to controls [7]. This effect persisted for 2 months after cessation of treatment, at which point tumor activity was stable. This study corroborates the efficacy of targeting the MAPK pathway, and it highlights the opportunity to intervene early in disease progression in order to prevent further irreversible damage to the RGCs and RNFL.

13.5 Differences Between Pediatric and Adult Patients

Briefly, OPGs are rare in adults but tend to be malignant when they do occur. Since 1973, approximately 70 cases of malignant optic pathway gliomas in adults have been reported, with a mean age of onset in the sixth decade [50]. While the pediatric population has a strong association with NF-1, adult OPGs arise sporadically [50]. Tissue biopsy is often necessary for diagnosis, with pathology most commonly demonstrating anaplastic astrocytoma (WHO grade III) or glioblastoma multiforme (WHO grade IV) [50]. For these histologies, treatment involves surgical resection, RT (54–60 Gy), and often chemotherapy [50]. Temozolomide, an alkylating agent, has been shown to be effective in targeting malignant gliomas [50]. Unlike pediatric patients, survival rates are poor and most patients die within a year of disease onset [50].

Key Points

1. OPGs arise sporadically or in conjunction with NF-1. Although they are benign and tend to be slow-growing, the clinical course is variable and may result in significant and debilitating vision loss.
2. Yearly screening with a thorough ophthalmologic exam is recommended for pediatric patients with NF-1 under 8 years of age.
3. Although consensus on a treatment regimen for OPGs is lacking, there is strong evidence to support the use of chemotherapy as a first-line approach for patients with symptomatic OPGs (carboplatin and vincristine).
4. Radiation can be highly effective but use is highly discouraged given acceptable efficacy of numerous chemotherapy regimens and availability of newer targeted agents. Surgery should be reserved for management of painful proptosis in an eye with no meaningful vision.
5. Molecularly targeted therapy is a promising future direction for the treatment of OPGS. MEK inhibitors have shown early success, though long-term studies are needed.

Acknowledgment This research did not receive any specific grant from funding agencies in the public, commercial, or not-for-profit sectors.

References

1. Farazdaghi MK, Katowitz WR, Avery RA. Current treatment of optic nerve gliomas. Curr Opin Ophthalmol. 2019;30(5):356–63.
2. Freret ME, Gutmann DH. Insights into optic pathway glioma vision loss from mouse models of neurofibromatosis type 1. J Neurosci Res. 2019;97(1):45–56.
3. Shofty B, Ben-Sira L, Kesler A, Jallo G, Groves ML, Iyer RR, et al. Isolated optic nerve gliomas: a multicenter historical cohort study. J Neurosurg Pediatr. 2017;20(6):549–55.
4. Fried I, Tabori U, Tihan T, Reginald A, Bouffet E. Optic pathway gliomas: a review. CNS Oncol. 2013;2(2):143–59.
5. Shapey J, Danesh-Meyer HV, Kaye AH. Diagnosis and management of optic nerve glioma. J Clin Neurosci. 2011;18(12):1585–91.
6. Czyzyk E, Jóźwiak S, Roszkowski M, Schwartz RA. Optic pathway gliomas in children with and without neurofibromatosis 1. J Child Neurol. 2003;18(7):471–8.
7. Toonen JA, Ma Y, Gutmann DH. Defining the temporal course of murine neurofibromatosis-1 optic gliomagenesis reveals a therapeutic window to attenuate retinal dysfunction. Neuro-Oncology. 2017;19(6):808–19.
8. Listernick R, Ferner RE, Liu GT, Gutmann DH. Optic pathway gliomas in neurofibromatosis-1: controversies and recommendations. Ann Neurol. 2007;61(3):189–98.
9. de Blank PMK, Fisher MJ, Liu GT, Gutmann DH, Listernick R, Ferner RE, et al. Optic pathway gliomas in neurofibromatosis type 1: an update: surveillance, treatment indications, and biomarkers of vision. J Neuroophthalmol. 2017;37(Suppl 1):S23–32.
10. Campen CJ, Gutmann DH. Optic pathway gliomas in neurofibromatosis type 1. J Child Neurol. 2018;33(1):73–81.

11. Karaconji T, Whist E, Jamieson RV, Flaherty MP, Grigg JRB. Neurofibromatosis type 1: review and update on emerging therapies. Asia-Pacific J Ophthalmol (Philadelphia, Pa). 2019;8(1):62–72.
12. Opocher E, Kremer LC, Da DL, van de Wetering MD, Viscardi E, Caron HN, et al. Prognostic factors for progression of childhood optic pathway glioma: a systematic review. Eur J Cancer. 2006;42(12):1807–16.
13. Hamideh D, Hoehn ME, Harreld JH, Klimo PD, Gajjar A, Qaddoumi I. Isolated optic nerve glioma in children with and without neurofibromatosis: retrospective characterization and analysis of outcomes. J Child Neurol. 2018;33(6):375–82.
14. Nair AG, Pathak RS, Iyer VR, Gandhi RA. Optic nerve glioma: an update. Int Ophthalmol. 2014;34(4):999–1005.
15. Listernick R, Charrow J, Greenwald M, Mets M. Natural history of optic pathway tumors in children with neurofibromatosis type 1: a longitudinal study. J Pediatr. 1994;125(1):63–6.
16. Dodgshun AJ, Elder JE, Hansford JR, Sullivan MJ. Long-term visual outcome after chemotherapy for optic pathway glioma in children: site and age are strongly predictive. Cancer. 2015;121(23):4190–6.
17. Chong AL, Pole JD, Scheinemann K, Hukin J, Tabori U, Huang A, et al. Optic pathway gliomas in adolescence—time to challenge treatment choices? Neuro-Oncology. 2013;15(3):391–400.
18. Toonen JA, Solga AC, Ma Y, Gutmann DH. Estrogen activation of microglia underlies the sexually dimorphic differences in Nf1 optic glioma-induced retinal pathology. J Exp Med. 2017;214(1):17–25.
19. Banerjee A, Jakacki RI, Onar-Thomas A, Wu S, Nicolaides T, Poussaint TY, et al. A phase I trial of the MEK inhibitor selumetinib (AZD6244) in pediatric patients with recurrent or refractory low-grade glioma: a pediatric brain tumor consortium (PBTC) study. Neuro-Oncology. 2017;19(8):1135–44.
20. Dodge HW Jr, Love JG, Craig WM, Dockerty MB, Kearns TP, Holman CB, et al. Gliomas of the optic nerves. AMA Arch Neurol Psychiatry. 1958;79(6):607–21.
21. Taylor T, Jaspan T, Milano G, Gregson R, Parker T, Ritzmann T, et al. Radiological classification of optic pathway gliomas: experience of a modified functional classification system. Br J Radiol. 2008;81(970):761–6.
22. Bergqvist C, Servy A, Valeyrie-Allanore L, Ferkal S, Combemale P, Wolkenstein P, et al. Neurofibromatosis 1 French national guidelines based on an extensive literature review since 1966. Orphanet J Rare Dis. 2020;15(1):33–7.
23. Grill J, Laithier V, Rodriguez D, Raquin MA, Pierre-Kahn A, Kalifa C. When do children with optic pathway tumours need treatment? An oncological perspective in 106 patients treated in a single Centre. Eur J Pediatr. 2000;159(9):692–6.
24. Ho CY, Deardorff R, Kralik SF, West JD, Wu YC, Shih CS. Comparison of multi-shot and single shot echo-planar diffusion tensor techniques for the optic pathway in patients with neurofibromatosis type 1. Neuroradiology. 2019;61(4):431–41.
25. Kruer MC, Kaplan AM Jr, Etzl MM Jr, Carpentieri DF, Dickman PS, Chen K, et al. The value of positron emission tomography and proliferation index in predicting progression in low-grade astrocytomas of childhood. J Neuro-Oncol. 2009;95(2):239–45.
26. Avery RA, Hwang EI, Ishikawa H, Acosta MT, Hutcheson KA, Santos D, et al. Handheld optical coherence tomography during sedation in young children with optic pathway gliomas. JAMA Ophthalmol. 2014;132(3):265–71.
27. Avery RA, Liu GT, Fisher MJ, Quinn GE, Belasco JB, Phillips PC, et al. Retinal nerve fiber layer thickness in children with optic pathway gliomas. Am J Ophthalmol. 2011;151(3):542–9.e2.
28. Moradi P, Robson AG, Rose GE, Holder GE. Electrophysiological monitoring in a patient with an optic nerve glioma. Doc Ophthalmol Ophthalmol. 2008;117(2):171–4.
29. Heidary G, Fisher MJ, Liu GT, Ferner RE, Gutmann DH, Listernick RH, et al. Visual field outcomes in children treated for neurofibromatosis type 1-associated optic pathway gliomas: a multicenter retrospective study. J AAPOS. 2020;24(6):349.e1–5.

30. Packer RJ, Lange B, Ater J, Nicholson HS, Allen J, Walker R, et al. Carboplatin and vincristine for recurrent and newly diagnosed low-grade gliomas of childhood. J Clin Oncol. 1993;11(5):850–6.
31. Ater JL, Zhou T, Holmes E, Mazewski CM, Booth TN, Freyer DR, Lazarus KH, Packer RJ, Prados M, Sposto R, Vezina G, Wisoff JH, Pollack IF. Randomized study of two chemotherapy regimens for treatment of low-grade glioma in young children: a report from the children's oncology group. J Clin Oncol. 2012;30(21):2641–7.
32. Lassaletta A, Scheinemann K, Zelcer SM, Hukin J, Wilson BA, Jabado N, Carret AS, Lafay-Cousin L, Larouche V, Hawkins CE, Pond GR, Poskitt K, Keene D, Johnston DL, Eisenstat DD, Krishnatry R, Mistry M, Arnoldo A, Ramaswamy V, Huang A, Bartels U, Tabori U, Bouffet E. Phase II weekly vinblastine for chemotherapy-Naïve children with progressive low-grade Glioma: a Canadian pediatric brain tumor consortium study. J Clin Oncol. 2016;34(29):3537–43.
33. Bouffet E, Jakacki R, Goldman S, Hargrave D, Hawkins C, Shroff M, Hukin J, Bartels U, Foreman N, Kellie S, Hilden J, Etzl M, Wilson B, Stephens D, Tabori U, Baruchel S. Phase II study of weekly vinblastine in recurrent or refractory pediatric low-grade glioma. J Clin Oncol. 2012;30(12):1358–63.
34. Banerjee A, Jakacki RI, Onar-Thomas A, Wu S, Nicolaides T, Young Poussaint T, Fangusaro J, Phillips J, Perry A, Turner D, Prados M, Packer RJ, Qaddoumi I, Gururangan S, Pollack IF, Goldman S, Doyle LA, Stewart CF, Boyett JM, Kun LE, Fouladi M. A phase I trial of the MEK inhibitor selumetinib (AZD6244) in pediatric patients with recurrent or refractory low-grade glioma: a pediatric brain tumor consortium (PBTC) study. Neuro-Oncology. 2017;19(8):1135–44.
35. Fangusaro J, Onar-Thomas A, Young Poussaint T, Wu S, Ligon AH, Lindeman N, Banerjee A, Packer RJ, Kilburn LB, Goldman S, Pollack IF, Qaddoumi I, Jakacki RI, Fisher PG, Dhall G, Baxter P, Kreissman SG, Stewart CF, Jones DTW, Pfister SM, Vezina G, Stern JS, Panigrahy A, Patay Z, Tamrazi B, Jones JY, Haque SS, Enterline DS, Cha S, Fisher MJ, Doyle LA, Smith M, Dunkel IJ, Fouladi M. Selumetinib in paediatric patients with BRAF-aberrant or neurofibromatosis type 1-associated recurrent, refractory, or progressive low-grade glioma: a multicentre, phase 2 trial. Lancet Oncol. 2019;20(7):1011–22.
36. Ronsley R, Hounjet CD, Cheng S, Rassekh SR, Duncan WJ, Dunham C, Gardiner J, Ghag A, Ludemann JP, Wensley D, Rehmus W, Sargent MA, Hukin J. Trametinib therapy for children with neurofibromatosis type 1 and life-threatening plexiform neurofibroma or treatment-refractory low-grade glioma. Cancer Med. 2021;10(11):3556–64.
37. Awada G, Serruys D, Schwarze JK, Van De Voorde L, Duerinck J, Neyns B. Durable complete response of a recurrent mesencephalic glioblastoma treated with trametinib and low-dose dabrafenib in a patient with neurofibromatosis type 1. Case Rep Oncol. 2020;13(2):1031–6.
38. Selt F, van Tilburg CM, Bison B, Sievers P, Harting I, Ecker J, Pajtler KW, Sahm F, Bahr A, Simon M, Jones DTW, Well L, Mautner VF, Capper D, Hernáiz Driever P, Gnekow A, Pfister SM, Witt O, Milde T. Response to trametinib treatment in progressive pediatric low-grade glioma patients. J Neuro-Oncol. 2020;149(3):499–510.
39. Manoharan N, Choi J, Chordas C, Zimmerman MA, Scully J, Clymer J, Filbin M, Ullrich NJ, Bandopadhayay P, Chi SN, Yeo KK. Trametinib for the treatment of recurrent/progressive pediatric low-grade glioma. J Neuro-Oncol. 2020;149(2):253–62.
40. Gururangan S, Cavazos CM, Ashley D, Herndon JE 2nd, Bruggers CS, Moghrabi A, Scarcella DL, Watral M, Tourt-Uhlig S, Reardon D, Friedman HS. Phase II study of carboplatin in children with progressive low-grade gliomas. J Clin Oncol. 2002;20(13):2951–8.
41. Wright KD, Yao X, London WB, Kao PC, Gore L, Hunger S, Geyer R, Cohen KJ, Allen JC, Katzenstein HM, Smith A, Boklan J, Nazemi K, Trippett T, Karajannis M, Herzog C, Destefano J, Direnzo J, Pietrantonio J, Greenspan L, Cassidy D, Schissel D, Perentesis J, Basu M, Mizuno T, Vinks AA, Prabhu SP, Chi SN, Kieran MW. A POETIC phase II study of continuous oral everolimus in recurrent, radiographically progressive pediatric low-grade glioma. Pediatr Blood Cancer. 2021;68(2):e28787.

42. Cappellano AM, Petrilli AS, da Silva NS, Silva FA, Paiva PM, Cavalheiro S, Bouffet E. Single agent vinorelbine in pediatric patients with progressive optic pathway glioma. J Neuro-Oncol. 2015;121(2):405–12.
43. Khaw SL, Coleman LT, Downie PA, Heath JA, Ashley DM. Temozolomide in pediatric low-grade glioma. Pediatr Blood Cancer. 2007;49(6):808–11.
44. Gururangan S, Fangusaro J, Poussaint TY, McLendon RE, Onar-Thomas A, Wu S, Packer RJ, Banerjee A, Gilbertson RJ, Fahey F, Vajapeyam S, Jakacki R, Gajjar A, Goldman S, Pollack IF, Friedman HS, Boyett JM, Fouladi M, Kun LE. Efficacy of bevacizumab plus irinotecan in children with recurrent low-grade gliomas—a Pediatric brain tumor consortium study. Neuro-Oncology. 2014;16(2):310–7.
45. Yamasaki F, Takano M, Yonezawa U, Taguchi A, Kolakshyapati M, Okumichi H, Kiuchi Y, Kurisu K. Bevacizumab for optic pathway glioma with worsening visual field in absence of imaging progression: 2 case reports and literature review. Childs Nerv Syst. 2020;36(3):635–9.
46. Avery RA, Hwang EI, Jakacki RI, Packer RJ. Marked recovery of vision in children with optic pathway gliomas treated with bevacizumab. JAMA Ophthalmol. 2014;132(1):111–4.
47. Awdeh RM, Kiehna EN, Drewry RD, Kerr NC, Haik BG, Wu S, et al. Visual outcomes in pediatric optic pathway glioma after conformal radiation therapy. Int J Radiat Oncol Biol Phys. 2012;84(1):46–51.
48. Hussain A, Wan M, DeAngelis D. Progressive optic nerve glioma: orbital biopsy technique using a surgical navigation system. Can J Ophthalmol. 2018;53(1):e18–22.
49. Fangusaro J, Onar-Thomas A, Poussaint TY, Wu S, Ligon AH, Lindeman N, Campagne O, Banerjee A, Gururangan S, Kilburn L, Goldman S, Qaddoumi I, Baxter P, Vezina G, Bregman C, Patay Z, Jones JY, Stewart CF, Fisher MJ, Doyle LA, Smith M, Dunkel IJ, Fouladi M. A phase 2 trial of selumetinib in children with recurrent optic pathway and hypothalamic low-grade glioma without NF1: a pediatric brain tumor consortium study. Neuro Oncol. 2021:noab047. https://doi.org/10.1093/neuonc/noab047. Epub ahead of print
50. Alabiad CR, Shah VS, Eatz TA, Sternau LL, Lam BL. Malignant optic nerve glioma in a young woman with 7 year follow up without recurrence. Am J Ophthalmol case reports. 2020;19:100862.

Update on Non-accidental Trauma

14

Helen H. Song and Samiksha Fouzdar Jain

14.1 Introduction

Abusive head trauma (AHT), also known as non-accidental head trauma, is among the leading causes of infant death and long-term morbidity secondary to abuse [1, 2]. The previously used term "shaken baby syndrome" represents a syndromic subset of AHT in which there is evidence of central nervous system (CNS) injury, with or without obvious external signs of trauma. Head injury, in these cases, may be primary or secondary, exhibiting diffuse unilateral or bilateral subdural hemorrhages, diffuse multiplanar retinal hemorrhages, and brain injuries such as diffuse axonal injury or other parenchymal injuries. These injuries are likely secondary to either rotational or blunt force trauma, which have been confirmed by perpetrator accounts [3]. However, the initial history provided is commonly a minor fall or injury or even a complete lack of trauma. In many cases, infants can present without external manifestations of trauma, and injuries are usually revealed during the workup. Eye findings are noted in approximately 85% of AHT cases [4–6]. Ophthalmic manifestations can vary from retinal or vitreous hemorrhages to retinoschisis, retinal detachment, choroidal rupture, hyphema, orbital fractures, or

H. H. Song
Department of Ophthalmology and Visual Sciences, Truhlsen Eye Institute, University of Nebraska Medical Center, Omaha, NE, USA
e-mail: Helen.song@unmc.edu

S. F. Jain (✉)
Department of Ophthalmology and Visual Sciences, Truhlsen Eye Institute, University of Nebraska Medical Center, Omaha, NE, USA

Pediatric Ophthalmology and Adult Strabismus, Children's Hospital & Medical Center, Omaha, NE, USA
e-mail: sjain@childrensomaha.org

A. Ramasubramanian (ed.), *Pediatric Ophthalmology*, Current Practices in Ophthalmology, https://doi.org/10.1007/978-981-19-4963-0_14

periorbital ecchymoses. Victims of AHT can have lifelong physical, psychological, and academic consequences [7]. Every healthcare professional in pediatric and emergency departments has a responsibility to identify child abuse cases.

14.2 Epidemiology/Differential Diagnosis

As per the National Child Abuse and Neglect Data System (NCANDS), there were 656,000 national reports of child abuse and neglect in 2019, with an estimated 1840 fatalities stemming from abuse and/or neglect [8]. 70.3% of those fatalities occurred in victims under the age of 3 years, and 45.4% occurred in victims under the age of one [8]. Incidence of AHT in the United States has been estimated to occur in 29.7 per 100,000 person-years in infants, resulting in as many as 80 deaths per year, with evidence of head trauma evident through clinical history or objective exam findings [8]. Measuring incidence worldwide is fraught with limitations and inconsistencies. However, when assessing studies regarding the statistical frequency of AHT abroad, similar incidence rates are evident when compared to the US [9].

The majority of victims of AHT are under the age of 3 [8]. Often, misdiagnosis of nonspecific complaints, including irritability, fussiness, lethargy, or poor appetite, precede an AHT diagnosis. Risk factors identified by NCANDS include prior episodes of abuse, low family socioeconomic status, unstable home environment, including single-parent households, substance/alcohol abuse, and prevalence of domestic abuse among parental figures [8]. Interestingly, one study revealed a 1493% increase in AHT cases over a 30-day period of nationally mandated quarantining during the COVID19 pandemic in the United Kingdom when compared to the incidence rate in the same 30-day period over the previous 3 years [10]. This suggests that times of national strife in a pandemic could have exacerbated many of the known risk factors of AHT, including increased substance use among caregivers, worsened financial instability, and delayed presentation to the hospital to avoid increased exposure to contracting COVID19.

Retinal hemorrhages (RH) are not exclusive to head injury secondary to abuse. The most compelling differential diagnosis of RH in neonates and infants is hemorrhages related to normal vaginal delivery. In one prospective study, the incidence of RH in normal, nonassisted vaginal deliveries was 30.4%, up to 77.8% in vacuum-assisted deliveries [11]. However, all RH seen were intraretinal, and the majority of eyes were completely resolved in less than 30 days [11]. Beyond a neonate's first month of life, the most common cause of RH in infants is abuse. Less common diagnoses include accidental trauma (including falls, motor vehicle crashes, crush, and blunt force), congenital coagulopathic or bleeding disorders (including blood-borne neoplastic processes, clotting factor/inhibitor deficiencies, myelodysplastic syndromes, and cytopenias), elevated intracranial or intrathoracic pressure, or meningitis/encephalitis. See Table 14.1 for a complete list of common differential diagnoses of RH in infants. Table 14.1 Causes of Retinal Hemorrhages in infants and young children [12].

Table 14.1 Common differential diagnoses of retinal hemorrhages in infants and young children

Condition	Frequency of RH	Hemorrhages	Clinical features
Abusive head trauma	50–100% of cases	Numerous, extending to periphery, multiple layers	History inconsistent with injuries; commonly associated with SDH, fractures, bruising, intraabdominal injury
Perinatal RH	20–30% of newborns examined within first 24 h; 10–15% of newborns examined within first 72 h	Numerous, extending to periphery, usually intraretinal	More common in vacuum-assisted deliveries, resolves in 4–6 weeks
Unintentional head injury	0–10% patients	Typically few in number, confined to posterior pole	Associated with severe mechanism of injury (MVC, fall from height)
Hematologic conditions			
Bleeding disorder (hemophilia, von Willebrand disease, vitamin K deficiency)	Unknown	All layers of retina, vitreous	Characteristic history of bleeding disorder, abnormal coagulation studies
Leukemia	Unknown; most patients have funduscopic changes at some point in disease	Usually at posterior pole in deep retinal layers, but may occur in all layers and in vitreous	Characteristic laboratory features (lymphoblasts on peripheral blood smear)
Anemia (juvenile pernicious, iron deficiency, sickle cell)	Unknown, more common in adults than children	Intraretinal dot, blot, flame, or splinter	Anemia
Metabolic conditions			
Glutaric aciduria type 1	Rare	Few in number, confined to posterior pole	Macrocephaly, characteristic basal ganglia findings, may present with subdural hematomas; absence of bony abnormalities
Galactosemia	Rare	Vitreous	Failure to thrive, cataracts
Infection			
Cerebral malaria	20–60% of children with severe cerebral malaria	Multiple white lesions	Travel history; fever, anemia, characteristic blood smear findings
Meningitis	Rare	Various	Fever, characteristic cerebrospinal fluid findings

(continued)

Table 14.1 (continued)

Condition	Frequency of RH	Hemorrhages	Clinical features
Retinal infection (CMV, HSV, toxoplasmosis, rickettsiae)	Rare	Small, intraretinal areas of retinal necrosis; may span all layers of necrotic retina	Systemic signs of infection may be present; immunodeficiency
Endocarditis	Rare	White-centered oval hemorrhages	Other characteristic features (cardiac murmur, fever, splinter hemorrhages in nail beds, Janeway lesions)
Primary retinal disease			
Retinopathy of prematurity	Rare	Small, usually intraretinal on surface of neovascular ridge; may extend to vitreous	History of prematurity; retinal neovascularization
Coats disease	Rare	Usually intraretinal but may extend to vitreous	Usually unilateral; subretinal exudate; telangiectatic vessels
Persistent fetal vasculature	Rare	May present with vitreous hemorrhage	Usually unilateral; may be associated with mild microphthalmos; intralenticular hemorrhage; retrolental membrane
Other			
Intracranial hemorrhage	Rare in absence of abusive head injury	May be extensive	Characteristic neuroradiographic features (aneurysm, arteriovenous malformation)
Chest compression			
Cardiopulmonary resuscitation	Rare if ever	Few in number, small in size	History of cardiopulmonary resuscitation
Thoracic crush injury	Rare	Superficial; white retinal patches	History of thoracic injury

The presence of ocular findings varies widely in reports of AHT; however, RH play a vital part in contributing to a convincing clinical picture if AHT is suspected. In a retrospective study of perpetrator-confessed inflicted brain injury, RH were prevalent in 83% of 81 reports [13]. Other studies reveal a prevalence of RH in nonaccidental head trauma cases to be upwards of 94%, with one study reporting 100% of cases with evidence of RH [2, 14]. Early identification can be lifesaving, and an ophthalmological exam is imperative as intraocular pathology may be the only clinical sign of possible abuse.

Observational studies have been conducted in which AHT was diagnosed by clinical findings, along with inclusive criteria consisting of perpetrator confession, legal conviction, autopsy data, or ancillary care team assessments. In a meta-analysis of these studies, intraocular (retinal or vitreous) hemorrhage had a sensitivity of 75%, and specificity of 94%, for AHT [15]. While intraretinal hemorrhages were found in both accidental and abusive groups, multilayered, numerous, and bilateral retinal hemorrhages were most specific for AHT [15]. Optic nerve sheath hemorrhages (ONSH) had a sensitivity of 72% and a specificity of 71% for AHT [15]. Lastly, retinoschisis and peri-macular folds were found only in cases associated with abuse, and not in the nonabuse head injury groups [15].

14.3 Pathophysiology

The pathophysiology of RH in AHT is not entirely understood. Vitreoretinal traction is widely accepted as the most likely mechanism for RH development. Other theories include repetitive acceleration-deceleration (with or without coup-contrecoup injury), increased intracranial pressure, intrathoracic pressure, hypoxia, coagulopathy, and intraorbital injury.

Force, and therefore pressure, at the vitreoretinal interface theoretically increases with repeated acceleration-deceleration. With vigorous shaking of an infant, vitreoretinal separation is most vulnerable at the posterior pole, along the retinal vasculature, and at the globe equator as tethering, areas which are subjected to greater shearing tangential forces [16]. In experimental studies, purely linear acceleration produced tenfold weaker tension stress than angular acceleration [16]. This differentiates the pathophysiological mechanism of a blunt force injury or purely linear acceleration that occurs along a single plane compared to tangential or angular forces seen during shaking.

Intracranial hemorrhage, and cerebral edema secondary to mechanical brain injury, can cause increased intracranial pressure (ICP). This pressure is purported to cause subsequent compression and downstream hemorrhages in the retinal vasculature due to increased venous congestion [17]. However, other entities that increase intracranial pressure do not present with the characteristic RH seen in AHT. In rare cases of increased ICP, RH are flame-shaped peripapillary intraretinal hemorrhages in conjunction with edematous optic nerves. Rarely do hemorrhages associated solely with increased ICP occur in the periphery, which are limited to the intraretinal pseudospace. In contrast, RH in AHT are usually described as multiplanar (i.e., evidence of subretinal, intraretinal, and preretinal) hemorrhages that can occur throughout the retina's panorama (Fig. 14.1) [18]. While the etiology of RH found throughout the retina layers is multifactorial. One study has shown that tangential shearing forces exert pressure on the retina transmitted throughout all layers with relatively congruent magnitude [16]. What is still not a consensus is if a rupture of the internal limiting membrane at the vitreoretinal interface is the instigator in permitting exaggerated pressure on the retina or if shaking causes enough localized pressure within all layers of the retina to cause internal limiting membrane rupture.

Increased intrathoracic pressure is also a proposed mechanism of ocular manifestations of AHT [17]. This theory assumes that AHT is accompanied by chest wall injury, including rib fractures, that would induce elevated intrathoracic pressure.

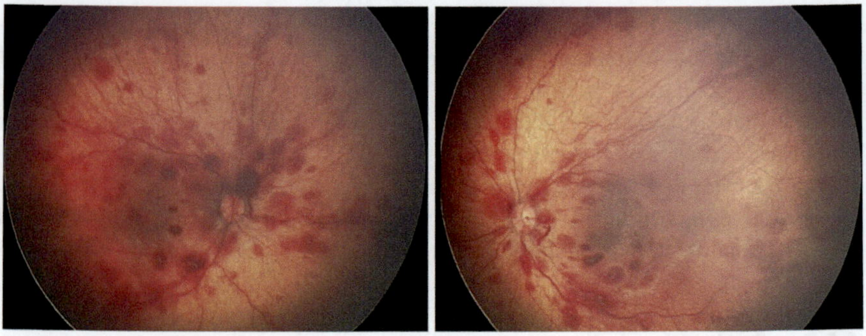

Fig. 14.1 Fundus photograph showing bilateral multiple Retinal Hemorrhages extending into the periphery

Acutely increased intrathoracic pressure is proposed to cause elevated retinal intravascular pressure, as seen in the Valsalva maneuver, or significant chest wall trauma, eponymously known as Purtscher retinopathy [19]. While Purtscher retinopathy was initially described by Otmar Purtscher in a man with head trauma secondary to falling from a tree, it is now more universally associated with pro-embolic systemic states. White retinal patches cotton-wool spots are seen in Purtscher retinopathy from vaso-occlusive processes, including fat emboli, circulating pancreatic enzymes during pancreatitis episodes, immune complex deposition, and also in disease states with decreased venous return, causing downstream retinal vein congestion. Purtscher retinopathy can be intrinsically associated with AHT, if superimposed by coagulopathy. However, it is more likely secondary to chest compressions performed during resuscitation events [20].

When shaking an infant, unique anatomical properties of the neonatal spinal cord and neck portend greater subjectivity to injury [21]. Spine ligaments have greater hydration, laxity, and elasticity, allowing greater displacement between vertebrae, and stretch significantly beyond subluxation limits of an adult without ligament rupture or spinal cord injury [22, 23]. Rigid limitations of mature bone provide a higher likelihood of spinal cord injury if repeatedly over-flexed and extended, and, thus, the infant's neck subtends a protective measure when shaking at low frequency, high displacement. Accordingly, spinal cord injuries may not be mutually inclusive with RH in AHT, and shaking does not requisitely lead to spinal cord injury in many cases.

Clotting disorders (Factor V Leiden, C/S deficiency, MTHFR mutation, homocysteinemia, etc., as well as conditions eliciting disseminated intravascular coagulation (DIC) response), could cause RH that may mimic those seen in AHT, given they may present with other systemic symptoms, including diffuse ecchymoses, erythema, swelling, and unlocalized pain [24]. Cytopenic or thrombophilic conditions superimposed on AHT may also complicate diagnosis.

The most common finding of abuse in postmortem autopsy examinations is subdural hemorrhages, and the presence of subdural hemorrhages has been reported in >70% of AHT victims [25–27]. RH are more commonly seen with subdural

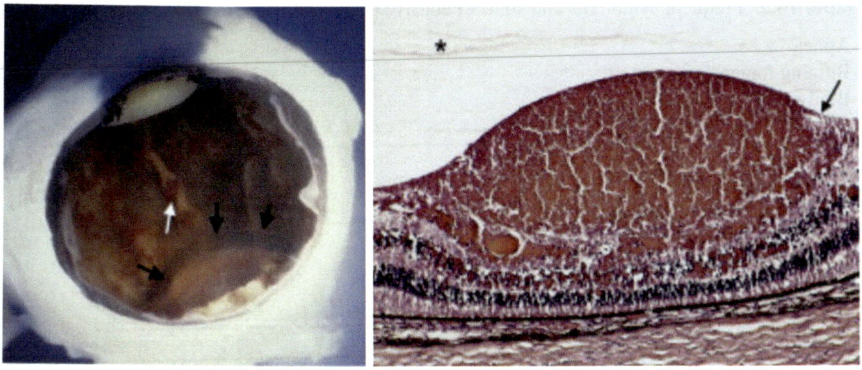

Fig. 14.2 Gross and histopathological section of eye post-shaking

hemorrhages (SDH), as both sequelae' mechanism depends on tangential and rotational inertia of the brain while shaking [28]. SDH develops as the bridging veins are sheared away from the arachnoid membrane with forceful rotational movement. Similarly, in the eye, histological evidence of internal limiting membrane (ILM) compromise suggests a shearing mechanism in which inertia of head contents produces a force that exceeds retinal adhesive composition. Erythrocyte extravasation through the ILM is the impetus for multilayered hemorrhages seen only with shearing forces, and, thus, a compelling diagnostic marker in this patient population. See Fig. 14.2 [29]

14.4 Clinical Presentation/Evaluation/Workup

Along with the physical signs and symptoms, presenting history is crucial for diagnosing AHT. Often, the account from caregivers is inconsistent or nonexistent, and a strong index of suspicion is required to make the diagnosis [30]. Initial presentation can vary widely, from minor nonspecific signs and symptoms to acute life-threatening complications. Often these signs can be mistaken for a virus or other minor illness. The presence of bruising in infants should alert a physician to the possibility of abuse. Examining physicians should pay particular attention to "TEN-4" bruising (bruising of the torso, ears, and neck in children younger than 4-years old or any bruising in an infant younger than 4 months) [31]. Findings such as apnea, retinal hemorrhages, and "TEN-4" bruising are much more common in abusive than accidental injury [31, 32]. A comprehensive medical evaluation includes a skin examination for bruising, a skeletal survey for fractures, head imaging for intracranial bleeds, and a prompt ophthalmology consultation scanning for retinal hemorrhages. This protocol remains the foundation of AHT assessments.

As mentioned above, the initial signs and symptoms of AHT can be nonspecific decreased interaction, lack of a social smile, including an acute decrease in the level of consciousness, poor feeding, vomiting, lethargy, hypothermia, increased sleeping, seizures, and failure to thrive, the latter of which is more chronic [33]. see Table 14.2.

Table 14.2 Frequent symptoms and signs of abusive head trauma (AHT)

Apnea
Bulging fontanel
Bradycardia
Cardiovascular collapse
Chills
Decreased interaction
Decreased level of consciousness
Failure to thrive
Hypothermia
Irritability
Increased sleeping
Lack of a social smile
Lethargy
Microcephaly
Poor feeding
Vomiting
Respiratory difficulty and arrest
Seizures

Rib, long bone, and complex skull fractures can support a diagnosis of AHT but are not required. However, in all cases, retinal and subdural hemorrhages are the most specific findings in AHT [1]. A study by Binenbaum et al. reported an association between severe retinal hemorrhage and the presence of hypoxic-ischemic brain injury (HII) patterns by diffusion-weighted magnetic resonance imaging (DW-MRI) in infants with AHT [34]. In addition, orbital and ocular injuries can be present secondary to blunt trauma. Periorbital ecchymosis, subconjunctival hemorrhages, traumatic hyphema, and traumatic cataracts are possible due to blunt trauma sequelae. Direct impact to the eye can also lead to corneal abrasions or lacerations, globe rupture, or damage to the iris. RH may occur with accidental head trauma. However, they are uncommon, seen in less than 10% of cases, often unilateral, and generally limited to the posterior pole adjacent to the optic nerve and macula, to a single layer of the retina [1].

14.4.1 Workup

14.4.1.1 Ophthalmic Examination

Often, the ophthalmic examination is imperative for any child presenting with visible trauma, altered mental status or consciousness, or laboratory or clinical signs of coagulopathy and problems with bleeding. Given the transient nature of RH, consultations should ideally be completed within 24 h of patient presentation; however, no later than 72 h to enumerate the full extent of RH that may be present due to trauma. Exams should begin with standard eye vitals, including pupil measurements, extraocular motility, and intraocular pressure, especially taking note of pupils for incongruent reflexes suggesting an afferent defect. Next, anterior segment assessment should follow for possible external signs of trauma or bleeding, followed by a dilated examination, ideally visualizing the fundus with indirect ophthalmoscopy. Ophthalmic consultation and fundus exam are helpful, even when dilated fundus exam is not feasible, especially in children who cannot undergo pupil dilation due to severe central nervous system injury.

When observing RH in the setting of suspected abuse, complete descriptions of the hemorrhages regarding location throughout the panorama and within which retinal layer(s), number, pattern, and bilaterality (if present in both eyes) is crucial to document. Fundus photographs may also be performed to aid in the characterization of RH. Intraretinal RH typically resolves more quickly than preretinal RH, the latter of which may last for a few days following the injury. Thus, it may be possible to roughly deduce the onset of injury—if there is a strong suspicion of abuse with the presence of preretinal RH but lack of intraretinal RH, it is reasonable to infer the incident occurred at least a few days to a week before the presentation [35].

14.4.2 Laboratory Tests

The laboratory evaluation aims to rule out medical conditions that may mimic AHT and evaluate for other abusive injuries. A list of workups can be seen in Table 14.3.

14.4.3 Imaging

A computerized head tomography (CT) scan is often the first study performed because it is easy and fast to complete; however, these scans are limited in evaluating cerebral injury. Therefore, a magnetic resonance imaging (MRI) examination of the brain and spine is recommended around 72 h post-injury [36, 37]. Cranial ultrasonography is an insufficient diagnostic neuroimaging modality in cases of suspected AHT [37].

A review by Kemp et al. looking at neuroimaging findings in children mostly over 3 years old has shown that multiple subdural hemorrhages (SDH) along the convexity, posterior fossa, interhemispheric location, hypoxic-ischemic injury (HII), and cerebral edema were significantly associated with AHT [38]. Chronic

Table 14.3 Blood workup for suspected abuse

CBC
CMP
Prothrombin time (PT)
Partial thromboplastin time (APTT)
Amylase
Lipase
Aspartate aminotransferase
Alanine aminotransferase
UA urinalysis

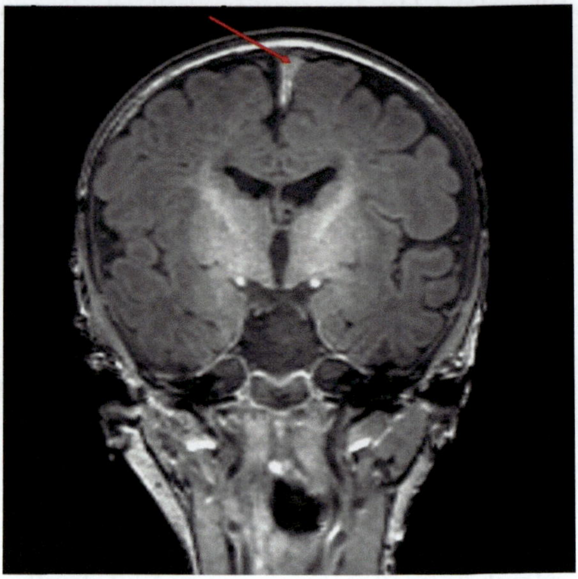

Fig. 14.3 MRI image showing Subdural Hematoma (SDH)

SDH appears specific for AHT, if not particularly sensitive, with less than half of identified AHT cases presenting with chronic SDH [38, 39] (Fig. 14.3).

A complete skeletal survey consisting of plain radiographs of the skull, spine, ribs, and long bones is performed in children younger than 2 years with concerns of AHT to rule out occult fractures. A limited skeletal survey (excluding the spine, pelvis, and skull) should be considered 2–3 weeks after initial presentation to assess for healing fractures that may not be apparent in the acute stage [40, 41].

Severe head injuries can rarely occur from a fall. Short falls (less than 1.5 m or 5 ft) generally do not cause a severe head injury. When the history of a short fall is provided for a child with a severe head injury, AHT should be considered in the differential diagnosis. Falling from a bed height is usually considered minor, although some children may suffer from a fractured arm, leg, or skull [42]. Vertical falls of 1–4 feet rarely cause severe head trauma or multiple injuries. One study evaluating children who died following a fall from that height found other concurrent evidence of abuse [43]. Even falls from 10 feet rarely result in death [44]. Generally however the greater the height, the greater likelihood of fractures and other injuries.

14.5 Management/Expected Sequelae or Complications/ Ancillary Consults

Management of AHT may involve the expertise of a number of medical specialists, including neurosurgery, trauma surgery, neurology, child abuse pediatrics, critical care physicians, and ophthalmology. The initial treatment of a patient with AHT should involve stabilizing the airway to support oxygenation, ventilation, hemodynamics, and mitigation of intracranial pathology. A more detailed evaluation for other abusive injuries of pathology can wait until the patient is stable.

Pediatricians' role in diagnosing and reporting abuse is crucial since often they are the first point of contact. Pediatricians must report suspected abuse or neglect to state child protective services. The diagnosis of abuse is sometimes straightforward but at times may not be informed or may often go unnoticed, especially when there are subtle signs and symptoms [33]. Sometimes, primary care physicians or pediatricians are not forthcoming in reporting all of the highly suspicious abuse cases. The decision to report is greatly influenced by the mechanism of injury, familiarity with family, and previous encounters with child protective services [45]. Pediatric practitioners should be aware of and must remain observant of the possibility of AHT in infants to protect and prevent any future cases. They must promptly inform relevant authorities of suspected abuse for further investigation.

Before making a diagnosis or reporting to the child protective agency, practitioners should consider various conditions that can present with findings indicative of AHT. Physicians should objectively communicate the findings and not overemphasize the impact of specific medical findings. Nevertheless, they should effectively convey child safety concerns. Early consultation with a child abuse physician may be sensible since verbal and written dialog with collaborative investigative agencies can be challenging.

In children with abusive head trauma, mortality rates ranges up to 35.7%. Forty-two to ninety-six percent of survivors suffer long-term neurologic morbidity [46]. High rates (72%) of any form of disability are commonly reported among the survivors, such as delayed psychomotor development; motor deficits (spastic hemiplegia or quadriplegia in 15–64%); epilepsy, often intractable (11–36%); microcephaly with corticosubcortical atrophy (61–100%); visual impairment (18–48%); language disorders (37–64%), and cognitive, behavioral, and sleep disorders, including intellectual deficits, agitation, aggression, tantrums, attention deficits, memory, inhibition or initiation deficits (23–59%) [7]. Due to significant short- and long-term complications, survivors, need to have frequent monitoring and prompt referral to a subspecialist to achieve the best possible outcomes. These sequelae may not manifest for years, as cognitive and behavioral consequences may only become apparent at school entry or later [47].

14.6 Primary/Secondary Prevention and Public/Parent Education

The diagnosis of abuse is intertwined with significant ramifications. Diagnosing AHT has severe legal and social implications, including for children who can be removed from their homes and adults imprisoned for their actions. However, missing a case of abuse can result in a child being returned to a potentially unsafe environment. Various strategies are implemented to decrease the incidence of AHT. Two primary areas include parental education about the crying infant and the risks of shaking a baby. Parents with newborn infants are provided with mandatory "shaken baby syndrome" education in some states. Dias et al. demonstrated success in reducing the number of AHT in a region of New York; however; similar results could not be replicated with statewide implementation of the education in Pennsylvania [48–50].

Another program is the Period of PURPLE Crying, where the acronym "PURPLE" stands for the characteristics of infant crying: P: Peak of crying, U: Unexpected, R: Resists soothing, P: Pain-like face, L: Long-lasting, E: Evening and late afternoon. This program provides parents and caregivers information about normal infant crying patterns and expected normal behavior in these infants based on scientific evidence. A three-step approach involves an in-hospital immediate postpartum education in the maternity ward to both parents, which provides written and video education, followed by public health nurses and annual community education in the second phase, public awareness and mass media promotion, as the third step. This program was successfully implemented in British Columbia. Still, performance in the state of North Carolina did not match up. It was not able to demonstrate a reduction in the incidence of AHT [51, 52]. Although it has been challenging to show a decrease in AHT rates with educational interventions consistently, some prevention programs have found self-reported, improved understanding of infant crying, improved emotional self-regulation, and increased parental knowledge of AHT [53]. Even though there has been no significant reduction in AHT rates with the Nurse-Family Partnership (an in-home visitation program), there has been a long-term decrease in child maltreatment reported, and this may be a helpful methodology in tackling AHT [54].

14.7 Ongoing New Research

Current research is ongoing to determine the force, frequency, pressure, and stress required to cause RH when shaking an infant. As noted in previous sections, research is underway to determine inciting factors that cause multilayered and distinctive RH patterns seen uniquely with AHT [16]. Several studies have been performed on dummy dolls or computer simulation models. However, the translation to animal and, eventually, human studies is complex and limited due to ethical concerns precluding the experimentation on in vivo subjects [55–58]. Autopsy data is limited, given an incomplete clinical picture and natural tissue decomposition postmortem [59, 60]. Early Ex vivo animal models have been developed in conjunction with more refined finite element (FE) eye simulated models since the initial description of FE eyes in 2014 [16, 61–63]. One preliminary study isolates the vitreoretinal interface in an intact globe and indirectly measures the force required to separate vitreous from the retina by pulling anchor points from opposite axes away from each other [16].

In addition to mechanistic studies, further research is currently being conducted to study long-term follow-up in infants who undergo ophthalmic intervention at the time of presentation, including corticosteroid therapy, hyperbaric oxygen, and surgery, such as pars plana vitrectomy [16]. Public health/epidemiologic studies are being undertaken to determine if a significant link exists between incidence and prevalence of brief unexplained events (BRUE), sudden infant death syndrome (SIDS), and shaken baby syndrome (SBS) [64]. While some have argued determining the exact mechanisms of ocular consequences post shaking may provide a theoretical manual for future perpetrators, the risk may outweigh the benefit of public education in showing how little force is required to overcome vitreoretinal adhesion.

The unifying goal of ongoing research about AHT is public education and determining primary and secondary prevention strategies to reduce rates and cases per year.

Key Points

1. Abusive head trauma in infants and children can be fatal. Even if they survive the trauma, children can have a substantial permanent disability.
2. Abusive head trauma can be missed initially or frequently misdiagnosed. Clinicians should remain mindful of infants with bruising or nonspecific symptoms, such as vomiting.
3. Children suspected to have abusive head trauma should undergo a thorough workup, including laboratory and imaging studies.
4. Child abuse patients will benefit from a multidisciplinary approach.

References

1. Maguire SA, Watts PO, Shaw AD, et al. Retinal haemorrhages and related findings in abusive and non-abusive head trauma: a systematic review. Eye. 2013;27(1):28–36. https://doi.org/10.1038/eye.2012.213.
2. Margolin EA, Dev LS, Trobe JD. Prevalence of retinal hemorrhages in perpetrator-confessed cases of abusive head trauma. Arch Ophthalmol. 2010;128(6):795. https://doi.org/10.1001/archophthalmol.2010.100.
3. Adamsbaum C, Grabar S, Mejean N, Rey-Salmon C. Abusive head trauma: judicial admissions highlight violent and repetitive shaking. Pediatrics. 2010;126(3):546–55. https://doi.org/10.1542/peds.2009-3647.
4. Gabaeff SC. Challenging the pathophysiologic connection between subdural hematoma, retinal hemorrhage and shaken baby syndrome. West J Emerg Med. 2011;12(2):144–58.
5. Kivlin JD, Simons KB, Lazoritz S, Ruttum MS. Shaken baby syndrome. Ophthalmology. 2000;107(7):1246–54.
6. Wright JN. CNS injuries in abusive head trauma. Am J Roentgenol. 2017;208(5):991–1001. https://doi.org/10.2214/AJR.16.17602.
7. Chevignard MP, Lind K. Long-term outcome of abusive head trauma. Pediatr Radiol. 2014;44(Suppl 4):S548–58. https://doi.org/10.1007/s00247-014-3169-8.
8. Kelly C, Street C, Building MES. Child Maltreatment 2019. Child maltreatment. Published online 2019:306.
9. Frasier LD, Kelly P, Al-Eissa M, Otterman GJ. International issues in abusive head trauma. Pediatr Radiol. 2014;44(Suppl 4):S647–53. https://doi.org/10.1007/s00247-014-3075-0.
10. Sidpra J, Abomeli D, Hameed B, Baker J, Mankad K. Rise in the incidence of abusive head trauma during the COVID-19 pandemic. Arch Dis Child. 2021;106(3):e14. https://doi.org/10.1136/archdischild-2020-319872.

11. Hughes LA, May K, Talbot JF, Parsons MA. Incidence, distribution, and duration of birth-related retinal hemorrhages: a prospective study. J AAPOS. 2006;10(2):102–6. https://doi.org/10.1016/j.jaapos.2005.12.005.
12. Child abuse: Anatomy and pathogenesis of retinal hemorrhages after abusive head trauma - UpToDate. https://www.uptodate.com/contents/child-abuse-anatomy-and-pathogenesis-of-retinal-hemorrhages-after-abusive-head-trauma?search=Child%20abuse:%20Anatomy%20and%20pathogenesis%20of%20retinal%20hemorrhaChild%20abuse:%20Anatomy%20and%20pathogenesis%20of%20retinal%20hemorrhages%20after%20abusive%20head%20traumages%20after%20abusive%20head%20trauma&source=search_result&selectedTitle=1~150&usage_type=default&display_rank=1. Accessed 11 Oct 2021.
13. Starling SP, Patel S, Burke BL, Sirotnak AP, Stronks S, Rosquist P. Analysis of perpetrator admissions to inflicted traumatic brain injury in children. Arch Pediatr Adolesc Med. 2004;158(5):454–8. https://doi.org/10.1001/archpedi.158.5.454.
14. Leestma JE. Case analysis of brain-injured admittedly shaken infants: 54 cases, 1969-2001. Am J Forensic Med Pathol. 2005;26(3):199–212. https://doi.org/10.1097/01.paf.0000164228.79784.5a.
15. Bhardwaj G, Chowdhury V, Jacobs MB, Moran KT, Martin FJ, Coroneo MT. A systematic review of the diagnostic accuracy of ocular signs in pediatric abusive head trauma. Ophthalmology. 2010;117(5):983–992.e17. https://doi.org/10.1016/j.ophtha.2009.09.040.
16. Suh DW, Song HH, Mozafari H, Thoreson WB. Determining the tractional forces on vitreoretinal Interface using a computer simulation model in abusive head trauma. Am J Ophthalmol. 2021;223:396–404. https://doi.org/10.1016/j.ajo.2020.06.020.
17. Levin AV. Ophthalmology of shaken baby syndrome. Neurosurg Clin N Am. 2002;13(2):201–11., vi. https://doi.org/10.1016/s1042-3680(02)00004-9.
18. Kim SY, Suh DW. Comparison of the characteristics of retinal hemorrhages in abusive head trauma versus normal vaginal delivery. JAAPOS. 2017;21(4):e24. https://doi.org/10.1016/j.jaapos.2017.07.079.
19. Tomasi LG, Rosman NP. Purtscher retinopathy in the battered child syndrome. Am J Dis Child. 1975;129(11):1335–7. https://doi.org/10.1001/archpedi.1975.02120480051012.
20. Budenz DL, Farber MG, Mirchandani HG, Park H, Rorke LB. Ocular and optic nerve hemorrhages in abused infants with intracranial injuries. Ophthalmology. 1994;101(3):559–65. https://doi.org/10.1016/s0161-6420(94)31300-5.
21. Garcia-Pires F, Jayappa S, Desai S, Ramakrishnaiah RH, Choudhary AK. Spinal subdural hemorrhage in abusive head trauma: a pictorial review. Pediatr Radiol. 2021;51(6):980–90. https://doi.org/10.1007/s00247-020-04931-7.
22. Guthkelch AN. Infantile subdural haematoma and its relationship to whiplash injuries. Br Med J. 1971;2(5759):430–1.
23. Committee on Child Abuse and Neglect. Shaken baby syndrome: rotational cranial injuries—technical report. Pediatrics. 2001;108(1):206–10. https://doi.org/10.1542/peds.108.1.206.
24. Thau A, Saffren B, Anderst JD, Carpenter SL, Levin AV. A review on clotting disorders and retinal hemorrhages: can they mimic abuse? Child Abuse Negl. 2021;118:105070. https://doi.org/10.1016/j.chiabu.2021.105070.
25. Piteau SJ, Ward MGK, Barrowman NJ, Plint AC. Clinical and radiographic characteristics associated with abusive and nonabusive head trauma: a systematic review. Pediatrics. 2012;130(2):315–23. https://doi.org/10.1542/peds.2011-1545.
26. Westrick AC, Moore M, Monk S, Greeno A, Shannon C. Identifying characteristics in abusive head trauma: a single-institution experience. Pediatr Neurosurg. 2015;50(4):179–86. https://doi.org/10.1159/000430846.
27. Roach JP, Acker SN, Bensard DD, Sirotnak AP, Karrer FM, Partrick DA. Head injury pattern in children can help differentiate accidental from non-accidental trauma. Pediatr Surg Int. 2014;30(11):1103–6. https://doi.org/10.1007/s00383-014-3598-3.
28. Maiese A, Iannaccone F, Scatena A, et al. Pediatric abusive head trauma: a systematic review. Diagnostics (Basel). 2021;11(4):734. https://doi.org/10.3390/diagnostics11040734.

29. Breazzano MP, Unkrich KH, Barker-Griffith AE. Clinicopathological findings in abusive head trauma: analysis of 110 infant autopsy eyes. Am J Ophthalmol. 2014;158(6):1146–1154.e2. https://doi.org/10.1016/j.ajo.2014.08.011.
30. Hymel KP, Lee G, Boos S, et al. Estimating the relevance of historical red flags in the diagnosis of abusive head trauma. J Pediatr. 2020;218:178–183.e2. https://doi.org/10.1016/j.jpeds.2019.11.010.
31. Pierce MC, Kaczor K, Aldridge S, O'Flynn J, Lorenz DJ. Bruising characteristics discriminating physical child abuse from accidental trauma. Pediatrics. 2010;125(1):67–74. https://doi.org/10.1542/peds.2008-3632.
32. Maguire S, Pickerd N, Farewell D, Mann M, Tempest V, Kemp AM. Which clinical features distinguish inflicted from non-inflicted brain injury? A systematic review. Arch Dis Child. 2009;94(11):860–7. https://doi.org/10.1136/adc.2008.150110.
33. Jenny C, Hymel KP, Ritzen A, Reinert SE, Hay TC. Analysis of missed cases of abusive head trauma. JAMA. 1999;281(7):621–6. https://doi.org/10.1001/jama.281.7.621.
34. Binenbaum G, Christian CW, Ichord RN, et al. Retinal hemorrhage and brain injury patterns on diffusion-weighted magnetic resonance imaging in children with head trauma. J AAPOS. 2013;17(6):603–8. https://doi.org/10.1016/j.jaapos.2013.09.002.
35. Binenbaum G, Chen W, Huang J, Ying G-S, Forbes BJ. The natural history of retinal hemorrhage in pediatric head trauma. J AAPOS. 2016;20(2):131–5. https://doi.org/10.1016/j.jaapos.2015.12.008.
36. Christian CW, Committee on Child Abuse and Neglect, American Academy of Pediatrics. The evaluation of suspected child physical abuse. Pediatrics. 2015;135(5):e1337–54. https://doi.org/10.1542/peds.2015-0356.
37. Kleinman PK. Diagnostic imaging of child abuse. Cambridge: Cambridge University Press; 2015.
38. Kemp AM, Jaspan T, Griffiths J, et al. Neuroimaging: what neuroradiological features distinguish abusive from non-abusive head trauma? A systematic review. Arch Dis Child. 2011;96(12):1103–12. https://doi.org/10.1136/archdischild-2011-300630.
39. Karibe H, Kameyama M, Hayashi T, Narisawa A, Tominaga T. Acute subdural hematoma in infants with abusive head trauma: a literature review. Neurol Med Chir (Tokyo). 2016;56(5):264–73. https://doi.org/10.2176/nmc.ra.2015-0308.
40. Keenan HT, Runyan DK, Marshall SW, Nocera MA, Merten DF. A population-based comparison of clinical and outcome characteristics of young children with serious inflicted and noninflicted traumatic brain injury. Pediatrics. 2004;114(3):633–9. https://doi.org/10.1542/peds.2003-1020-L.
41. Bradford R, Choudhary AK, Dias MS. Serial neuroimaging in infants with abusive head trauma: timing abusive injuries. J Neurosurg Pediatr. 2013;12(2):110–9. https://doi.org/10.3171/2013.4.PEDS12596.
42. Chadwick DL, Bertocci G, Castillo E, et al. Annual risk of death resulting from short falls among young children: less than 1 in 1 million. Pediatrics. 2008;121(6):1213–24. https://doi.org/10.1542/peds.2007-2281.
43. Chadwick DL, Chin S, Salerno C, Landsverk J, Kitchen L. Deaths from falls in children: how far is fatal? J Trauma. 1991;31(10):1353–5. https://doi.org/10.1097/00005373-199110000-00006.
44. Plunkett J. Fatal pediatric head injuries caused by short-distance falls. Am J Forensic Med Pathol. 2001;22(1):1–12. https://doi.org/10.1097/00000433-200103000-00001.
45. Jones R, Flaherty EG, Binns HJ, et al. Clinicians' description of factors influencing their reporting of suspected child abuse: report of the child abuse reporting experience study research group. Pediatrics. 2008;122(2):259–66. https://doi.org/10.1542/peds.2007-2312.
46. Shein SL, Bell MJ, Kochanek PM, et al. Risk factors for mortality in children with abusive head trauma. J Pediatr. 2012;161(4):716–722.e1. https://doi.org/10.1016/j.jpeds.2012.03.046.
47. Flaherty E, Legano L, Idzerda S, Council On Child Abuse and Neglect. Ongoing pediatric health care for the child who has been maltreated. Pediatrics. 2019;143(4):e20190284. https://doi.org/10.1542/peds.2019-0284.

48. Dias MS, Smith K, DeGuehery K, Mazur P, Li V, Shaffer ML. Preventing abusive head trauma among infants and young children: a hospital-based, parent education program. Pediatrics. 2005;115(4):e470–7. https://doi.org/10.1542/peds.2004-1896.
49. Altman RL, Canter J, Patrick PA, Daley N, Butt NK, Brand DA. Parent education by maternity nurses and prevention of abusive head trauma. Pediatrics. 2011;128(5):e1164–72. https://doi.org/10.1542/peds.2010-3260.
50. Dias MS, Rottmund CM, Cappos KM, et al. Association of a postnatal parent education program for abusive head trauma with subsequent pediatric abusive head trauma hospitalization rates. JAMA Pediatr. 2017;171(3):223–9. https://doi.org/10.1001/jamapediatrics.2016.4218.
51. Barr RG, Barr M, Rajabali F, et al. Eight-year outcome of implementation of abusive head trauma prevention. Child Abuse Negl. 2018;84:106–14. https://doi.org/10.1016/j.chiabu.2018.07.004.
52. Zolotor AJ, Runyan DK, Shanahan M, et al. Effectiveness of a statewide abusive head trauma prevention program in North Carolina. JAMA Pediatr. 2015;169(12):1126–31. https://doi.org/10.1001/jamapediatrics.2015.2690.
53. Lopes NRL, de Albuquerque Williams LC. Pediatric abusive head trauma prevention initiatives: a literature review. Trauma Violence Abuse. 2018;19(5):555–66. https://doi.org/10.1177/1524838016675479.
54. Eckenrode J, Campa MI, Morris PA, et al. The prevention of child maltreatment through the nurse family partnership program: mediating effects in a long-term follow-up study. Child Maltreat. 2017;22(2):92–9. https://doi.org/10.1177/1077559516685185.
55. Bandak FA. Shaken baby syndrome: a biomechanics analysis of injury mechanisms. Forensic Sci Int. 2005;151(1):71–9. https://doi.org/10.1016/j.forsciint.2005.02.033.
56. Yamazaki J, Yoshida M, Mizunuma H. Experimental analyses of the retinal and subretinal haemorrhages accompanied by shaken baby syndrome/abusive head trauma using a dummy doll. Injury. 2014;45(8):1196–206. https://doi.org/10.1016/j.injury.2014.04.014.
57. Bonfiglio A, Lagazzo A, Repetto R, Stocchino A. An experimental model of vitreous motion induced by eye rotations. Eye Vis (Lond). 2015;2:10. https://doi.org/10.1186/s40662-015-0020-8.
58. Uchio E, Ohno S, Kudoh J, Aoki K, Kisielewicz LT. Simulation model of an eyeball based on finite element analysis on a supercomputer. Br J Ophthalmol. 1999;83(10):1106–11.
59. Lantz PE, Stanton, CA. Postmortem detection and evaluation of retinal hemorrhages. Presented at the: AAFS annual meeting; February 2006; Seattle, WA.
60. Wygnanski-Jaffe T, Levin AV, Shafiq A, et al. Postmortem orbital findings in shaken baby syndrome. Am J Ophthalmol. 2006;142(2):233–40. https://doi.org/10.1016/j.ajo.2006.03.038.
61. Roth S, Raul J-S, Ludes B, Willinger R. Finite element analysis of impact and shaking inflicted to a child. Int J Legal Med. 2007;121(3):223–8. https://doi.org/10.1007/s00414-006-0129-3.
62. Hans SA, Bawab SY, Woodhouse ML. A finite element infant eye model to investigate retinal forces in shaken baby syndrome. Graefes Arch Clin Exp Ophthalmol. 2009;247(4):561–71. https://doi.org/10.1007/s00417-008-0994-1.
63. Rangarajan N, Kamalakkannan SB, Hasija V, et al. Finite element model of ocular injury in abusive head trauma. JAAPOS. 2009;13(4):364–9. https://doi.org/10.1016/j.jaapos.2008.11.006.
64. Lynøe N, Eriksson A. Is there a common denominator for brief resolved unexplained events, sudden infant death syndrome, and alleged shaken baby syndrome? Med Hypotheses. 2020;144:109939. https://doi.org/10.1016/j.mehy.2020.109939.

GPSR Compliance

The European Union's (EU) General Product Safety Regulation (GPSR) is a set of rules that requires consumer products to be safe and our obligations to ensure this.

If you have any concerns about our products, you can contact us on ProductSafety@springernature.com

In case Publisher is established outside the EU, the EU authorized representative is:

Springer Nature Customer Service Center GmbH
Europaplatz 3
69115 Heidelberg, Germany

Batch number: 10726135

Printed by Printforce, the Netherlands